Rheumatoid Arthritis

An Illustrated Guide to Pathology, Diagnosis, and Management

H. Ralph Schumacher, MD

Professor, Department of Internal Medicine
University of Pennsylvania School of Medicine
Director, Arthritis-Immunology Center
Veterans Administration Medical Center
Philadelphia, Pennsylvania

Eric P. Gall, MD, FACP

Professor, Department of Internal Medicine and
Department of Surgery (Orthopedics)
Professor, Department of Family and Community Medicine
Chief, Section of Rheumatology, Allergy, and Immunology
College of Medicine, University of Arizona
Medical Director, University of Arizona Arthritis Center
Tucson, Arizona

J. B. Lippincott Company · Philadelphia
Gower Medical Publishing · New York · London

Distributed in the USA and Canada by
J.B. Lippincott Company
East Washington Square, Philadelphia, PA 19105, USA

Distributed in all countries except the USA and Canada
by Harper and Row Publishers Inc., International Division
East Washington Square, Philadelphia, PA 19105, USA

ISBN 397-44653-5

Library of Congress Cataloging-in-Publication Data
Rheumatoid arthritis.
   Includes bibliographies and index.
   1. Rheumatoid arthritis.   2. Rheumatoid
arthritis—Atlases.   I. Schumacher, H. Ralph,
1933–   .   II. Gall, Eric P. (Eric Papineau),
1940–   .   [DNLM: 1. Arthritis,
Rheumatoid—diagnosis—atlases.
2. Arthritis, Rheumatoid—pathology—atlases.
WE 17 R4725]
RC933.R427   1988   616.7'22   87-30144
ISBN 0-397-44653-5 (Lippincott)

British Library Cataloguing in Publication Data
Schumacher, H. Ralph
   Rheumatoid arthritis : an illustrated
   guide to pathogenesis, diagnosis and
   management.
   1. Man. Joints. Rheumatoid arthritis
   I. Title   II. Gall, Eric P.
   616.7'22
   ISBN 0-397-44653-5

Editor: Kristin Robie
Art Director: Jill L. Feltham
Illustrator: Carol Kalafatić
Designer: Romi Dorsey

10 9 8 7 6 5 4 3 2 1

Printed in Singapore by Imago Productions (FE) PTE Ltd

To my family: my wife, Liz, my daughters, Heidi and
Kaethe, and my parents, Dorothy and Ralph Sr. whose
love and encouragement have made all facets of life,
including writing this book, a delight.
H.R.S.

To my wife, Kathy, and my children, Gretchen and
Michael, who supported and encouraged me during
the many long, extra hours that it took to edit and put
together this book; to my mentors, who instilled a
curiosity and wonderment about the field of arthritis,
Joe Hollander, H. Ralph Schumacher, and Allen Myers;
and finally, to my parents, Edward and Phyllis Gall,
who encouraged my pursuits and nurtured them all
my life.
E.P.G.

FOREWORD

After more than fifty years in rheumatology, it has been a pleasure and a privilege as well as a singular honor to have been invited by the editors of this unique and superb presentation to write a foreword. Most who have been aware of my own previous writings and comments in this field know that I am not given to superlatives, particularly when describing the accomplishments of others. This, however, is the exception that proves my long-established rule.

Never before, during my long career of reading and editing, have I been as delighted to review the proofs and illustrations of any forthcoming work as I have with this superb description and splendidly and bountifully illustrated "state of the art" summary of knowledge of rheumatoid arthritis.

There are several excellent textbooks and monographs on rheumatoid arthritis available, and the illustrations in the ARA slide collection are particularly good, but here is a combination of succinct and authoritative text plus the best collection of color illustrations of the disease and its complications to be found anywhere in the world. The reproductions of x-ray films supersedes in clarity and completeness any I

have seen. The tables are well-composed and beautifully presented. Unique and practical are the chapters dealing with rheumatoid involvement of individual joints, with numerous illustrations of deformities to be prevented or corrected. The bibliographies at the end of each chapter are well-chosen and up-to-date.

All the contributors to this book are to be congratulated on the splendid job they have accomplished, but Eric Gall and Ralph Schumacher have distinguished themselves in conceiving, organizing, collecting x-rays and illustrations, collating, editing and executing this real landmark in rheumatologic literature. I cannot find words adequately to express my enthusiasm in recommending this ATLAS to all physicians with any interest in rheumatoid arthritis.

Joseph Lee Hollander, MD
Master, American College of Physicians
Master, American Rheumatism Association
Emeritus Professor of Medicine,
School of Medicine, University of Pennsylvania
Emeritus Editor, ARTHRITIS AND ALLIED
CONDITIONS

ACKNOWLEDGEMENTS

I thank my teachers, co-workers (many of whom have also contributed chapters to this book), trainees, and students whose questions and comments over the years have encouraged development of some of the original approaches in this book. I thank the staff at Gower for their promptness and committment to excellence. At this time however I specifically want to acknowledge members of my long suffering laboratory and office staff, who have been with me now for 9 or more years. Mary Ellen Maguire, my Program Assistant, has handled all the coordination of this book in addition to her usual heavy duties. Susan Rothfuss, Gilda Clayburne, and Marie Sieck have helped gather laboratory material and have assumed unaccustomed burdens to keep our research going when some of my effort was temporarily diverted. I and the Philadelphia Veterans Administration Medical Center—University of Pennsylvania Arthritis-Immunology Center could not function without these wonderful loyal people.

H.R.S.

My deepest gratitude goes to my Administrative Assistant, Cynthia Stein, who has spent many hours typing, retyping, correcting, editing, tracking down photographs, arranging and suggesting changes, and dealing with authors, editors, and many conflicting tasks that had to be taken care of at the same time as the book was put together.

Acknowledgement is given also to the Rheumatology/Allergy and Immunology faculty who participated, helped and gave me ideas for this book, including Jack Boyer, MD, David Yocum, MD, Paul Alepa, MD, Michael Maricic, MD, and Margaret Miller, MD. To the many individuals who helped by contributing photographs, all of whom are acknowledged in this book. My Department Chairman, Rubin Bressler, who has allowed me to develop and shape interest in arthritis here at the University of Arizona, has helped me put together a Section and an Arthritis Center which gives us the opportunity to devote time to such important endeavors as this book.

I am grateful to my co-Editor, H. Ralph Schumacher, MD, who has been my mentor, colleague, and friend for many, many years and without whom I never would have entered into the development of this book; and to Kristin Robie, the Editor, who did such a superb job of making sure that all the needs for this book were met, and who cajoled, called, and kindly needled me into making sure everything was done and done correctly.

E.P.G.

PREFACE

The term "rheumatoid arthritis," coined by AB Garrod in the late 19th century replaced previous designations such as "atrophic arthritis" and "rheumatic gout" for patients with similar chronic erosive polyarthritis. The term "rheumatoid" was meant to imply similarities to "rheumatism" or rheumatic fever, and to more clearly distinguish it from gout. "Rheum," meaning "flowing," was not intended to suggest any modern concept of pathogenesis, so "rheumatoid arthritis" is still felt to be an appropriate name for this disease or group of syndromes of unknown cause.

Rheumatoid arthritis is a common disease whose course can be most unpredictable. Some patients appear to do well with little intervention, but for many other patients it often becomes a cause of a major alteration in lifestyle, or even of early mortality. Most patients with rheumatoid arthritis in the United States are still managed by primary care and general physicians despite the complexity involved in both accurate assessment and comprehensive disease management. Although rheumatoid arthritis is certainly addressed in most medical and rheumatologic texts, there is rarely the in-depth consideration that is needed. This book is our attempt to fill that gap while keeping the size and style to that which will be readable, and not only a reference source. As with any text there must be areas of relatively greater emphasis. Detailed clinical description of rheumatoid involvement and differential diagnosis of disease at individual joints has not been provided in most texts. Section II is devoted entirely to reviewing the clinical involvement at the various joints. The opportunity to use many color figures, beautifully reproduced radiographs, tables, and schematics, we believe will increase the value of these chapters. Because rheumatoid arthritis is still often a diagnosis of exclusion and a source of potential over and under diagnosis we have emphasized diseases and local syndromes that must be distinguished from it; some of these conditions have much more effective or specific therapy than is available for rheumatoid arthritis.

The authors are from two medical centers, the University of Pennsylvania and Arthritis-Immunology Center at the Philadelphia VA Hospital, and the Arthritis Center of the University of Arizona in Tucson. This permitted some consistency of the material but, at the same time, we have not stifled controversial or some conflicting interpretations. Awareness of the fact that there are many unclear and controversial areas is one of the points that must be appreciated in diagnosing and treating patients with rheumatoid arthritis. Some repetition between chapters occurs when it is important to the integrity and clarity of the individual chapters.

Treatment and management are addressed as the principal subject of only one chapter (Chapter 15), even though it is recognized that drug and comprehensive team therapies could be the subject of books on their own. We have documented the current state of therapy and provided extensive references for further reading in all chapters. In Chapters 6 through 13 about specific joints we have focused on certain therapeutic problems and opportunities for local care. Important aspects of clinical diagnosis and methods to use to follow and evaluate treatment responses are provided in our description of general clinical features (Chapter 1). The basis, value, and limitations of most laboratory tests are reviewed in Chapter 2. Diagnosis is largely clinical in rheumatoid arthritis but the important role of synovial fluid analysis is emphasized and illustrated in Chapter 4.

A tight production and editing schedule has allowed us to produce a very up-to-date text that reflects the complexity of mechanisms recognized to be involved in pathogenesis (Chapter 5) and shows the newest developments in radiologic imaging (Chapter 3). With the advantage of color illustrations we have been able to review and document pathology (Chapter 4) and systemic features (Chapter 14) in unusual detail and to provide a chapter on complications of rheumatoid arthritis (Chapter 16).

This book is directed at students and teachers in order to impart practical information that can facilitate instruction about known aspects of this common disease. At the same time, it is also intended to encourage those in either group with inquisitive minds to consider further investigation into the many puzzles that remain in this disease of unknown cause. Certainly more clinical and basic research into the disease's cause(s) or perpetuating mechanisms is needed before we can have truly effective treatment or prevention. We welcome discussion and hope that this and future editions will provide a format for state-of-the-art teaching in this important disease.

H. Ralph Schumacher, Jr, MD and
Eric P. Gall, MD

CONTRIBUTORS

SUZANNE ALGEO, MD
Rheumatology Fellow
University of Pennsylvania School of Medicine
Arthritis-Immunology Center, VAMC
Philadelphia, Pennsylvania

DANIEL G. BAKER, MD
Associate Professor of Medicine
Medical College of Pennsylvania
Adjunct Assistant Professor of Medicine
University of Pennsylvania School of Medicine
Arthritis-Immunology Center, VAMC
Philadelphia, Pennsylvania

JOHN S. BOMALASKI, MD
Assistant Professor of Medicine
Medical College of Pennsylvania
Adjunct Assistant Professor of Medicine
University of Pennsylvania School of Medicine
Arthritis-Immunology Center, VAMC
Philadelphia, Pennsylvania

GINGER CONSTANTINE, MD
Rheumatology Fellow
University of Pennsylvania School of Medicine
Arthritis-Immunology Center, VAMC
Philadelphia, Pennsylvania

MURRAY DALINKA, MD
Professor of Radiology
University of Pennsylvania School of Medicine
Philadelphia, Pennsylvania

BRUCE FREUNDLICH, MD
Assistant Professor of Medicine
University of Pennsylvania School of Medicine
Philadelphia, Pennsylvania

ERIC P. GALL, MD
Chief, Rheumatology, Allergy and Immunology
  Section
Professor, Department of Internal Medical and
  Department of Surgery (Orthopedics)
Professor, Department of Family and Community
  Medicine
University of Arizona College of Medicine
Medical Director, University of Arizona Arthritis
  Center
Tucson, Arizona

BRIAN F. MANDELL, PhD, MD
Assistant Professor of Medicine
University of Pennsylvania School of Medicine
Philadelphia, Pennsylvania

MICHAEL J. MARICIC, MD
Clinical Instructor, Department of Internal Medicine
Rheumatology, Allergy and Immunology Section
University of Arizona College of Medicine
Tucson, Arizona

MARGARET M. MILLER, MD
Assistant Clinical Professor, Department of Internal
  Medicine
Rheumatology, Allergy and Immunology Section
University of Arizona College of Medicine
Tucson, Arizona

H. RALPH SCHUMACHER, Jr, MD
Professor of Medicine
University of Pennsylvania School of Medicine
Director, Arthritis-Immunology Center, VAMC
Philadelphia, Pennsylvania

JOSEPH TSAI, MD
Resident in Radiology
Hospital of University of Pennsylvania School of
  Medicine
Philadelphia, Pennsylvania

DAVID E. YOCUM, MD
Assistant Professor, Department of Internal
  Medicine
Rheumatology, Allergy and Immunology Section
University of Arizona College of Medicine
Tucson, Arizona

CONTENTS

SECTION II

1

GENERAL FEATURES AND PATHOGENESIS

This Section describes the general clinical, laboratory, radiographic, and pathologic features of rheumatoid arthritis. It seems likely that as the pathogenesis of this disease is better understood, varying initiating agents and important differences in perpetuating mechanisms will emerge that will distinguish features within what is now called rheumatoid arthritis. For now, the many features patients with this disease have in common allow a ready diagnosis of most cases. The new criteria for diagnosis proposed by the American Rheumatism Association are included, and promise to be less cumbersome than outdated ones. Emphasis in this Section is placed on the importance of synovial fluid analysis in differential diagnosis and on the nonspecific information obtained from most procedures used in evaluation. The complex factors involved in pathogenesis should serve as a reminder of why there is much difficulty in the practical management of this disease.

CHAPTER 1

GENERAL FEATURES OF RHEUMATOID ARTHRITIS

ERIC P. GALL, MD

Rheumatoid arthritis is a common, inflammatory polyarthritis affecting approximately 1% to 3% of the population in the United States. Most but not all authors agree that it is a disease of modern man, beginning to appear worldwide around the time of the industrial revolution (Short, 1974). This is in sharp contrast to other common rheumatic diseases, such as osteoarthritis, gout, and ankylosing spondylitis, that have been definitively identified in skeletal remains dating back to the Egyptian pyramids and before (Fig. 1.1).

DEFINITION

Early descriptions of the disease are confusing. Differentiation of rheumatoid arthritis from degenerative arthritis, rheumatic fever, gout, and nonspecific rheumatism is difficult based on the literature. Attempts to define this entity in the writings of Sydenham in the mid-1600s and other authors of that time are quite vague. Indeed, confusion in clinical descriptions and proposed etiology often have led to equally confusing and changing treatments over time. As more is learned about its pathogenesis, changes in treatment and more precise explanations for the efficacy of some medications that were used empirically for the wrong reasons will be-

come more defined. Examples of these treatments and their relation to pathogenetic mechanisms will be discussed in Section 3.

The term "rheumatoid arthritis" was first used by Alfred Garrod in his treatise of 1876 (Garrod, 1876). Landre-Beauvais in his doctoral thesis of 1800 gave the first good clinical description of this disorder. Osler (1892) used the term "arthritis deformans" and "chronic rheumatism" in his first textbook of medicine. These terms actually referred to a conglomeration of many types of arthritis. Standardized criteria for the diagnosis of rheumatoid arthritis were not developed until 1958 by the American Rheumatism Association (Ropes, 1958) and, despite flaws, have been in use until now. New criteria is being developed.

Cecil in 1931 recognized that serum from patients with rheumatoid arthritis caused agglutination of streptococci leading to the speculation of an infectious etiology for this disease. In 1948, Rose and colleagues found that this clumping was caused by an antibody to gamma globulin which had coated the organisms, and that the carrier was not a specific pathogen, thus first describing the rheumatoid factor (Figure 1.2). This led to an explosion of work which continues today regarding the complex pathogenesis of rheumatoid arthritis (see Chapter 5).

A standard definition of rheumatoid arthritis is difficult to come by and most major rheumatology texts avoid the issue, giving only the accepted diagnostic criteria. Short et al in 1957 defined it as "a chronic systemic inflammatory disorder of unknown etiology characterized by the manner in which it involves the joint." This is probably as close to a definitive description as possible at this time (Fig. 1.3). While this disease is defined by joint involvement, the tendon sheath is also commonly involved with tenosynovitis causing loosening of tendons and potential rupture (Fig. 1.4). Periarticular muscle pain and stiffness frequently occurs along with systemic symptoms.

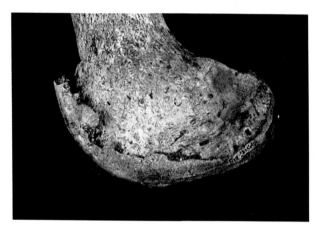

Figure 1.1 Skeletal remains from Arizona Indian ruins shows femoral head with osteoarthritis. (Courtesy of Michael Pitt, MD).

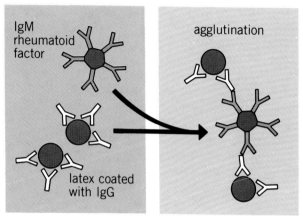

Figure 1.2 Rheumatoid factor test by agglutination of latex particles coated with heat aggregated IgG. Serum is mixed in serial dilution with a prepared latex particle. Serum from patients with IgM rheumatoid factor will agglutinate such particles. The agglutination reaction is then read under the microscope and titered.

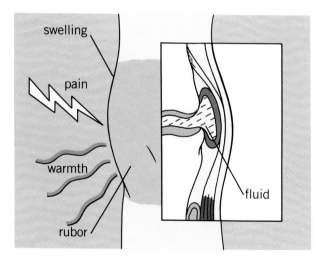

Figure 1.3 Inflammation of rheumatoid arthritic joints is characterized by redness, swelling, pain, tenderness, and effusion.

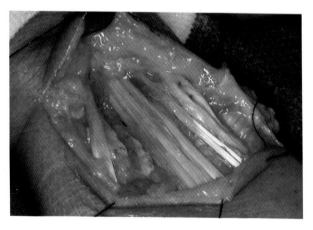

Figure 1.4 Intraoperative view of wrist with rheumatoid arthritis. Pinkish synovium surrounds the tendons which have been partially dissected out. The synovium is filled with inflammatory cells and eventually will erode the tendons, leading to deformity and tendon rupture.

EPIDEMIOLOGY

Given the difficulty of definition, it is not surprising that there are differing estimates of incidence and prevalence of rheumatoid arthritis. Suffice it to say, the disease is common in most populations.

In a review of multiple studies, the estimate of prevalence of definite and classical rheumatoid arthritis using the American Rheumatism Association criteria (thus ignoring the common instances of possible and probable rheumatoid arthritis) is at a level of 0.3% to 1.5% (Wolfe, 1968). The incidence is conservatively estimated at 100,000 to 200,000 new cases a year in the United States (Harris, 1985).

There is a marked age differentiation in the incidence. One study suggested rheumatoid arthritis symptoms began at age 5 to 14 in 0.3% of the population while the incidence

of the onset of symptoms at age 65 was 2% (Lawrence, 1977). Onset can occur at any age and in females there seems to be a steady progression of onset with increasing age. Males may show two peaks, first in early adulthood (ages 24 to 34) and after age 65 (Fig. 1.5).

In North America there appears to be an increased incidence during winter months, twice that of the rest of the year. The reason for this has not been pinpointed although increased viral upper respiratory infections, the proximity of individuals during cold weather, and the effect of cold weather on symptoms have all been implicated. Climate has not been shown to have any specific effect on rheumatoid arthritis although good studies have not been done.

There is a clear female predominance in the disease, usually thought to be about 3:1 (female:male), particularly in young adults

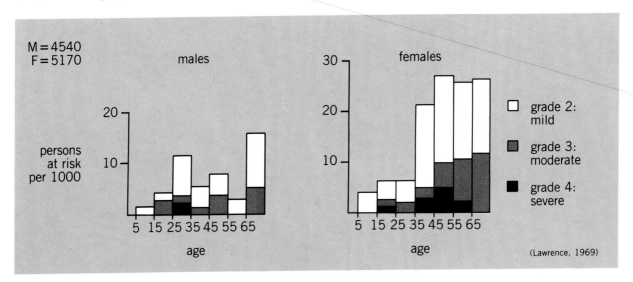

Figure 1.5   Age of onset of rheumatoid arthritis. Based on anamnesis in 1954–1959.

(up to 5:1). This is tempered by a marked increase in male onset over the age of 60 resulting in a female:male ratio of 2:1 (Lawrence, 1977).

There have been many ethnic, racial, and geographic studies. Extremely low incidences of rheumatoid arthritis have been reported in Japan (0.2%) (Shichikwi, 1966) and Puerto Rico (Mendez, 1964). Looking at the age-sex adjusted ratios for different ethnic groups revals marked differences (Fig. 1.6). Studies comparing rural and urban incidence of rheumatoid arthritis do not show remarkable differences. Social class, occupation, and similar factors show no consistent special risk factors. Prevalence rates for blacks and whites in the United States are similar (McCarty, 1979). Latitude, longitude, and altitude have no known influence (Kelsey, 1982).

While it was previously reported that no genetic and familial inheritance of rheumatoid arthritis occurs, recent data suggests this not to be true. Rheumatoid arthritis appears to have an expressed female dominance although the incidence at onset of rheumatoid arthritis may be 1:1 (Fleming, 1976). This control of expression may be hormonal or through some sex-linked influence.

Recent advances in tissue typing have shown the cell surface antigen HLA-Dw4 to be related to the incidence of rheumatoid arthritis (Silver, 1985). There is also a similar association with HLA-DR4 and a lesser association with HLA-Cw3. Only a small number of individuals with the HLA-Dw4 type actually contract rheumatoid arthritis and the correlation is far from complete, suggesting a multifactorial pathogenesis (see Chapter 5).

ETHNIC DISTRIBUTION OF RHEUMATOID ARTHRITIS

Study	Total	Male	Female
Israel	1.7%	0.8%	2.6%
USA National Health Survey	3.0%	1.7%	4.4%
Great Britain (Leigh and Wensleydale)	4.2%	2.8%	5.6%
American Indians (Blackfeet and Pima)	5.1%	4.5%	5.8%

(Cobb, 1971)

Figure 1.6 Ethnic distribution of rheumatoid arthritis. Age-sex adjusted rates per 100 persons age 35–64 for probable and definite cases of rheumatoid arthritis by ARA criteria, from selected large studies. Adjusted to the United States 1940 population.

ECONOMIC AND SOCIAL IMPACT

Economic costs of rheumatoid arthritis were estimated for 245,730 persons developing the disease in the United States in 1977 (Stone, 1984). Total lifetime costs were 5 billion dollars or $20,412 per person; direct costs comprising one fifth of the total and indirect costs (eg, productivity) four fifths. For men under 45 years the cost was about $60,000; for women it was $26,000. Younger people had higher costs because of longer life expectancy. Average cost covers patients with milder disease; more serious disease entails far higher costs. Costs were similar to those estimated for heart disease and stroke (Fig. 1.7).

MORTALITY

A prospective study of 1196 rheumatoid arthritis patients treated at the University of Saskatchewan between 1966–1974 was done. Of the 805 patients who were observed for an average of 12 years, 233 died and survival was 50% of the control population. The rheumatoid arthritis patients showed a marked increase in deaths from sepsis, rheumatoid arthritis itself (vasculitis, rheumatoid lung, amyloid, cervical spine subluxation) and gastrointestinal causes (hemorrhage and perforation). Treatment had no discernible effect on mortality (Mitchell, 1986). Multiple other studies confirm that rheumatoid arthritis patients have excess mortality rates and reduced life expectancy ranging from 3

LIFETIME COSTS OF RHEUMATOID ARTHRITIS FOR 3 HYPOTHETICAL PATIENTS

Cost Category	Patient A	Patient B	Patient C
Physician visits, drugs, aids	$4,320	$15,560	$66,000
Hospitalization	$0	$6,000	$67,500
Nursing care (home)	$0	$32,620	$238,464
Nursing care (private)			$40,000
Total direct costs	**$0**	**$54,180**	**$411,964**
Lost employment income	$0	$24,200	$320,780
Activity limitations after retirement	$0	$37,350	$100,000
Total indirect costs	**$0**	**$61,550**	**$420,780**
Total costs	**$4,320**	**$115,730**	**$832,744**

Patient A: Onset of disease at age 50. Mild, intermittent symptoms. Person remains self-sufficient.
Patient B: Onset of disease at age 40. More frequent physician treatments. Disease necessitates part-time work after age 60 and spending last 5 years of life in a nursing home.

Patient C: Onset of disease at age 30. Destructive and disabling disease. Employment impossible after age 40. Extensive medical treatment needed. Confined to a nursing home after age 55.

(Straszheim, 1985)

Figure 1.7   Lifetime costs of rheumatoid arthritis for three hypothetical patients.

to 18 years (Vanderbroecke, 1984; Reah, 1963). Studies looking at the overall causes estimated 20% of the deaths were due to rheumatoid arthritis itself and 25% due to therapy (Scott, 1986). Drugs are a dual-edged sword, delaying mortality in some cases and hastening it in others.

CLINICAL ONSET

The onset of rheumatoid arthritis varies from acute to insidious. The most common site of onset is in the hands and feet accounting for 70% of cases (Fig. 1.8). In one study of 102 pa-

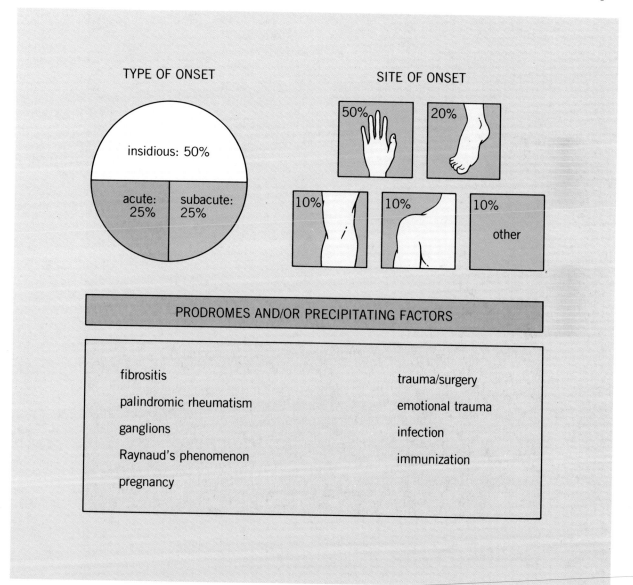

Figure 1.8 Common characteristics of onset of rheumatoid arthritis.

tients with early rheumatoid arthritis 36% presented with hand and wrist arthritis, 29% with multiple joints, 19% with foot or ankle, and 16% with other joints (Fleming, 1976). While episodes of pain and stiffness often precede the onset of frank arthritis, there are no clear precipitating causes. The relationship to trauma, infection, and other proposed inciting events may be coincidental.

Some interesting prospective studies have shown that when rheumatoid arthritis diagnosed within one year of onset is followed for

FEATURES INDICATING POOR PROGNOSIS

Significant Features	Nonsignificant Features
Subcutaneous nodules	Morning stiffness
*Muscle atrophy in hand	Pain and/or swelling in one joint
Lymphadenopathy	Swelling in second joint
*Positive latex test	Symmetrical swelling
*Punched out areas on radiograph	Mean number of joints affected
Significant anemia	Weight loss
*CRP positive	Moist palms
Insidious onset	Osteoporosis
*Onset limited to hands and feet	Elevated ESR
	Elevated WBC
	Increased protein and γ globulin

*P < .001
All others P > .05

(Wawryrnska, 1970)

Figure 1.9 A comparison of features found at early diagnosis of rheumatoid arthritis. Significant and nonsignificant indicators of poor prognosis when the disease was confirmed radiographically at two year follow-up are listed.

up to 7 years, the disease is either no longer present (40% of patients) (Mikkelson, 1969) or has changed at follow-up (6 of 15 patients) (Berkowitz, 1968). In another study of all patients with the most definitive diagnosis of rheumatoid arthritis, 37% had no discernible symptomatic disease four years later, although 40% had developed a variety of other rheumatic diseases. Also, of 105 patients without symptoms but with a positive rheumatoid factor, only 10% developed symptoms over four years (Mikkelson, 1969).

A study in Poland tried to determine which signs, symptoms, laboratory and radiograph findings had poor prognostic results over a two year period (Fig. 1.9). The most significant poor prognostic features included hand muscle atrophy, positive latex fixation, erosions on radiograph, and onset limited to the hands and feet. Surprisingly nonsignificant prognostic factors included many acute phase reactants in serum, symmetric arthritis and the mean number of joints at onset.

CLINICAL FEATURES

Rheumatoid arthritis has articular and systemic clinical complaints. Understanding the clinical picture and the supporting laboratory studies is essential to the diagnosis and management of the disease, particularly because of the problem with exact definition and diagnosis of rheumatoid arthritis. There is no single diagnostic clinical picture or exact physical finding or laboratory test which precisely defines this clinical entity. The disease is multifactorial and thus the clinical picture varies widely both in severity, course, extent of involvement, and in the clinical symptoms that it manifests (Fig. 1.10).

When taking the medical history the physician must take a good general history and focus on specifics that help define the diagnosis, its severity, the extra-articular features and symptoms that may differentiate rheu-

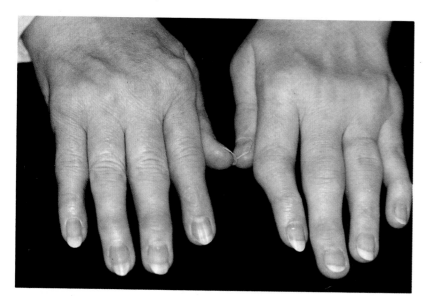 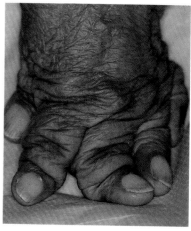

Figure 1.10 A comparison of disease progression over the same period of time. (*Left*) Rheumatoid arthritis with swelling of the MCP and PIP joints. Early deformity is seen at some of the interphalangeal joints. Disease duration of 10 years. (*Right*) Advanced rheumatoid changes in the hand. Telescoping of the digits with phalangeal resorption. Subluxation is severe. Disease duration of 10 years.

matoid arthritis from other common arthritides (Fig. 1.11).

An explosive onset may not predict a poor prognosis; many such cases undergo spontaneous remission. On the other hand, a few such cases progress quickly and relentlessly, leading to rapid joint destruction and occasionally death. An insidious onset often

FACTORS IN ESTABLISHING DIAGNOSIS OF RHEUMATOID ARTHRITIS

Onset

Prodromal Symptoms
Inciting Factors (eg, immunization, trauma,
   pregnancy)
Involved Joints
   Hands: PIP, MCP, not DP
   Symmetry
   Inflammatory nature
   Progressive
Previous Diagnosis
Response to Medication (to establish dose)

Systemic Manifestations

Nodules **(Fig. 1.12)**
Vasculitis **(Fig. 1.13)**
   Skin
   Neuropathy
   CNS
   Gangrene
Eyes
   Episcleritis, melting cornea **(Fig. 1.14)**
Fever, Malaise
Compression Neuropathy
   Headache, weakness, paresthesia,
   bladder dysfunction
Amyloidosis **(Fig. 1.15)**
Felty's Syndrome (infection, splenomegaly)
Anemia
Sjögrens Syndrome (dry eyes, mouth)
   (Fig. 1.16)
Pulmonary Fibrosis, Effusion **(Fig. 1.17)**
Cardiac Valve Pathology, Pericarditis
Muscle Wasting
Osteopenia **(Fig. 1.18)**

Course of Rheumatoid Arthritis and Other Diseases

Progressive (typical of rheumatoid arthritis)
Migratory (typical of rheumatic fever, gout,
   gonococcal arthritis)
Intermittent
   Palindromic rheumatism (inflammatory)
   Intermittent hydrarthrosis (noninflammatory)
   Early onset rheumatoid arthritis

Differentiation From Other Rheumatic Diseases

SLE
   Sun sensitivity
   Renal, neurologic, hematologic tests
   Serologic tests
Spondyloarthropathies
   Sacroiliac and spinal involvement
Psoriasis
Inflammatory Bowel Disease
Reiter's syndrome
   Urethrititis, conjuntivitis, keratoderma
Other Collagen Diseases
   Myopathy
   Scleroderma

General Review of Systems

Figure 1.11   Factors in establishing diagnosis of rheumatoid arthritis.

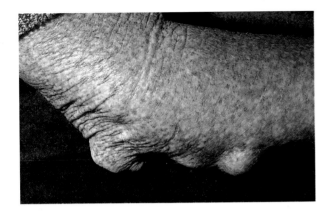

Figure 1.12 Rheumatoid nodules on the elbow.

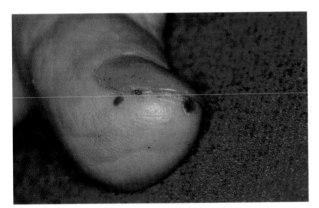

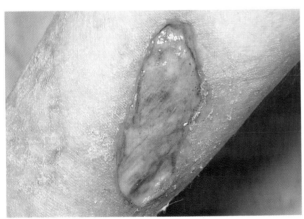

Figure 1.13 Small vessel abnormalities (*top*) at the tips of a digit of a patient with active rheumatoid arthritis. Vascular abnormalities in the distal extremity of a patient with rheumatoid arthritis lead to a typical rheumatoid ulceration (*bottom*).

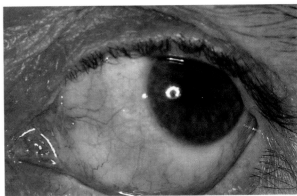

Figure 1.14 Scleromalacia. Episcleritis (inflammation over the sclera) leads to thinning and blue discoloration surrounding the iris, and can lead to perforation of the eye (scleromalacia perforans).

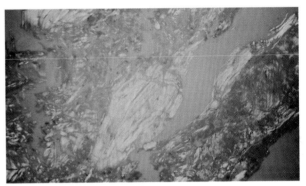

Figure 1.15 Amyloid deposits in the synovium. Synovium stained with Congo red shows typical apple-green birefringence seen under polarized light.

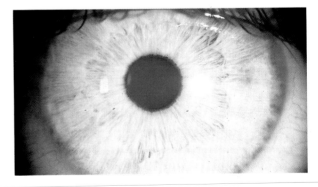

Figure 1.16 Sjögren's syndrome. Loss of epithelium over the cornea in the dry eyes associated with Sjögren's syndrome and rheumatoid arthritis.

indicates a slow but steadily progressive disease course.

The disease is usually polyarticular and involves multiple joints symmetrically. The most commonly involved joints are the hands and wrist, foot and ankle, and the knee. The pattern of joints affected may aid in differential diagnosis (Fig. 1.19). In some rheumatoid patients who chronically overuse one hand, the deformity may be more pronounced in that hand, leading to asymmetric involvement rather than the more typical symmetric in-

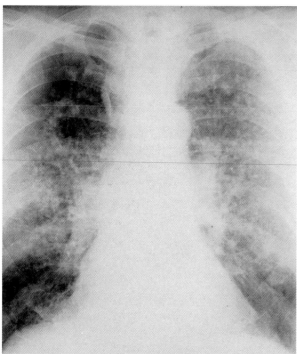

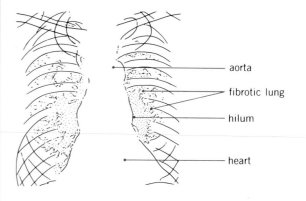

Figure 1.17 Rheumatoid lung. Interstitial fibrosis of the lung in a patient with rheumatoid arthritis.

— aorta

— fibrotic lung

— hilum

— heart

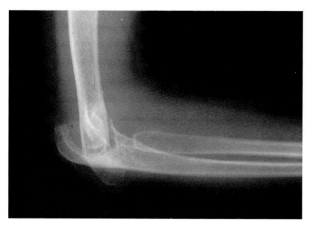

Figure 1.18 Severe elbow subluxation and erosion of osteopenic bone, leading to ulnar nerve entrapment.

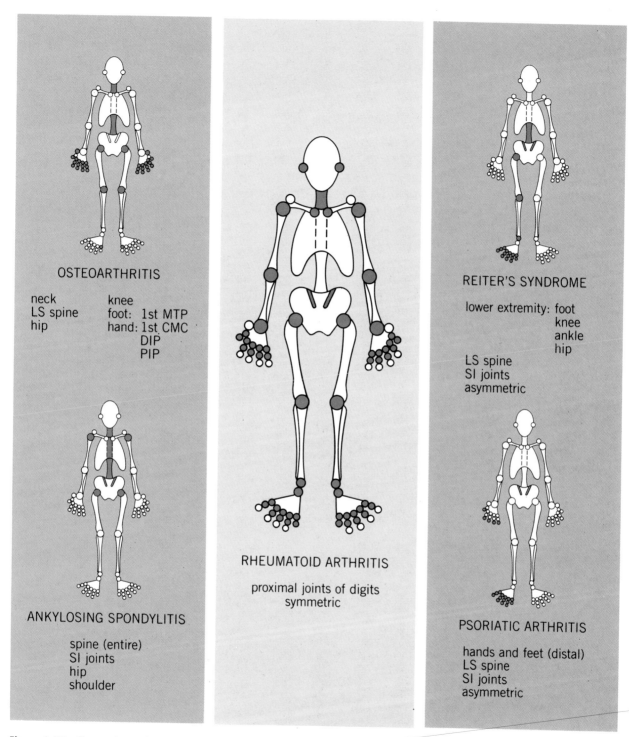

OSTEOARTHRITIS

neck
LS spine
hip

knee
foot: 1st MTP
hand: 1st CMC
      DIP
      PIP

ANKYLOSING SPONDYLITIS

spine (entire)
SI joints
hip
shoulder

RHEUMATOID ARTHRITIS

proximal joints of digits
symmetric

REITER'S SYNDROME

lower extremity: foot
                 knee
                 ankle
                 hip

LS spine
SI joints
asymmetric

PSORIATIC ARTHRITIS

hands and feet (distal)
LS spine
SI joints
asymmetric

Figure 1.19 Comparison of affected joints in different rheumatic diseases.

volvement (Fig. 1.20). For some reason the distal joints of the involved extremity are relatively spared as are the thoracic and lumbar spine. The specifics of joint involvement are covered in individual chapters on specific joints (see Section 2).

Many cases of what might be rheumatoid arthritis may never be diagnosed. Some disease could be relatively subclinical with aches and fatigue and no definitive objective findings. In others a single episode of the disease occurs and spontaneous remission ensues which may be permanent or may separate exacerbations by weeks, months, or years (Fig. 1.21). These spontaneous and/or drug associated exacerbations and remissions in the progressive course of the disease force the clinician to be wary of reports of drug efficacy or "miraculous" cures. Only through large, multicenter controlled treatment trials can efficacy of therapy be established since the manifestations of the disease are protean and highly variable. Finally, there are some patients whose disease rapidly progresses with or without aggressive treatment to severe joint destruction, severe systemic manifestations, and ultimately death from the disease itself or from complications of therapy.

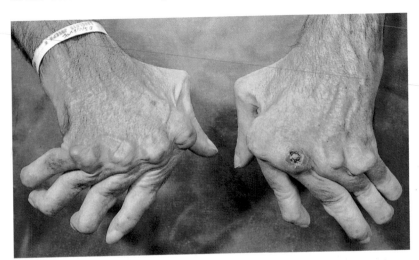

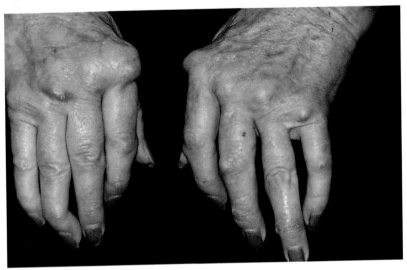

Figure 1.20 Subluxation and ulnar deviation are common in rheumatoid arthritis. The deformities are caused by joint, ligament, and tendon destruction as well as by physical forces. Severe subluxation, ulnar drift, and swan-neck deformity in a typically symmetric pattern is seen (*top*). Asymmetric disease can also be seen (*bottom*); in this case deformity is greater in the left hand. This is often caused by repetitive forces using one side of the body and suggests that joint protection can prevent deformity.

PHYSICAL EXAMINATION

Like the history, a thorough physical examination is necessary for several reasons. Rheumatoid arthritis does not occur as an isolated entity, and patients may have other unrelated and undetected disorders (ie, hypertension, ASHD, etc). Rheumatoid arthritis is, as previously noted, a systemic disease and a general physical examination may reveal additional findings. The discovery of some systemic problems may lead the clinician to discover that the symptoms, while mimicking rheumatoid arthritis, is not rheumatoid arthritis, ie, psoriatic skin and nail changes in psoriatric arthritis (Fig. 1.22), or tophi in chronic polyarticular gout (Fig. 1.23).

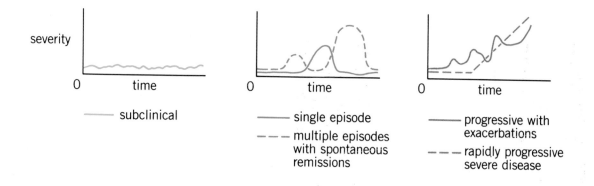

severity — time

—— subclinical

—— single episode
--- multiple episodes with spontaneous remissions

—— progressive with exacerbations
--- rapidly progressive severe disease

Figure 1.21 Various possible courses of rheumatoid disease over time.

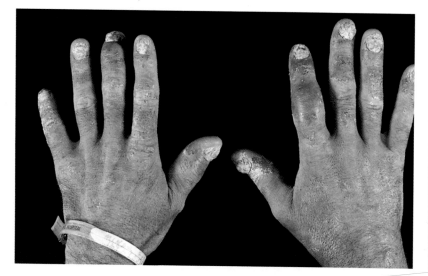

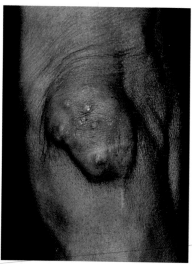

Figure 1.22 Psoriatic arthritis. Note the plaques of psoriasis on the hands, the onycholysis and the sausage swelling of the PIP joints. Asymmetric and distal joint involvement is seen.

Figure 1.23 Gout with gouty tophus evident around the joint.

The joints are swollen (Fig. 1.24) and may be dramatically red (Fig. 1.25), warm, tender, and show fluid and synovial thickening (Fig. 1.26). Severe swelling may lead to compression of the median nerve and the carpal tunnel syndrome (Fig. 1.27). The joint feels doughy; the fluid may be detected by a fluid wave (bulge sign), transillumination in a dark room, or ballottement. Swelling and heat may be subtle and comparison with contralateral or another normal joint may be helpful. The finding of heat is subjective and is sometimes best felt with the fingertip or palm of the hand being held over the joint and then in the midpart of the extremity away from the joint. Palpation may reveal tenderness along the joint margin and the supporting ligaments. If cartilaginous damage has occurred crepitus can be felt with joint motion. Loose bodies or tendon nodules may cause clicking with joint motion or may cause sudden cessation of joint excursion. Noting the location and signs of inflammation on a series of "stickman figures" records disease progression and the effect of medication (Fig. 1.28). Selected joints should be measured for

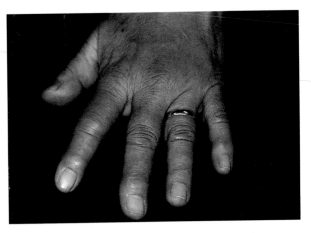

Figure 1.24 Inflammation with soft tissue swelling around the MCP and PIP joints of a patient with rheumatoid arthritis.

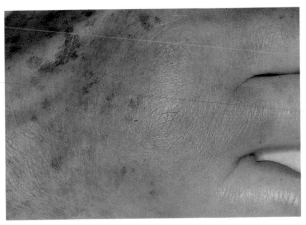

Figure 1.25 Acute synovitis of the MCP joint with swelling, synovial thickening, and redness.

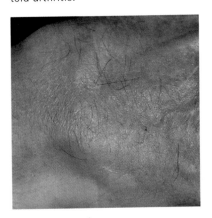

Figure 1.26 Severe synovitis of the MCP joint. Aspirated synovial fluid revealed no crystals, ruling out crystal-induced arthritis.

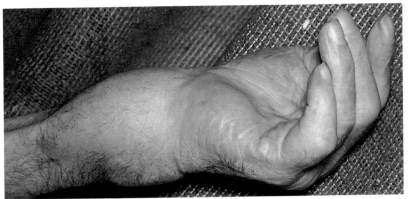

Figure 1.27 Marked swelling of the wrist with compression of the median nerve causing carpal tunnel syndrome.

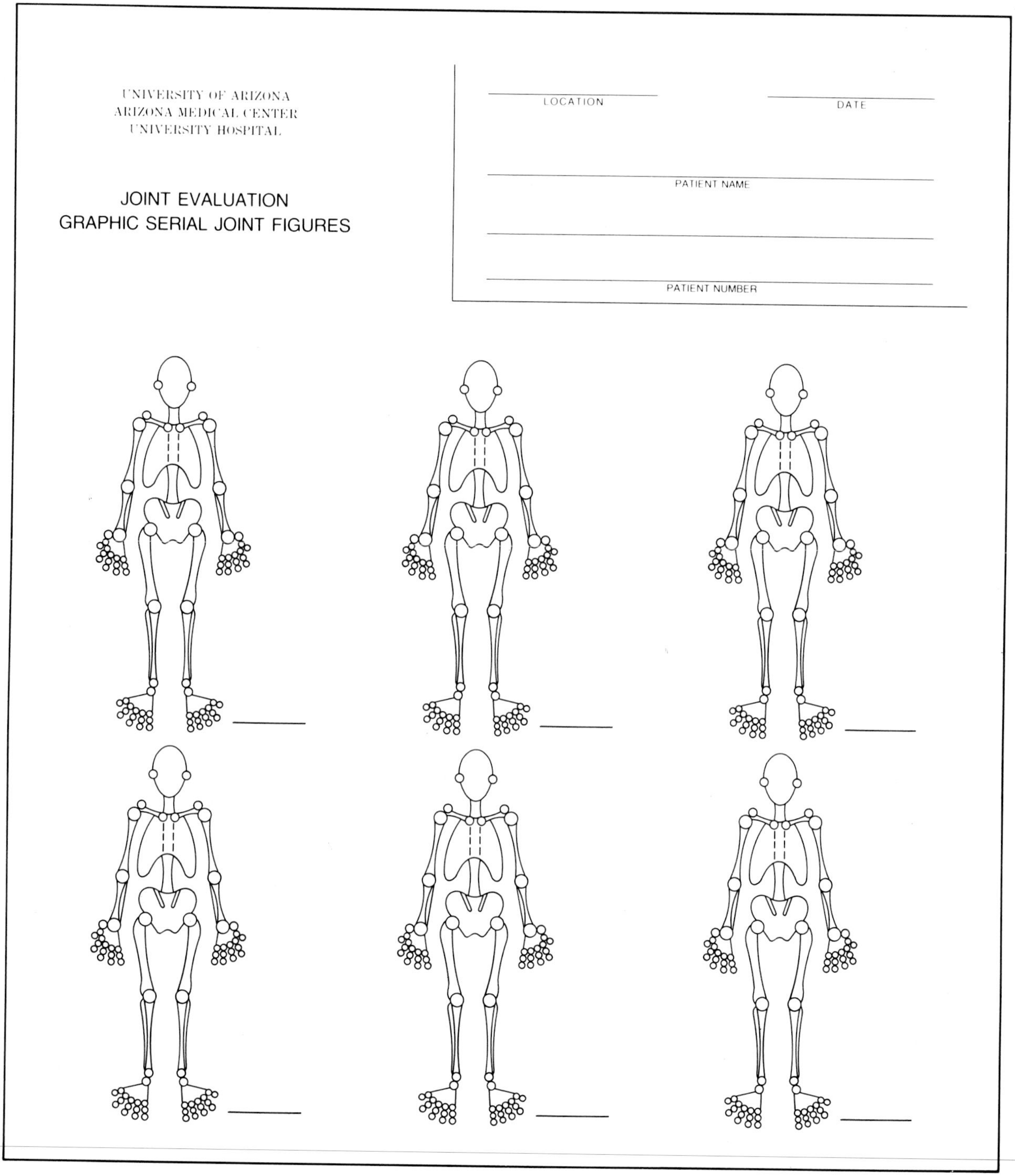
UNIVERSITY OF ARIZONA
ARIZONA MEDICAL CENTER
UNIVERSITY HOSPITAL

JOINT EVALUATION
GRAPHIC SERIAL JOINT FIGURES

LOCATION

DATE

PATIENT NAME

PATIENT NUMBER

Figure 1.28 Joint evaluation using graphic serial joint figures. (Courtesy of University of Arizona Medical Center).

range of motion by goniometer (Fig. 1.29) or by function (eg, grip, strength, fine motor function, walking times). Subjective, semi-quantitative estimation of pain or well-being (perhaps using a linear or curvilinear analog scale) and the amount of analgesic medication required complete the data needed for the diagnosis and to adequately follow the disease. Various indices of activity have been used to assess pain and progression of joint involvement including simple joint counts, the Lansbury scale, and the Ritchie scale (Figs. 1.30 and 1.31).

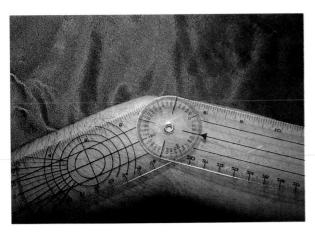

Figure 1.29 Measuring elbow flexion contracture using a goniometer over the joint.

THE LANSBURY SCALE

Joint	Value
Knuckles, Toes, Jaw and Acromioclavicular	1 Each
Bunion	2 Each
Sternoclavicular	3 Each
Wrist	4 Each
Carpals, Chopart's joint, and Subastragalar	5 Each
Ankle and Tarsals	9 Each
Elbow and Shoulder	12 Each
Knee and Hip	25 Each

(Lansbury, 1958)

Figure 1.30 The Lansbury Scale. Examine all peripheral joints for tenderness and/or pain on forced, passive motion. Write down the numerical value for each joint that is "positive." Add these up. This is the Articular Index. When one is not sure whether the joint is active or not, a half value may be given. When a joint has rest pain, or marked heat and fluid accumulation, it may be given an extra half value. Most joints are in the "average" range. When fleeting pain is said to be present without objective evidence of arthritis (eg, thickening) do not count it. Old, painless deformities also do not count.

RITCHIE SCALE

Joints Examined	Left Joint	Right Joint
Temporomandibular		
Cervical Spine*		
Sternoclavicular		
Acromioclavicular		
Shoulder		
Elbow		
Wrist		
MCP		
PIP		
Hip		
Knee		
Ankle		
Talocalcaneal*		
Midtarsal*		
Metatarsal		
TOTAL:		

KEY: 0 = not tender   3 = tender, winced, and withdrew
1 = tender
2 = tender and winced   *move, instead of press

(Ritchie, 1968)

Figure 1.31 The Ritchie Scale. To assess pain and tenderness, press each of the joints listed. Those indicated by an * should be moved instead of pressed. Record a value from 0 to 3 for each joint.

DIFFERENTIAL DIAGNOSIS

Rheumatoid arthritis sometimes may overlap with other related rheumatic disorders, such as systemic lupus erythematosus (SLE), polymyositis, scleroderma, or polyarteritis, and patients should be assessed for manifestations of these diseases. SLE has different organ systems involved and often has reversible hand deformities (Fig. 1.32). Polymyositis, while often having joint problems, will have muscle weakness and soreness as the most prominent symptoms. In scleroderma skin tightness is almost uniformly present while polyarteritis has vascular disease usually without significant arthritis. Rheumatoid arthritis and SLE may share many findings and occasionally the patient may manifest both or shift from one disease to the other ("rhupus"). This also may be true of many of the diseases mentioned earlier. Some diseses which overlap have been characterized clinically and serologically. "Mixed connective tissue disease" is one such syndrome. Treatment is directed toward the predominant clinical problem.

Intermittent syndromes are sometimes hard to diagnose. Intermittent hydroarthrosis is a problem of young women who have recurrent noninflammatory knee effusions often related to their menstrual periods. Palindromic rheumatism is also an episodic disease but the joint fluid is inflammatory in nature. When followed for years a number of these cases develop rheumatoid arthritis.

Viral syndromes, such as hepatitis, rubella, mumps, and immunizations for the latter two, may have an arthritis associated with them that resembles early rheumatoid arthritis. Proof of their nature comes with a permanent remission of the arthritis over time or with clinical manifestations typical of the viral illness itself.

The so-called "rheumatoid variants" have characteristics differentiating them from rheumatoid arthritis and these are summarized in Figure 1.33. Many of these differences will be discussed in subsequent chapters.

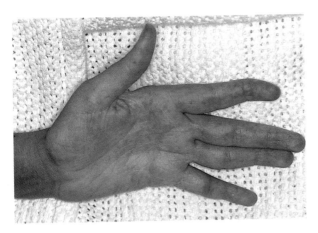

Figure 1.32 Hand with systemic lupus erythematosus. There is some palmar rash and redness of the distal digits (periungual distal erythema). Deformities are present which are readily reducible by placing the hand on a firm surface.

A COMPARISON OF CHARACTERISTICS OF ARTHRITIC CONDITIONS

	Rheumatoid Arthritis	Ankylosing Spondylosis	Enteropathic Syndromes	Psoriatic Arthritis	Reiter's Syndrome
Male/Female Occurence	1:3	20:1	1:1	1:1	20:1
Frequency in Population	1% to 3%	0.2%	< 0.1%	< 0.1%	< 0.1%
Genetic	Weak + HLA-DR4 in 50% to 60%	90% HLA-B27	↑ HLA-B27 only with Spondylitis	↑ HLA-B27 only with Spondylitis	↑ HLA-B27 in all cases
Joint Distribution	Peripheral Symmetrical	Axial and pauciarticular Symmetrical **(Fig. 1.34)**	Axial and pauciarticular Symmetrical	DIP* and Axial Asymmetrical	DIP* and Axial Asymmetrical **(Fig. 1.35)**
Conjunctivitis	0	0	0	0	+
Iritis (Acute)	0	+	0	0	+
Urethritis	0	0	0	0	+
Diarrhea	0	0	+	0	+/−
Psoriasiform Rash	0	0	0	+	+/−
Syndesmo-phytes	0	Thin, longitudinal Symmetrical	Thin, longitudinal Symmetrical	Heavy, transverse Asymmetrical	Heavy, transverse Asymmetrical
Nodules/ Rheumatoid factor/ ↓ in joint complement	+	0	0	0	0
Synovial Pro-liferation/ Joint Erosion	+	+	+	+	+
Response to Anti-Inflam-matory Drugs	+	+	+	+	+
Other Drug Treatment (remittive)	Gold, Antimalarial drugs	0	Drugs for bowel disease (ie, sulphasalizine)	Gold	0

Key: + = usually present
     +/− = sometimes present
     ↑ = elevated or increased incidence
     ↓ = decreased incidence
     0 = none

* Characteristically DIP, but not always

Figure 1.33 A comparison of characteristics of arthritic conditions.

RADIOLOGIC AND LABORATORY FINDINGS

The clinical diagnosis is modified by laboratory and radiologic findings. Appropriate baseline laboratory work might include those listed in Figure 1.36. The failure to obtain some baseline studies often leads to difficulty in diagnosis, treatment, and following the disease progression. For instance, the finding of typical marginal erosions on hand radiograph helps confirm the diagnosis, aids in making a decision as to whether to prescribe early remittive agents, and provides a baseline for following the progression of the disease (Fig. 1.38). Serum and fluid studies provide important diagnostic information,

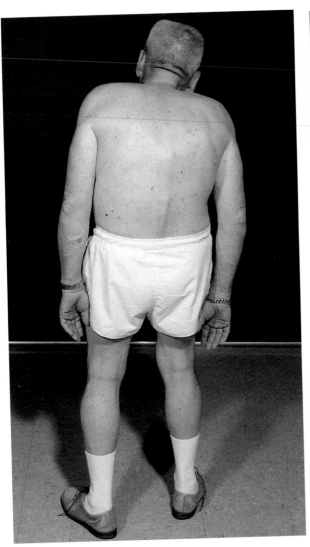

Figure 1.34 Ankylosing spondylitis with severe involvement of the spine. The distal joints are relatively spared.

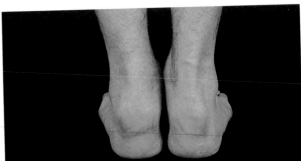

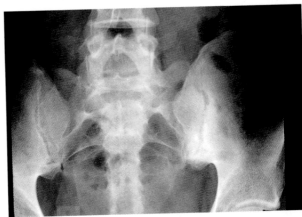

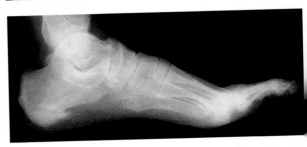

Figure 1.35 Reiter's syndrome, characterized by (*top*) Achilles tendinitis, (*middle*) asymmetric sacroiliac changes with erosion and reactive new bone. Reactive new bone formation with heel spur (*bottom*).

BASELINE LABORATORY WORKUP FOR RHEUMATOID ARTHRITIS

Blood

Complete blood count with differential and
  platelet count
Sedimentation rate (Westergren)
Rheumatoid factor with titer
Chemistry profile
Other tests in selected cases:
  antinuclear factor
  complement (C3, C4, CH50)
  special immunologic tests

Urine

Complete urinalysis with microscopic analysis

Synovial Fluid

Qualitative color, turbidity, and viscosity
Cell count, differential analysis
Crystal analysis under polarized light
Other tests in selected cases:
  complement with concomittent serum level
  sugar with concommitent serum level
  culture and sensitivity
  synovial biopsy

Radiographic Studies (Fig. 1.37)

Baseline radiographs of selected joints:
  knee radiographs with weightbearing views
  hands/feet likely to show early changes
  "joint survey," if available as a cost saving
    package
Radioisotope joint scan in selected cases

Figure 1.36 Baseline laboratory workup for rheumatoid arthritis.

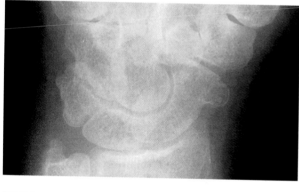

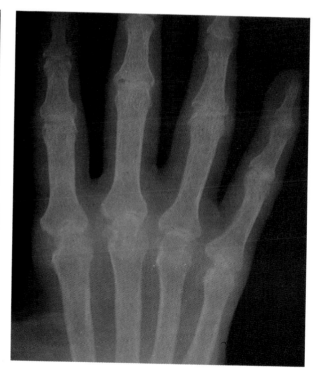

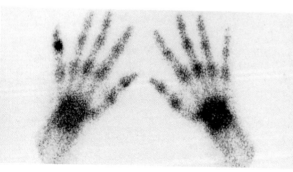

Figure 1.37 Note narrowing of radiocarpal joint and re-sorption of the ulnar styloid process (*top*). In scan (*bottom*) increased uptake in wrists, MCP, most PIP joints is symmetric, favoring rheumatoid arthritis diagnosis.

Figure 1.38 Early subluxation of the MCP joints and multiple marginal erosions are evident.

which, while not definitive, assist in establishing the diagnosis. Studies such as CAT scans, MRIs, angiography, and arthroscopy provide special anatomic information not available by less expensive, complicated, or invasive means (see Chapters 2, 3 and 4).

DIAGNOSTIC CRITERIA FOR RHEUMATOID ARTHRITIS (REVISED, 1958)

1. Morning stiffness.
2. Pain on motion or tenderness in at least one joint (observed by a physician).
3. Swelling in at least one joint that represents soft tissue thickening or fluid, not bony overgrowth alone (observed by a physician).
4. Swelling of at least one other joint (observed by a physician). An interval free of joint symptoms between the two joint involvements may not be more than 3 months.
5. Symmetrical joint swelling with simultaneous involvement of midphalangeal, metacarpophalangeal, or metatarsophalangeal joints is acceptable without absolute symmetry (observed by a physician). Terminal phalangeal joint involvement does not satisfy this criterion.
6. Subcutaneous nodules over bone prominences, on extensor surfaces or in juxta-articular regions (observed by a physician).
7. Radiographic changes typical of rheumatoid arthritis, which must include at least bony decalcification localized to or greatest around the involved joint and not just degenerative changes. Degenerative changes do not exclude patients from any group classified as rheumatoid arthritis.
8. Positive agglutination test: demonstration of the "rheumatoid factor" by any method that has been positive in not over 5% of normal controls in two laboratories, or from positive streptococcal agglutination test.
9. Poor mucin precipitate from synovial fluid with shreds and cloudy solution.
10. Characteristic histologic changes in synovial membrane with three or more of the following: marked villous hypertrophy; proliferation of superficial synovial cells, often with pali-

sading; marked infiltration of chronic inflammatory cells (lymphocytes or plasma cells predominating), with tendency to form "lymphoid nodules"; deposition of compact fibrin, either on surface or interstitially; foci of necrosis.
11. Characteristic histologic changes in nodules showing granulomatous foci with central zones of cell necrosis, surrounded by a palisade of proliferated mononuclear cell, peripheral fibrosis and chronic inflammatory cell infiltration

The diagnosis of classic rheumatoid arthritis requires 7 of the above criteria. The diagnosis for definite rheumatoid arthritis requires 5 of the above criteria. The diagnosis for probable rheumatoid arthritis requires 3 of the above criteria. For all three categories, in at least one of criteria 1 through 5 the joint signs or symptoms must be continuous for at least 6 weeks.

1. Morning stiffness
2. Tenderness or pain on motion with history of recurrence or persistence for 3 weeks (observed by a physician).
3. History or observation of joint swelling.
4. Subcutaneous nodules (observed by a physician).
5. Elevated sedimentation rate or C-reactive protein.
6. Iritis (of dubious value as a criterion except in juvenile arthritis).

The diagnosis for possible rheumatoid arthritis requires 2 of the above criteria and total duration of joint symptoms must be at least 3 months.

Figure 1.39 Diagnostic criteria for rheumatoid arthritis (revised).

DIAGNOSTIC CRITERIA

For many years the diagnosis of rheumatoid arthritis has been made by utilizing the 1958 modified diagnostic criteria of the American Rheumatism Association (Fig. 1.39). It is important to note the need for multiple exclusions. New criteria have been proposed

DIAGNOSTIC CRITERIA FOR RHEUMATOID ARTHRITIS (cont.)

Any of the following features will exclude a patient from all categories of rheumatoid arthritis.

Exclusions

1. The typical rash of systemic lupus erythematosus (with butterfly distribution, follicle plugging, and areas of atrophy).
2. High concentration of lupus erythematosus cells (1 or more in 2 smears prepared from heparinized blood incubated not over 2 hours) or other clear-cut evidence of systemic lupus erythematosus.
3. Histologic evidence of periarteritis nodosa with segmental necrosis of arteries associated with nodular leukocytic infiltration extending perivascularly and tending to include many eosinophils.
4. Weakness of neck, trunk and pharyngeal muscles or persistent muscle swelling or dermatomyositis.
5. Definite scleroderma, not limited to the fingers. (This is an arguable point.)
6. A clinical picture characteristic of rheumatic fever with migratory joint involvement and evidence of endocarditis, especially if accompanied by subcutaneous nodules or erythema marginatum or chorea. (An elevated anti-streptolysin titer will not rule out the diagnosis of rheumatoid arthritis.)
7. A clinical picture characteristic of gouty arthritis with acute attacks of swelling, redness, and pain in one or more joints, especially if relieved by colchicine, or accompanied by urate crystals.
8. Tophi.
9. A clinical picture characteristic of acute infectious arthritis of bacterial or viral origin with: an acute focus of infection or in close association with a disease of known infectious origin; chills; fever; and an acute joint involvement, usually migratory initially (especially if there are organisms in the joint fluid or there is a response to antibiotic therapy).
10. Tubercule bacilli in the joints or histologic evidence of joint tuberculosis.
11. A clinical picture characteristic of Reiter's syndrome with urethritis and conjunctivitis associated with acute joint involvement, usually migratory initially.
12. A clinical picture characteristic of the shoulder-hand syndrome, with unilateral involvement of shoulder and hand and diffuse swelling of the hand followed by atrophy and contractures.
13. A clinical picture characteristic of hypertrophic pulmonary osteoparthropathy with clubbing of fingers or hypertrophic periostitis along the shafts of the long bones, especially if an intrapulmonary lesion is present.
14. A clinical picture characteristic of neuroarthropathy, with condensation and destruction of bones of involved joints and with associated neurologic findings.
15. Homogentisic acid in the urine detectable grossly with alkalinization.
16. Histologic evidence of sarcoid or a positive Kveim test.
17. Multiple myeloma, as evidenced by a marked increase in plasma cells in the bone marrow or Bence Jones protein in the urine.
18. Characteristic skin lesions of erythema nodosum.
19. Leukemia or lymphoma with characteristic cells in peripheral blood, bone marrow, or tissues.
20. Agammaglobulinemia.

(Ropes, 1958)

(Arnett et al, 1987) and are undergoing testing. In these criteria there is no distinction between classic and definite disease and probable disease is deleted. There are seven criteria and any four are about 93% sensitive and 90% specific for rheumatoid arthritis. The criteria are: 1) morning stiffness for at least an hour for 6 or more weeks; 2) swelling of three or more joints for six or more weeks; 3) swelling of wrist, MCP, or PIP joint(s) for six or more weeks; 4) symmetrical swelling; 5) hand radiograph changes; 6) subcutaneous nodules; and 7) rheumatoid factor.

Only by putting together multiple criteria and ruling out other rheumatic disease can the diagnosis be made with a reasonable amount of certainty. The greatest use of the American Rheumatism Association (ARA) criteria is to assist the physician through an orderly diagnostic approach and ensure that studies of rheumatoid arthritis utilize a well-defined group of patients.

Various long-term follow-up studies have shown that these diagnostic criteria, even in the case of classical rheumatoid arthritis, are not foolproof. The first step to differentiate rheumatoid arthritis from other diseases is to determine whether the pain is articular rather than nonarticular. If the pain is in the joint, then one must determine if it is inflamma-

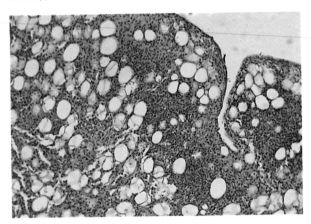

Figure 1.40 Severely inflamed synovium in rheumatoid arthritis. Thickening of the synovial lining cell layer and infiltrate with inflammatory cells can be seen.

CLASSIFICATION OF FUNCTIONAL CAPACITY IN RHEUMATOID ARTHRITIS

Class I Complete functional capacity with ability to carry on all usual duties without handicaps.

Class II Functional capacity adequate to conduct normal activities despite discomfort or limited mobility of one or more joints.

Class III Functional capacity adequate to perform few or none of the duties of usual occupation or self-care.

Class IV Total or almost total incapacitation, with patient bedridden or confined to wheelchair, able to perform little or no self-care.

Steinbrocker, 1949

Figure 1.41 Classification of functional capacity in rheumatoid arthritis.

tory. This is best done by synovial fluid examination which at the same time may be helpful in ruling out infection or crystal-induced disease. Histologic examination of the synovium shows chronic inflammatory cells, increased vascularity, and synovial lining cells but is nonspecific for the diagnosis (Fig. 1.40). The histology can help confirm the diagnosis and rule out tumor, infection, and crystal deposition disease. Once this is done, other rheumatic diseases are ruled out systemically by history, physical examination, and laboratory tests.

After the diagnosis of rheumatoid arthritis is made, the level of confidence is determined as possible, probable, definite, or classical, by ARA criteria. A functional classification then can be applied to the patient according to the ability of patients to perform the activities of daily living (Fig. 1.41). Accompanying this classification is a classification of rheumatoid arthritis progression using radiographic findings (Fig. 1.42). Despite being over 35 years old these two classifications are still widely used to stratify patients for epidemiologic and therapeutic studies (Steinbrocker, 1949).

Two more sophisticated descriptions of functional assessment that are widely used are the Arthritis Impact Measurement Scale (AIMS) from Boston Univesity and the Stanford Health Assessment Questionnaire (HAQ)

RADIOGRAPHIC CLASSIFICATION OF PROGRESSION OF RHEUMATOID ARTHRITIS

Stage I: Early

*No destructive changes on radiographic examination.
Radiographic evidence of osteoporosis may be present.

Stage II: Moderate

*Radiographic evidence of osteoporosis, with or without slight subchondral bone destruction. Slight cartilage destruction may be present.
*No joint deformities, although limitation of joint mobility may be present.
Adjacent muscle atrophy.
Extra-articular soft tissue lesions, such as nodules and tenosynovitis, may be present.

Stage III: Severe

*Radiographic evidence of cartilage and bone destruction, in addition to osteoporosis.
*Joint deformity, such as subluxation, ulnar deviation, or hyperextension, without fibrous or bone ankylosis.
Extensive muscle atrophy.
Extra-articular soft tissue lesions, such as nodules and tenosynovitis, may be present.

Stage IV: Terminal

*Fibrous or bony ankylosis.
Criteria of stage III.

*Primary criteria that must be met to permit classification of a patient in any particular stage grade.

Steinbrocker, 1949

Figure 1.42 Radiographic classification of progression of rheumatoid arthritis.

which utilize physical, social, and psychologic parameters (Fig. 1.43). These two instruments measure disability and correlate well with one another (correlation coefficient 0.91) (Brown, 1982). There are numerous other useful scales available.

Once the diagnosis has been made and functional capacity has been assessed, it is

STANFORD HEALTH ASSESSMENT QUESTIONNAIRE

	Without difficulty?	With difficulty?	With some help from another person?	Unable to do?

Dressing and Grooming
Able to:
   get your clothes out of the closet and drawers?
   dress yourself including handling of closures (buttons, zippers, snaps)?
   shampoo your hair?				

Arising Able to: stand up from a straight chair without using your arms for support?				

Eating
Able to:
   cut your meat?
   lift a full cup or glass to your mouth?				

Walking Able to: walk outdoors on flat ground?				

Hygiene
Able to:
   wash and dry your entire body?
   use the bathtub?
   turn faucets on and off?
   get on and off the toilet?				

Reach
Able to:
   comb your hair?
   reach and get down a 5 lb bag of sugar which is above your head?				

Figure 1.43 Stanford Health Assessment Questionnaire.

useful to determine if the disease has gone into either a natural or therapeutically-induced remission. Such an event has been written about frequently but not defined until recently (Fig. 1.44). These criteria are useful in determining medication effects as well as the natural history of the disease.

STANFORD HEALTH ASSESSMENT QUESTIONNAIRE (cont.)

	Without difficulty?	With difficulty?	With some help from another person?	Unable to do?

Grip
Able to:
   open push-button car doors?
   open jars which have been
      previously opened?
   use a pen or pencil?				

Activity
Able to:
   drive a car?
      (for reasons other than arthritis
      I do not drive _____)
   run errands and shop?				

Sex
Able to:
   have sex?
      (I am not involved in a sexual
      relationship _____)				

(Fries, 1980)

CRITERIA FOR REMISSION OF RHEUMATOID ARTHRITIS

Five or more of the following criteria must be fulfilled for at least two consecutive months:

1. Duration of morning stiffness not exceeding 15 minutes.
2. No fatigue.
3. No joint pain (by history).
4. No joint tenderness or pain on motion.
5. No soft tissue swelling in joints or tendon sheaths.
6. Erythrocyte sedimentation rate (Westergren method) less than 30 mm/hour for a female or 20 mm/hour for a male.

(Pinals, 1981)

Figure 1.44 Criteria apply to spontaneous remission or drug-induced suppression simulating spontaneous remission. Patient must have met criteria for definite or classic rheumatoid arthritis at some time. No alternative explanation allowable for not meeting a particular requirement. Exclusions: Clinical manifestations of active vasculitis, pericarditis, pleuritis or myositis, or an unexplained weight loss or fever attributable to rheumatoid arthritis.

REFERENCES

Arnett FC, Edworthy S, Bloch DA, McShane DJ, Fries JF and the ARA Rheumatoid Arthritis Criteria Subcommittee: The 1987 revised ARA criteria for rheumatoid arthritis. *Arthritis Rheum* 1987; 30:S17.

Berkowitz SS, Guariglia E, Laurian S, Steinbrocker O: Follow-up study of early arthropathies. *Hosp for Joint Dis Bulletin* 1968;29:65–76.

Brown JH, Kasis LE, Spitz PW, Gertman PM, Fries JF, Meenan RF: The dimension of health outcomes: A cross-validated examination of health status measurements. *Arthritis Rheum* 1982; 25(suppl): S149.

Cecil RL, Nichollis EE, Stainsby WI: The etiology of rheumatoid arthritis. *Am J Med Sci* 1931;181:12–25.

Cobb S: *The Frequency of Rheumatic Diseases.* Cambridge, Harvard University Press, 1971, p 29.

Fleming A, Crown JM, Corbett M: Early rheumatoid arthritis. *Ann Rheum Dis* 1976;35:357–360.

Fries JF, Spitz PW, Kraines RG, Holman HR: Measurement of patient outcome in arthritis. *Arthritis Rheum* 1980;23:137–145.

Garrod AB: A treatise on gout and rheumatic gout (rheumatoid arthritis), 3 ed, London, Longman, Green, 1876.

Harris ED Jr: Rheumatoid arthritis: The clinical spectrum, in Kelly WN, Harris ED, Ruddy S, Sledge CB: *Textbook of Rheumatology*, ed 2. Philadelphia, Saunders, 1985, pp 915–950.

Kelsey JL: *Epidemiology of Musculoskeletal Disorders: Monographs and Epidemiology in Biostatistics.* New York, Oxford University Press, 1982.

Landre-Beauvais AJ: Doit-ou admettre un nouvelle aspiece te goutte sous la denomination de goutte asthenique primitive? Paris, Brisson An. VIII, 1800.

Lansbury J: Report of a three year study of systemic and articular indexes in rheumatoid arthritis. *Arthritis Rheum* 1958;1:505–522.

Lawrence, JS: The epidemiology and genetics of rheumatoid arthritis, in *Rheumatology.* Basel, S. Krager, 1969.

Lawrence, JS: Rheumatism and populations, in Lawrence JS (ed): *Rheumatoid Arthritis.* London, William Heinemann, 1977.

McCarty DJ: *Arthritis and Allied Conditions: Textbook of Rheumatology*, ed 9. Philadelphia, Lea & Febiger, 1979.

Meenan RF, Gertman PM, Mason JH: Measuring health status in arthritis: The arthritis impact measurement scales. *Arthritis Rheum* 1980;23:146–152.

Mendez R, Gonzales-Alcover R, Roger L: Rheumatoid arthritis prevalence in a tropical area. *Arthritis Rheum* 1964;7:171–176.

Mikkelson WM, Dodge H: A four year follow-up of suspected rheumatoid arthritis. *Arthritis Rheum* 1969;12:87–91.

Mitchell DM, Spitz PW, Young DY, Bloch DA, McShane DJ, Fries JF: Survival, prognosis and causes of death in rheumatoid arthritis. *Arthritis Rheum* 1986;29:709–714.

Osler W: *The Principles and Practice of Medicine.* New York, D. Appleton & Co, 1892.

Pinals RS, Masi AT, Larsen RA and Subcommittee for the Criteria of Remission of the American Rheumatism Association Diagnostic Criteria Committee: Preliminary criteria for clinical remission in rheumatoid arthritis. *Arthritis Rheum* 1981;24:1308–1315.

Reah TG: The prognosis of rheumatoid arthritis. *Proc R Soc Med* 1963;56:813–817.

Ritchie DM, Boyle JA, McInnes JM, et al: Clinical studies with an articular index for the assessment of joint tenderness in patients with rheumatoid arthritis. *Qtrly J Med* 1968; 37:393–406.

Ropes MW, Bennett GA, Cobb S, Jacox R, Jesser RA: 1958 revision of criteria for rheumatoid arthritis. *Bull Rheum Dis* 1958;9:175–176.

Rose HM, Regan C, Pearce E, Lippman MO: Differential agglutination of sheep arthrocytes. *Proc Soc Exp Biol Med* 1948;68:1–6.

Scott DL, Symmons DPM: The mortality of rheumatoid arthritis, in *Reports on Rheumatic Disease, Series 2.* London, Arthritis & Rheumatism Council, 1986.

Shichikwi I, Mayeda A, Komat, Subara Y, et al: Rheumatic complaints in urban and rural populations in Osaka. *Ann Rheum Dis* 1966;25:25–31.

Short CL: The antiquity of rheumatoid arthritis. *Arthritis Rheum* 1974;17:193–205.

Short CL, Bauer W, Reynolds WS: *Rheumatoid Arthritis.* Cambridge, Harvard University Press, 1957.

Steinbrocker O, Traegey CH, Bateman RC: Therapeutic criteria in rheumatoid arthritis. *JAMA* 1949;140:659–662.

Stone CE: The lifetime economic cost of rheumatoid arthritis. *J Rheumatol* 1984;11:819–827.

Straszheim M: Economic costs, in Utsinger PA, Zvaifler NJ, Ehrlich G: *Rheumatoid Arthritis:* Philadelphia, JB Lippincott Co, 1985; pp 845-857.

Vanderbroecke JP, Hazevoet HM, Cats A: Survival and
cause of death in rheumatoid arthritis: A 25 year
prospective follow-up. *J Rheumatol* 1984;11:158–161.

Wawyrynska T, Pagowski J, Brezezinska M, Brzo-
zowskia D, et al: Observations on the signs and
symptoms of early rheumatoid arthritis in a prospective study. *Acta Rheum Scand* 1970;16:99–105.

Wolfe AM: The epidemiology of rheumatoid arthritis:
A review. *Bull Rheum Dis* 1968;19:518.

CHAPTER 2

LABORATORY FINDINGS IN RHEUMATOID ARTHRITIS

BRIAN F. MANDELL PhD, MD

Although joint symptoms are the predominant feature of rheumatoid arthritis, the high prevalence of fatigue and occasional fever, weight loss, and visceral involvement is evidence of the systemic nature of the disease. Several abnormalities in frequently-performed laboratory tests reflect this fact as well. Anemia, elevated acute phase reactants, and positive serologic tests are commonly observed.

ACUTE PHASE REACTANTS AND THE ERYTHROCYTE SEDIMENTATION RATE

Tissue injury and the resultant inflammation elicits a systemic reaction known as the acute phase response. The injury and inflammation can be anatomically localized (bacterial pneumonia, bone fracture, myocardial infarction) or generalized (rheumatoid arthritis, tuberculosis, metastatic cancer). The response, which is characterized by the rapid induction of specific protein synthesis by hepatocytes, is also seen in normal pregnancy after the first trimester. The acute phase reaction can be demonstrated in many animals as well as man, and has been presumed to have evolved as a defense mechanism to help ward off potential pathogens, and perhaps aid in the reparative response.

The liver, stimulated by intercellular immune modulators (including interleukin-1), rapidly produces increasing amounts of several plasma proteins (Fig. 2.1). Some of the

SOME COMPONENTS OF THE ACUTE PHASE RESPONSE

Protein	Extent of Increase
Ceruloplasmin	50%
Complement component C3	50%
α-1-antitrypsin	2 to 3X > normal
Haptoglobin	2 to 3X > normal
Fibrinogen*	2 to 3X > normal
Ferritin	2 to 20X > normal
C-reactive protein	100 to 1000X > normal
Serum amyloid-A protein	100 to 1000X > normal

*Major contributor to elevated erythrocyte sedimentation rate.

Figure 2.1 Some components of the acute phase response.

acute phase reactants, such as C-reactive protein, have been shown to participate in various phases of the inflammatory response, including complement activation (Kushner et al, 1981). Concomitant with this selective increased synthesis, there is a slight depression in the relative amount of albumin production. The increased synthesis of acute phase reactants occurs within a very short time of the in vivo noxious stimulus. The rate at which the peak serum levels of reactants are reached is almost entirely dependent upon the degradative rate of the individual proteins. These proteins, although released synchronously, may thus reach their maximal levels at various times. The absolute protein level attained in the serum is dependent upon the rate of both synthesis and degradation. Experimental studies using constant stimulation have demonstrated increasing hepatocyte recruitment over time, with each cell synthesizing C-reactive protein at an elevated rate. Likewise, the rate at which these proteins return to normal after the inciting trigger is removed is primarily dependent upon the individual protein degradation rates. In summary, the acute phase response is a complicated process with the levels of individual serum components exhibiting specific patterns of rise and fall.

Easier than measuring levels of specific components of the acute phase response is the measurement of the erythrocyte sedimentation rate. Recently reviewed by Bedell and Bush (1985), the erythrocyte sedimentation rate is dependent upon the balance between red blood cell repulsive and adhesive forces which influence the stacking of red cells termed rouleaux formation. Factors which enhance rouleaux, and thus increase the rate of sedimentation, include primarily the serum fibrinogen level, and to a lesser extent, gamma globulins and cholesterol. Other factors which can alter the erythrocyte sedimentation rate include anemia (hematocrits lower than 30% slightly raise the erythrocyte sedimentation rate), duration of time that the blood stands before the assay is run (passage of time lowers the erythrocyte sedimentation rate) and red blood cell shape (spherocytes and sickled cells settle more slowly). The erythrocyte sedimentation rate is slightly higher in the elderly and in females, decreased in hyperviscosity states, and dependent upon specific laboratory technique (such as anticoagulant, tube size, blood dilution).

The method generally used for determination of the sedimentation rate is that of Westergren (Fig. 2.2). This technique, characterized by the use of long tubes of narrow diameter has been found to be highly reliable over a wide range of values. The alternative Wintrobe method is rarely utilized as it gives a narrower range of values and provides less discrimination between higher values.

Acute phase reactants tend to be elevated in the vast majority of patients with rheumatoid disease. There has been a general sense that the erythrocyte sedimentation rate is higher in patients with more active or more severe disease. A normal erythrocyte sedimentation rate (0 to 20mm/hr in men and 0 to 30mm/hr in women) has also been listed as a criterion for remission (Pinals et al, 1981). Studies have indeed shown broad correlations between disease activity and erythrocyte sedimentation rate (Mallya et al, 1982). Others have shown depression of erythrocyte sedimentation rate with prednisone (Walsh et al, 1979), but not with nonsteroidal therapy (McConkey et al, 1973), despite the lack of evidence demonstrating a remittive effect of corticosteroids on disease progression and bone destruction. A minority of patients with active rheumatoid arthritis have normal erythrocyte sedimentation rates. A rare complication of rheumatoid disease, the hyperviscosity syndrome, would be expected to dramatically depress the erythrocyte sedimentation rate. In such cases, the quantitative level of C-reactive protein would still be elevated. Some authors believe C-reactive protein, measured by quantitative nephelometry, is generally a better correlate of disease activity than the erythrocyte sedimentation rate. This has not been rigorously demonstrated and *quantitative* C-reactive protein measurement is not uniformly available. Interestingly, some drugs influence these laboratory parameters in a manner discrepant from their clinical effect on disease activity (Dixon et al, 1985), and affect one acute phase reactant more than others.

Erythrocyte sedimentation rate and C-reactive protein measurements clearly cannot be utilized in all patients as firm indicators of disease activity or response to therapy. This has also recently been demonstrated in patients with ankylosing spondylitis (Nashel et al, 1986). A marked elevation in acute phase reactants is not expected, however, in uncomplicated osteoarthritis, but can be seen in other causes of arthritis (such as crystal-induced arthropathies), and in polymyalgia rheumatica. The utility of following any of these tests as disease activity markers must, therefore, be individualized. Certainly an elevated sedimentation rate alone, in the absence of clinical symptoms or findings, cannot be used reliably as an indication for treatment intensification. The sedimentation rate tends to increase slightly with age, and this too must be kept in mind when following patients over a long period of time.

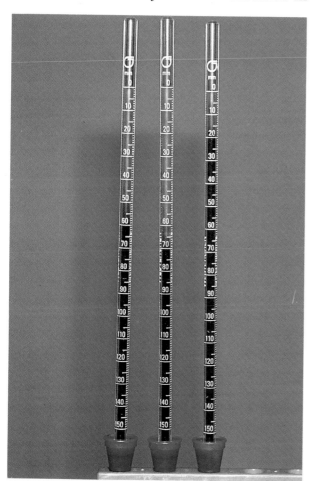

Figure 2.2 Three Westergren sedimentation rate tubes are shown. The distance that the erythrocytes have settled at 1 hour shows three different rates of sedimentation.

HEMATOLOGIC PARAMETERS

The majority of patients with rheumatoid disease who have significant involvement have anemia. As in all patients with a chronic systemic disease, the anemia may be multifactorial. Dietary or malabsorptive etiologies must be considered, as must iron deficiency secondary to iatrogenic gastrointestinal complications. By far the most common identified cause is the "anemia of chronic disease." This form of anemia is characterized by a hematocrit in the range of 30%, with automated red blood cell indices showing normal mean cell size and hemoglobin content. Peripheral blood smears often show a mild degree of cell heterogeneity with minimal microcytosis and hypochromicity. Bone marrow examination most commonly reveals normal erythroid maturation, no megaloblastoid changes, and slight to marked intracellular nonerythroid iron. Other laboratory concommitants include normal serum folate and B_{12} levels, low iron, low or normal total iron binding capacity, and a low (sometimes very low) percent iron saturation. Serum ferritin levels are variable. The degree of anemia does not necessarily correlate with severity of disease (Mallya et al, 1982), and even severe erosive disease can occasionally occur in its absence.

The pathogenesis of the anemia of chronic disease is still controversial, despite extensive studies in experimental animals and man. Marrow examination reveals normal or excess iron stores with redistribution into nonerythroid cells, leading to the suggestion that an iron transport defect is a primary etiology. Iron absorption is generally normal in rheumatoid arthritis patients (Weinstein, 1959), and only slight alterations in free iron clearance and cellular iron reutilization (Temple and Stuckey, 1986) have been described. Erythrocyte survival is slightly shortened. A mean survival of 80 days (range, 43 to 122 days) was found in one study (Cavill et al, 1977) and this has been previously documented by other investigators (Miller et al, 1956; Weinstein, 1959). However, this mild decrease in erythrocyte survival is not likely to be sufficient by itself to account for the anemia if marrow production is normal. Inappropriately depressed erythroprotein production has been observed in rats with experimentally induced anemia secondary to adjuvant arthritis (Lukens, 1973). Thus, the full explanation for the anemia in rheumatoid disease may include inappropriately low erythropoietin levels, relative marrow failure with resistance to stimulation by erythropoietin, low-grade hemolysis, and altered iron distribution.

Since the anemia of chronic disease is present in many of the same situations which trigger the acute reactant response, the two processes may be intimately connected. The anemia may result from the effect of one of the acute phase reactants. The availability of genetically engineered erythropoietin may allow, in the near future, for attempts to treat the anemia with high concentrations of this hormone, and to resolve the issue of marrow resistance.

A common problem encountered when treating patients with rheumatoid disease is distinguishing between the anemia of chronic disease and iron deficiency anemia (Fig. 2.3), and recognizing that the two conditions can coexist. Iron deficiency anemia may be more common in rheumatoid arthritis patients, but because of its high prevalence among age and sex-matched controls—usually menstruating women—this has not been conclusively demonstrated. It is predictable that the use of nonsteroidal anti-inflammatory drugs would contribute to iron deficiency by causing chronic low-grade gastrointestinal blood loss. Additionally, the antiplatelet effects of these drugs can enhance bleeding from other lesions. Hence, the physican should fully evaluate gastrointestinal blood loss in patients with rheumatoid disease, and not assume it to be secondary to the ulcerogenic effects of drug therapy.

Iron deficiency anemia is definitively diagnosed only by examination of bone marrow iron stores. The classic findings in patients with well-developed iron deficiency anemia, in the absence of an underlying inflammatory disease, include microcytic-hypochromic red blood cells on smear examination, low iron, high total iron binding capacity, low percent saturation, and a low serum ferritin level.

The last finding has been touted as a sensitive and fairly specific indicator of total body iron stores (Finch et al, 1986). However, since ferritin is an acute phase reactant and is thus commonly elevated in patients with rheumatoid disease, normal levels are not applicable (Blake and Bacon, 1981). In one study of randomly selected rheumatoid patients with anemia, 21 of 38 patients had iron deficiency by marrow aspirate. A serum ferritin level of less than 60 mcg/L was 86% sensitive and 88% specific for the diagnosis of iron deficiency (Hansen et al, 1983). In a

ANEMIA OF CHRONIC DISEASE v UNCOMPLICATED IRON DEFICIENCY ANEMIA

	CHRONIC DISEASE ANEMIA	IRON DEFICIENCY ANEMIA
Hemoglobin	Rarely < 9.0 g/dL	May be very low
Red cell morphology	Normal by automated indices*	Hypochromic, microcytic**
Serum iron	Low	Low
Total iron binding capacity	Low or normal	Normal or high
% Saturation	Low or normal	Low
Ferritin	Often high	Low or normal
Bone marrow iron	Normal with redistribution	Absent

*but often mixed normal and mild hypochromic, microcytic cells by microscopy
**although may be normal at onset

Figure 2.3 Anemia of chronic disease versus uncomplicated iron deficiency anemia

second study, a trial of iron therapy was given to 67 patients with rheumatoid disease and anemia; 83% of patients with a ferritin level less than 60 mcg/L responded (Hansen and Hansen, 1986). Therefore, although a low serum ferritin level is suggestive, it is not sufficient evidence to establish the diagnosis of iron deficiency in all patients. The incidence of falsely depressed ferritin values indicating a diagnosis of iron deficiency in a large rheumatoid population is not known. Marrow examination thus remains the diagnostic "gold standard."

Other nonerythroid blood cell lines are also affected in rheumatoid arthritis. Platelets are commonly elevated and the degree of thrombocytosis has been correlated by some authors with the erythrocyte sedimentation rate and articular index (Hutchinson et al, 1976; Farr et al, 1983). Interestingly, both of these studies, plus a third one (Colli et al, 1982), revealed elevated rates of platelet turnover. The possible association of the thrombocytosis with coexistent iron deficiency in these patients was not commented upon. Eosinophilia of variable degree has been reported in patients with rheumatoid disease, even in the absence of any drug reaction (Short et al, 1957; Sylvester and Pinals, 1970). Some authors have described patients with eosinophilia as having worse disease and an increased incidence of nodules, vasculitis, and episcleritis (Winchester et al, 1971; Panush et al, 1971). Leukocytosis has been reported with acute onset of disease. Leukopenia (neutropenia) is a major diagnostic component of Felty's syndrome, which occasionally also includes other components of hypersplenism.

IMMUNOLOGIC PARAMETERS

Features consistent with an autoimmune disorder are often found in patients with rheumatoid disease. Hypergammaglobulinemia and circulating immune complexes are extremely common. Delayed hypersensitivity is often depressed; one study demonstrated cutaneous anergy in 12 of 50 rheumatoid patients and 0 of 50 controls (Helliwell et al, 1984). Whether anergic patients exhibit specific clinical characteristics or respond differently to therapy has yet to be fully evaluated.

The HLA marker DR4 is common in seropositive rheumatoid arthritis patients (55% to 69%), but it is also present in 14% to 31% of normal people (Dinant et al, 1980; Scherak et al, 1980; Alarcon et al, 1982). Thus, it can hardly be used as a diagnostic marker. Alarcon et al (1982) have suggested a worse prognosis in rheumatoid factor negative (seronegative) patients who are DR4 positive, as compared to rheumatoid factor and DR4 negative patients with clinical rheumatoid disease. Preliminary studies have suggested that detection of specific DNA sequences within the DR4 region may further enhance the potential diagnostic utility of haplotype assessment. Patients carrying the DR3 marker have been reported by some investigators to be more susceptible to certain complications of gold and penicillamine therapy, including renal and hematologic toxicity.

Approximately 20% of rheumatoid patients may have low titer antinuclear antibodies (Fig. 2.4). Antibodies to single stranded DNA are common but antibodies to double stranded DNA are unusual. The latter are more commonly found (70%) in patients with systemic lupus erythematosus. Patients with rheumatoid arthritis may have anti-Ro or anti-La antibodies, but these are usually seen in conjunction with Sjögren's syndrome. Mothers with anti-Ro are at risk for giving birth to infants with congenital complete heart block.

Rheumatoid Factor

The best known laboratory test associated with rheumatoid arthritis is for the rheumatoid factor. It is the only serologic test listed among the American Rheumatism Association's criteria for the diagnosis of rheumatoid arthritis. Most large studies of rheumatoid arthritis indicate that 70% to 80% of patients fulfilling the clinical criteria for diagnosis have circulating rheumatoid factor as identified by agglutination tests. It is tempting to speculate that rheumatoid factor plays a role in the pathogenesis of rheumatoid disease.

Yet, despite statistically milder systemic disease (less vasculitis and nodules) and altered patterns of erosive disease (more asymmetry and wrist involvement) in seronegative patients, there is a great deal of clinical overlap between individual rheumatoid arthritis patients with or without circulating rheumatoid factors (Alarcon et al, 1982; Burns and Calin, 1983; Masi et al, 1976).

Whether seronegative patients have rheumatoid factor-producing cells in their synovium is still an open question. Masi et al (1976) noted more erosions in a female rheumatoid arthritis population aged 16 to 44 years old who were seropositive at the time of diagnosis than in similar seronegative patients. Interestingly, rheumatoid factor positivity was persistent in only 45% of these patients, but the outcome was correlated only with the initial presence or absence of rheumatoid factor.

Generally, patients who will produce rheumatoid factor do so within the first two years of disease. In a study of the efficacy of penicillamine, a drug which can dissociate IgM rheumatoid factor in vitro (Wernick et al,

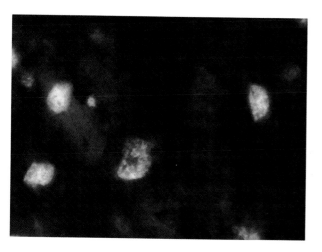

Figure 2.4 A speckled pattern of antinuclear antibody is nonspecific, certainly does not establish a diagnosis of systemic lupus erythematosus, and may be seen in many patients with rheumatoid arthritis.

1983), there was no association between levels of circulating IgM or IgG rheumatoid factors and clinical disease activity.

The presence of rheumatoid factor is not specific for rheumatoid arthritis (Fig. 2.5). Low to moderate titers develop with normal aging; in population studies, more normal people than rheumatoid patients were seropositive (Mikkelson et al, 1967; Cathcart and O'Sullivan, 1969). Another argument against the direct participation of circulating rheumatoid factor in the pathogenesis of rheumatoid disease is the finding that high rheumatoid factor titers can be seen in patients with subacute bacterial endocarditis and other chronic infections, as well as in primary Sjögren's syndrome, without the development of erosive arthritis. The issue of distinct molecular types of rheumatoid factor in these different situations is discussed below. It has generally been felt that rheumatoid vasculitis is more likely to develop in patients with a history of nodules and erosive arthritis in association with high titers of rheumatoid factor. Serum complement levels are often normal or elevated in rheumatoid arthritis, although with the development of systemic vasculitis or high titer cryoglobulinemia hypocomplementemia (C3, C4) can be observed. Hypocomplementemia with rheumatoid vasculitis is not a universal finding, and is not a prerequisite for diagnosis.

SOME DISEASES ASSOCIATED WITH RHEUMATOID FACTOR

Autoimmune Disease	Infection	Idiopathic
Rheumatoid arthritis	Bacterial endocarditis	Aging
Sjögren's syndrome	Chronic invasive parasitic diseases	Sarcoidosis
Systemic lupus erythematosus	Infectious mononucleosis	Interstitial lung disease
	Influenza	Tissue destruction (neoplasms following therapy)
Intensive Vaccination Regimens	Mycobacterial diseases	
	Spirochetal diseases	
	Chronic hepatitis	
	Salmonellosis	

Figure 2.5   Some diseases associated with rheumatoid factor.

Rheumatoid factors are autoantibodies which react, by definition, with the constant (Fc) portion of IgG. Anti-idiotype antibodies, which react with the antigen reactive moiety of the immunoglobulin protein, are therefore not considered to be rheumatoid factors. Because of the nature of most rheumatoid factor assays (agglutination techniques), the rheumatoid factors most commonly detected in clinical tests are of the IgM class. These IgM rheumatoid factors react only weakly with native IgG which is not heat aggregated, or in the form of antigen-IgG complexes. In 1956 Singer and Plotz described an assay which utilized latex beads coated with IgG as a suitable substrate for detecting agglutinating substances (Fig. 2.6). In serum, heat-treated to inactivate complement, the most commonly reacting substance is polymeric IgM. Studies using sheep erythrocytes coated with rabbit anti-sheep IgG (Rose-Waaler technique) instead of human IgG coated latex beads, demonstrated that IgM rheumatoid factors from different diseases could be differentiated. Sera from patients with seropositive (by latex) rheumatoid disease retained their reactivity, while patients with even high titers of rheumatoid factor as a result of endocarditis showed decreased or absent reactivity (Williams and Kunkel, 1962). Greater reactivity with human IgG than rabbit IgG has been seen in rheumatoid factors from patients with sarcoidosis, leprosy, and syphilis (Williams and Kunkel, 1963). The Rose-Waaler test is, however, a more cumbersome assay to perform, and is not in general clinical use.

Rheumatoid factors react preferentially with IgG of subclasses 1, 2, and 4 and can precipitate preformed immune complexes containing these IgGs. These subclasses, but not IgG_3, share the heavy chain genetic marker Ga. Rheumatoid factors are not monospecific; one well-described monoclonal rheumatoid factor was shown to cross react with DNA-nucleoprotein (Agnello et al, 1980). It is not clear whether this type of phenomenon explains the incidence of positive antinuclear antibodies in patients with rheumatoid arthritis or the 25% incidence of rheumatoid factors seen in patients with systemic lupus erythematosus.

Rheumatoid factors can be found in synovial fluids of patients with rheumatoid arthritis, even in the absence of detectable circulating rheumatoid factor activity (Munthe and Natvig, 1971). The demonstration of lo-

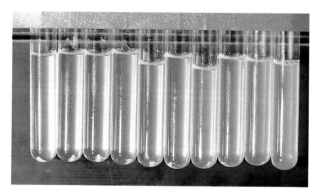

Figure 2.6 Tube dilutions of the latex fixation test are needed to determine titers of rheumatoid factor that are likely to be of significance.

calized production of rheumatoid factor in these few cases raises the following questions: Is the autoimmune response limited to the synovial membrane because lymphoid cells capable of producing rheumatoid factor are selectively drawn to the synovium by the presence of a specific antigen? Or does the local environment in the rheumatoid joint favor increased rheumatoid factor production by resident cells via selective stimulation and/or loss of tolerance? Isolated rheumatoid synovial membranes in vitro produced greater amounts of IgG than "normal" synovium, but amounts of IgG similar to normal spleen or lymph nodes (Smiley et al, 1968). Yet, response to specific antigenic challenge with tetanus toxoid, given systemically or locally, was far less than in peripheral cells (Herman et al, 1971). This suggests that the synovial lymphocyte population was committed to production of other antibodies, presumably including those with rheumatoid factor specificities.

Peripheral mononuclear cells from seropositive rheumatoid patients spontaneously elaborate rheumatoid factor. Peripheral blood cells from 8 of 22 seronegative patients secreted rheumatoid factor, detected by ra-dioimmunoassay, after (but not before) stimulation with pokeweed mitogen (Alarcon et al, 1982). The ability to make rheumatoid factor was independent of DR4 status, and since cells of some normal controls could also make rheumatoid factor, this further suggests that some exogenous (possibly intra-articular) trigger is necessary for rheumatoid factor production. Normal peripheral blood lymphocytes express rheumatoid factor upon stimulation with pokeweed mitogen or infection with Epstein-Barr virus (Slaughter et al, 1978). Perhaps as an in vivo correlate of this, 50% of patients with subacute bacterial endocarditis have detectable serum rheumatoid factor (Williams and Kunkel, 1962).

These results, plus recent studies using monoclonal antibodies (Fong et al, 1986), are consistent with the existence of a preserved, possibly germ line gene for rheumatoid factor which can be activated by systemic or local stimulation. The specific antigenic stimulus in rheumatoid arthritis is not known, but it has not been conclusively demonstrated to be aggregated IgG. The potential pathogenic role that rheumatoid factors play in rheumatoid arthritis remains to be elucidated.

REFERENCES

Agnello V, Arbetter A, de Kasep GI, et al: Evidence for a subset of rheumatoid factors that cross-react with DNA-histone and have a distinct cross-idiotype. *J Exp Med* 1980;151:1514–1527.

Alarcon GS, Koopman, WJ, Schrohenloher RE: Differential patterns of *in vitro* rheumatoid factor synthesis in seronegative and seropositive rheumatoid arthritis. *Arthritis Rheum* 1982;25:150–155.

Alarcon GS, Koopman WJ, Acton RT, et al: Seronegative rheumatoid arthritis: A distinct immunogenetic disease? *Arthritis Rheum* 1982;25:502–507.

Bedell SE, Bush BT: Erythrocyte sedimentation rate: From folklore to facts. *Am J Med* 1985;78:1001–1009.

Blake DR, Bacon PM: Serum ferritin and rheumatoid disease. *Br Med J* 1981;282:1273–1274.

Burns, TM, Calin, A: The hand radiograph as a diagnostic discriminant between seropositive and seronegative 'rheumatoid arthritis': A controlled study. *Ann Rheum Dis* 1983;42:605–12.

Cathcart ES, O'Sullivan JB: A longitudinal study of rheumatoid factors in a New England town. *Ann NY Acad Sci* 1969;168:41–50.

Cavill J, Ricketts C, Napier J: Erythropoiesis in the anemia of chronic disease. *Scand J Haematol* 1977;19:509–512.

Colli S, Maderna P, Tremoli E et al: Platelet function in rheumatoid arthritis. *Scand J Rheum* 1982;11:139–43.

Dinant HJ, Muller WH, van den Bergloonen EM, et al: HLA-DRw4 in Felty's syndrome (letter). *Arthritis Rheum* 1980;23:1336.

Dixon JS, Bird HA, Martin MFR, et al: Biochemical and clinical changes occurring during the treatment of rheumatoid arthritis with novel antirheumatoid drugs. *Int J Clin Pharmacol Res* 1985;5:25–33.

Farr M, Scott DL, Constable TJ et al: Thrombocytosis of active rheumatoid disease. *Ann Rheum Dis* 1983;42:545–549.

Finch CA, Bellotti V, Stray S, et al: Plasma ferritin determination as a diagnostic tool. *West J Med* 1986;145:657–663.

Fong S, Chen PP, Gilbertson TA, et al: Expression of three cross-reactive idiotypes on rheumatoid factor autoantibodies from patients with autoimmune diseases and seropositive adults. *J Immunol* 1986;137:122–128.

Hansen TM, Hansen NE, Birgens HS, et al: Serum ferritin and the assessment of iron deficiency in rheumatoid arthritis. *Scand J Rheumatol* 1983;12:353–359.

Hansen TM, Hansen NE: Serum ferritin as indicator of iron responsive anemia in patients with rheumatoid arthritis. *Ann Rheum Dis* 1986;45:596–602.

Helliwell MG, Panayi GS, Unger A: Delayed cutaneous hypersensitivity in rheumatoid arthritis: The influence of nutrition and drug therapy. *Clin Rheumatol* 1984;3:39–45.

Herman JH, Bradley J, Ziff M, et al: Response of the rheumatoid synovial membrane to exogenous immunization. *J Clin Invest* 1971;50:266–273.

Hutchinson RM, Davis P, Jayson MIV: Thrombocytosis in rheumatoid arthritis. *Ann Rheum Dis* 1976;35:138–142.

Kushner I, Gewurz H, Benson MD: C-reactive protein and the acute-phase response. *J Lab Clin Med* 1981;97:739–749.

Lukens JH: Control of erythropoiesis in rats with adjuvant induced chronic inflammation. *Blood* 1973;41:37–44.

Mallya RH, deBeer FC, Berry H, et al: Correlation of clinical parameters of disease activity in rheumatoid arthritis with serum concentrations of C-reactive protein and erythrocyte sedimentation rate. *J Rheumatol* 1982;9:224–228.

Masi AT, Muldonado-Cocco JA, Kaplan SB, et al: Prospective study of the early course of rheumatoid arthritis in young adults: Comparison of patients with and without rheumatoid factor positivity at entry and identification of variables correlating with outcome. *Semin Arthritis Rheum* 1976;5:299–326.

McConkey B, Crockson RA, Crockson AP, et al: The effects of some anti-inflammatory drugs on the acute phase proteins in rheumatoid arthritis. *Q J Med* 1973;42:785–791.

Mikkelsen WM, Dodge HJ, Duff IF, et al: Estimates of the prevalence of rheumatic disease in the population of Tecumseh, Michigan, 1959–1960. *J Chronic Dis* 1967;20:351–369.

Miller A, Chodos RB, Emerson CP, et al: Studies of the anemia and iron metabolism in cancer. *J Clin Invest* 1956;35:1248–1262.

Munthe E, Natvig JB: Characterization of IgG complexes in elevates from rheumatoid tissue. *Clin Exp Immunol* 1971;8:249–262.

Nashel DJ, Petrone DL, Ulmer CC, et al: C-reactive protein: A marker for disease activity in ankylosing spondylitis and Reiter's syndrome. *J Rheumatol* 1986;13:364–367.

Panush RS, Franco AE, Schur PH: Rheumatoid arthritis associated with eosinophilia. *Ann Int Med* 1971;75:199–205.

Pinals RS, Masi AT, Larsen RA, et al: Preliminary criteria for clinical remission in rheumatoid arthritis. *Arthritis Rheum* 1981;24:1308–1315.

Scherak O, Smolen JS, Mayr WR: Rheumatoid arthritis and B lymphocyte alloantigen HLA-DRw4. *J Rheumatol* 1980;7:9–12.

Short CS, Bauer W, Reynolds WE: *Rheumatoid Arthritis*. Cambridge, Harvard University Press, 1957, p 355.

Singer JM, Plotz CM: The latex fixation test. I. Application to the serologic diagnosis of rheumatoid arthritis. *Am J Med* 1956;21:888–892.

Slaughter L, Carson DA, Jensen FC, et al: In vitro effects of Epstein-Barr virus on the peripheral blood mononuclear cells from patients with rheumatoid arthritis and normal subjects. *J Exp Med* 1978;148:1429–1434.

Smiley JD, Sachs C, Ziff M: *In vitro* synthesis of immunoglobulin by rheumatoid synovial membrane. *J Clin Invest* 1968;47:624–632.

Sylvester RA, Pinals RS: Eosinophilia in rheumatoid arthritis. *Ann Allergy* 1970;28:565–568.

Temple JT, Stuckey WJ: Mechanisms contributing to the anemia associated with a localized solid tumor. *Am J Med Sci* 1986;292:277–281.

Walsh L, Davies P, McConkey B: Relationship between erythrocyte sedimentation rate and serum C-reactive protein in rheumatoid arthritis. *Ann Rheum Dis* 1979;38:362–363.

Weinstein IM, A correlative study of the erythrokinetics and disturbances in iron metabolism associated with the anemia of rheumatoid arthritis: *Blood* 1959;14:950–966.

Wernick R, Merryman P, Jaffe I, et al: IgG and IgM rheumatoid factors in rheumatoid arthritis: Quantitative response to penicillamine therapy and relationship to disease activity. *Arthritis Rheum* 1983;26:593–598.

Williams RC, Kunkel HG: Rheumatoid factor, complement and conglutinin aberrations in patients with subacute bacterial endocarditis. *J Clin Invest* 1962;41:666–675.

Williams RC, Kunkel HG: Separation of rheumatoid factors of different specificities using columns conjugated with gammaglobulin. *Arthritis Rheum* 1963;6:665–675.

Winchester RJ, Litwin SD, Koffler D, et al: Observations on the eosinophilia of certain patients with rheumatoid arthritis. *Arthritis Rheum* 1971;14:650–665.

CHAPTER 3

RADIOLOGIC FINDINGS IN RHEUMATOID ARTHRITIS

JOSEPH TSAI, MD AND MURRAY K. DALINKA, MD

Routine radiology has an important role in the initial diagnosis as well as the monitoring of disease activity in rheumatoid arthritis. This chapter reviews the radiographic findings typical of patients with rheumatoid arthritis. In addition, the roles of other imaging modalities such as arthrography, thermography, bone scintigraphy, ultrasonography, computed tomography, and magnetic resonance are discussed.

JOINT DISTRIBUTION

While rheumatoid arthritis is classically described as a symmetric arthritis involving the diarthrodial joints, its initial manifestations are often unilateral (Fleming et al, 1976; Halla et al, 1986). As rheumatoid arthritis progresses, joint involvement usually becomes more symmetric. Initially rheumatoid arthritis most commonly involves the small joints of the hand, wrist, and foot. Larger joints including the hip, shoulder, elbow, and knee may be also affected. Cervical spine involvement is usually accompanied by advanced disease in the extremities, although it may occur early in the course of disease (Bland et al, 1963). Rheumatoid arthritis less commonly affects the manubrium sterni

(Kelly et al, 1986; Perrin et al, 1977; Sebes and Salazar, 1982), temporomandibular (Martis and Karakasis, 1973), and cricoarytenoid (Brazeau-Lamontagne et al, 1986; Montgomery and Goodman, 1980) joints. Interestingly, in patients with a neurologic deficit and rheumatoid arthritis, the neurologically affected extremity may be spared by rheumatoid arthritis (Yaghmai et al, 1977).

PATHOLOGIC CORRELATION

Radiographic findings correlate directly with the underlying pathology. Proliferation and inflammation of the synovium is manifested radiographically by soft tissue swelling. Juxta-articular osteoporosis frequently accompanies soft tissue swelling as a consequence of hyperemia and subsequent increased bone resorption.

Soft tissue manifestations visible on radiographs include rheumatoid nodules and lymphedema. Rheumatoid nodules are most often located in the subcutaneous tissue of extensor surfaces. Occasionally, these nodules may erode adjacent bone, even in the absence of active joint rheumatoid arthritis

(Dalinka and Wunder, 1970; Dorfman et al, 1970; Kreel and Urquhart, 1963). Lymphedema of the upper extremities in the absence of cardiac or venous disease has been described in rheumatoid arthritis (DeSilva et al, 1980; Wu et al, 1982). The lymphedema has been hypothesized to result from the extension of inflammation from the synovium to the lymphatics leading to lymphatic obstruction.

Early in the course of disease, bony erosions may occur in the "bare areas" of the joint; these occur at sites within the synovial cavity not covered by articular cartilage. In the wrist, the ulnar styloid process may be involved early. Erosions of the ulnar styloid occur in three major locations (Resnick, 1974): at the tip, caused by inflammatory pannus involving the prestyloid recess (Fig. 3.1); on the ulnar side of the distal ulna secondary to inflammation about the extensor carpi ulnaris tendon (Fig. 3.2); and at the distal ulnar surface secondary to involvement of the triangular fibrocartilage (Fig. 3.3). Occasionally, periosteal reaction can be seen adjacent to acutely inflamed joints, but this reaction is seldom seen in chronic rheumatoid arthritis.

As the disease progresses, the articular cartilage is destroyed, leading to joint narrowing. Inflammation or destruction of the cartilage, ligaments, and tendons may lead to muscular or tendinous imbalance causing joint deformity (Fig. 3.4) or tendon rupture (Fig. 3.5). Ulnar deviation is the most common manifestation of tendon imbalance (Fig. 3.6) and is often accompanied by subluxation of the proximal phalanges.

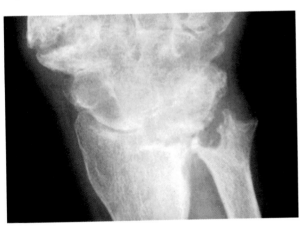

Figure 3.1 Erosion of the tip of the ulna styloid process secondary to pannus in the prestyloid recess. Erosions of the distal ulna and radius secondary to destruction of the triangular fibrocartilage are visible. The intercarpal joints are partially fused and the unfused articulations are narrowed.

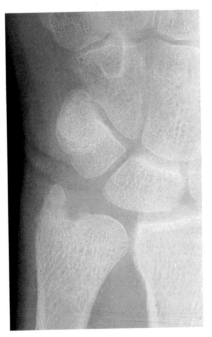

Figure 3.2 View of the ulna styloid showing erosion of the distal ulna adjacent to the base of the ulna styloid process and another smaller ill-defined erosion on the ulnar aspect of the styloid process secondary to erosion by the inflammatory change in the extensor carpilunaris tendon.

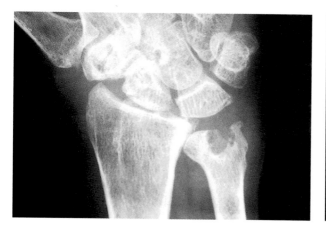

Figure 3.3 A large erosion is present in the distal ulna beneath the triangular fibrocartilage, and another is on the ulna side of the distal ulna. Soft tissue swelling is present in the region of the ulna styloid process.

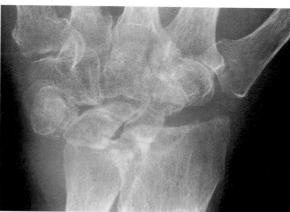

Figure 3.4 Ulna translocation. Wrist instability is present with the carpel bones displaced away from the radius towards the ulna. There is destruction of the distal ulna and soft tissue swelling over the ulna side of the wrist. The triangular fibrocartilage is disrupted, as are the ligamentous attachments between the radius and the scaphoid.

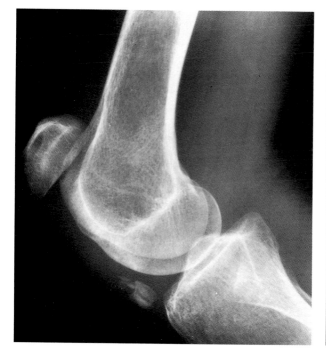

Figure 3.5 Patella tendon rupture. The patella is retracted superiorly by the quadriceps tendon. There is swelling in the infrapatellar region with multiple small bony fragments representing bony avulsions from the tibial tubercle.

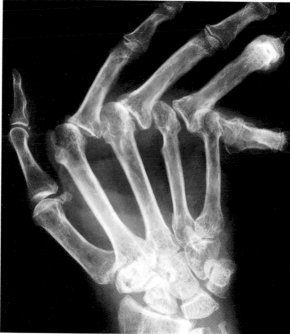

Figure 3.6 Ulnar deviation of the metacarpophalangeal joints of the second through fifth digits. A large pressure erosion is present on the radial side of the metacarpal head of the fourth digit. Flexion deformities are present at the fourth and fifth digits. The fourth digit exhibits a swan-neck deformity.

As a consequence of osteoporosis and malalignment, pressure erosions may occur. Pressure erosions appear as shallow, smooth cortical defects at sites of abutting bone (Monsees et al, 1985; Monsees and Murphy, 1985) (see also Fig. 3.6). In severe rheumatoid arthritis a pencil and cup deformity may occur at various sites, most often at the metacarpalphalangeal (MCP) joints (Fig. 3.7). This deformity represents an erosion of the metacarpal head into the proximal phalange. Similarly, a protrusio acetabuli deformity occurs when the femoral head protrudes into a softened acetabulum (Fig. 3.8).

Inflammation at the atlantoaxial joint may result in subluxation of C-1 on C-2, which is the most common manifestation of rheumatoid arthritis in the cervical spine (Cabot and Becker, 1978) (Fig. 3.9). Anterior subluxation is secondary to inflammation or rupture of the transverse atlantoaxial ligament, which surrounds the odontoid process posteriorly. Anterior subluxation may also occur as a result of erosion or fracture of the odontoid process. Occasionally, anterior subluxation may only be apparent with the patient's neck fully flexed. Posterior, vertical, lateral, or rotatory subluxation at the atlantoaxial joint oc-

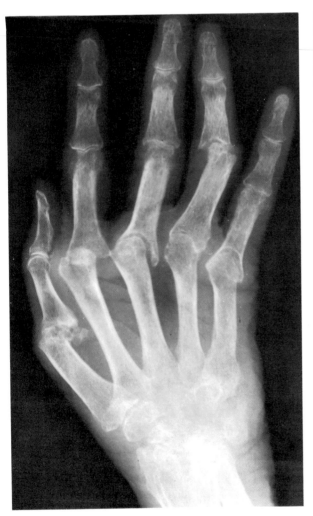

Figure 3.7 Ulnar deviation and pencil and cup deformities. There is remodeling of the bases of the proximal phalanges with mild ulnar subluxation at the second MCP joint. The overgrowth of the proximal phalangeal articular surfaces are particularly well demonstrated in the third digit. This has been called the "pencil and cup" deformity which may be associated with resorption and narrowing of the metacarpal head. Carpal fusions are present with destruction of the distal ulna and the radial styloid process. PIP involvement and diffuse osteopenia are also present.

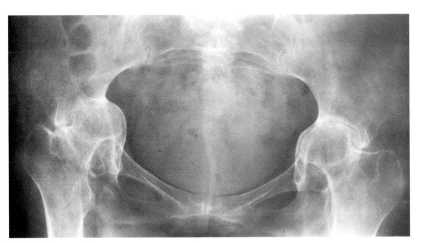

Figure 3.8 Protrusio acetabuli. There is marked central narrowing of both hip joints with protrusion of the femoral heads and medial wall of the acetabulum into the pelvis.

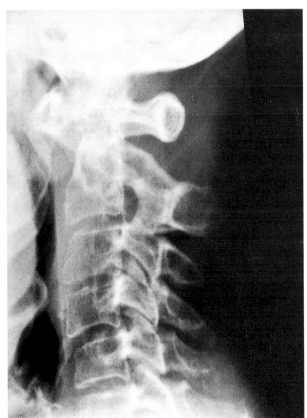

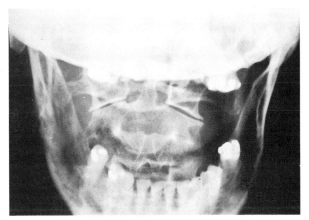

Figure 3.9 Atlantoaxial subluxation with odontoid erosions (*left*) lateral view of the cervical spine revealing anterior displacement of 8 mm of C-1 on C-2. Note the displacement of the spinal laminar line anteriorly. Anteroposterior open-mouth view (*right*) on the same patient revealing multiple erosions of the odontoid process.

cur less frequently.

Other important radiologic abnormalities of the cervical spine include cranial settling (Fig. 3.10) and multiple subaxial subluxations (Fig. 3.11). Cranial settling or atlantoaxial impaction, occurs when the articular relationships between the occiput, C-1, and C-2 are disrupted. This causes the cranium to articulate with the cervical spine below the level of C-2 and the odontoid to protrude into the foramen magnum (El-Khoury et al, 1980). Subaxial subluxations occur secondary to instability of the synovial-lined apophyseal joints.

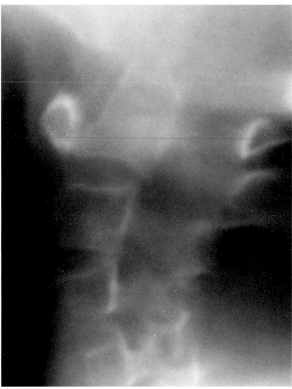

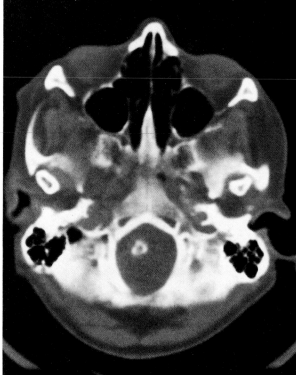

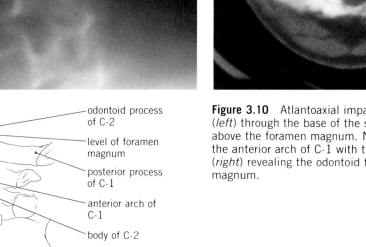

odontoid process of C-2

level of foramen magnum

posterior process of C-1

anterior arch of C-1

body of C-2

C-3

C-4

C-5

Figure 3.10 Atlantoaxial impaction. Lateral tomogram (*left*) through the base of the skull showing the odontoid above the foramen magnum. Note the low articulation of the anterior arch of C-1 with the body of C-2. CAT scan (*right*) revealing the odontoid to be within the foramen magnum.

RADIOGRAPHIC FEATURES OF SOME CLINICAL "SUBTYPES"

In many respects, rheumatoid arthritis represents a spectrum of disease manifestations, with several interesting clinical subtypes or closely related diseases that may have different radiographic features.

Seronegative Rheumatoid Arthritis

Ten percent to 30% of patients who are presumed to have rheumatoid arthritis do not have measurable rheumatoid factor in the serum. Several authors have suggested that patients with seronegative rheumatoid arthritis have milder radiographic progression of disease and are less likely to have rheumatoid nodules (DeCarvalho and Graudal, 1980; Sharp et al, 1971; Terkeltaub et al, 1983). One investigator has reported more frequent involvement of the metacarpophalangeal and metatarsophalangeal joints in seropositive patients compared to seronegative patients (Bland, 1963). No other differences in joint distribution or radiographic appearance were seen.

Adult Onset Still's Disease

Still's disease is a form of juvenile chronic polyarthritis which presents as a systemic disease in which joint features may not be prominent initially. When the onset of this

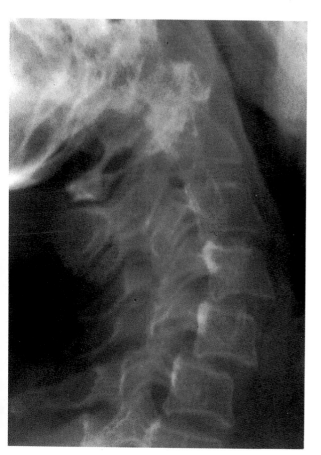

Figure 3.11 Multiple subaxial subluxations. Lateral view of cervical spine demonstrating multiple subluxations most marked anteriorly at C4-5 and C5-6.

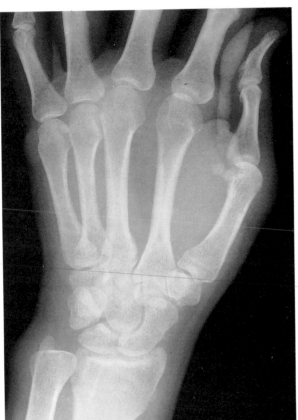

disease is beyond the age of 15 years, it is called adult onset Still's disease. Disease manifestations include fever, constitutional symptoms, an erythematous rash, lymphadenopathy, and arthralgia. An elevated white blood cell count is common as are lymphadenopathy and splenomegaly. Pleuritis, pericarditis, pneumonitis, and pharyngitis also occur in at least 25% of patients (Esdaile et al, 1980). In a study of seven adults and 53 cases from the literature (Del Paine and Leek, 1983), it was reported that the median age of onset was 28 years with five patients over the age of 50. In this series, two patients presented without a rash. The arthritis was commonly chronic and progressive.

A distinctive radiographic pattern of wrist disease has been reported in patients with Still's arthritis (Medsger and Christy, 1977). This consists of narrowing of the carpometacarpal and midcarpal compartments without erosions and may result in bony ankylosis. The second and third carpometacarpal joints are often selectively involved.

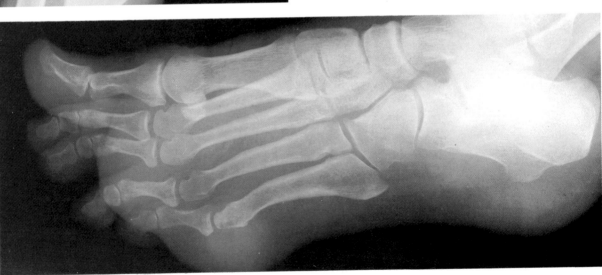

Figure 3.12 Oblique view (*top*) of hand revealing large nodules in the region of the ulna styloid process and the fifth metacarpal. Right foot in same patient (*bottom*) revealing large nodule around the undersurface region of the fifth metatarsal with bony erosion.

Rheumatoid Nodulosis

Several authors (Brower et al, 1977; Burry et al, 1979; Ginsberg et al, 1975; Snow et al 1979; Wisnieski and Askari, 1981) have described a clinical subtype of rheumatoid arthritis in which patients have extensive rheumatoid nodules (Fig. 3.12), high titers of rheumatoid factor, and subchondral bone cysts. They have little clinical evidence of active synovitis or systemic disease. This clinical syndrome can be confused with gout or xanthomatosis.

Robust-Type Rheumatism

An unusual group of nine men and one woman with classic rheumatoid arthritis who were largely asymptomatic from their disease has been described (DeHaas et al, 1974). These patients remained active, usually doing heavy manual work. They complained of brief periods of joint pain, mainly in the shoulder, requiring little if any analgesics. All the patients had multiple rheumatoid nod-ules and high serum titers of rheumatoid factor. The primary radiographic findings were osteoporosis and moderately-sized erosions, without evidence of large cysts. These patients may also develop intra-articular loose bodies secondary to the trauma of continued activity which is superimposed upon pannus and cartilage erosion (Moldofsky and Dalinka, 1979) (Fig. 3.13).

Fistulous Rheumatism

Occasionally, patients with rheumatoid arthritis develop cutaneous fistulas which usually occur adjacent to severely affected joints. Shapiro et al (1975) described several possible mechanisms for the development of these fistulas. Cutaneous fistulas may occur when bone fragments extruded from the diseased joint subsequently rupture through the skin (Resnick and Gmelich, 1975). Cutaneous fistulas also may develop as complications of synovial cyst rupture, septic arthritis, or iatrogenic aspiration of synovial cysts (Shapiro et al, 1975).

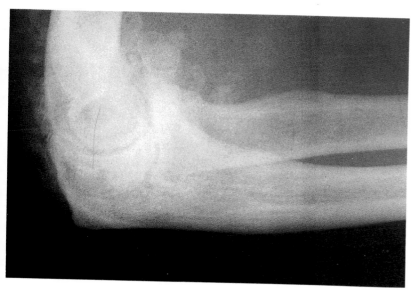

Figure 3.13 Lateral view of elbow in patient with rheumatoid arthritis and multiple loose bodies.

RADIOGRAPHIC DETECTION OF DISEASE COMPLICATIONS

Radiographically detectable complications of rheumatoid arthritis include ischemic necrosis, infection, insufficiency fracture, rotator cuff tear, tendon rupture, periarticular cysts, and geode formation.

Ischemic Necrosis

Most patients with ischemic necrosis and rheumatoid arthritis have been on long-term high-dose corticosteroid therapy. Ischemic necrosis may also possibly occur secondary to intra-articular steroid therapy and, very rarely, in association with vasculitis in the absence of steroids. Ischemic necrosis occurs most commonly in the hips and shoulders. Radiographic findings include the presence of a subchondral crescent, cyst formation, mottled sclerosis, flattening of the articular surface, and secondary degenerative joint disease. Magnetic resonance imaging is the primary method of early diagnosis.

Infection

There is an increased risk of septic arthritis in patients with rheumatoid arthritis, especially those on long-term corticosteroid treatment and following intra-articular steroids (Gelman and Ward, 1977; Good et al, 1978; Kartén, 1969; Resnick, 1975). This diagnosis should be suspected in a patient who exhibits a dramatic new asymmetric joint effusion or has disproportionate pain (Resnick, 1975). The differential diagnosis includes flares of the rheumatoid arthritis or trauma to the joint. Early diagnosis is made by aspiration with culture of joint fluid, rather than radiographically. Baseline radiographs should be obtained to search for new cortical defects or signs of osteomyelitis on follow-up.

Insufficiency Fracture

Rheumatoid arthritis patients are at increased risk for fractures secondary to osteoporosis, malalignment, and corticosteroid therapy. Spontaneous fractures, in the absence of significant trauma, most commonly occur in the lower extremities (Fig. 3.14). Fractures have also been reported to occur in the odontoid process (Martel and Bole, 1968; Resnick and Cone, 1984), olecranon (Rappoport et al, 1976), and pelvis (Taylor et al, 1971). These fractures often occur in association with abnormal alignment or may follow total joint replacement (Schneider and Kaye, 1975). Malalignment creates abnormal stress with weightbearing. Joint replacement increases the stress on the diseased bone by enabling the patient to use the abnormal extremity in a more normal way, so increasing the risk of insufficiency fractures in previously immobile patients.

Rotator Cuff Tears

Chronic synovitis may cause thinning or tearing of the rotator cuff. These patients may present with increased shoulder pain and joint immobility. Plain film findings include proximal migration of the humeral head, cystic changes in the humeral head, and irregularity and sclerosis of the undersurface of the acromion. The diagnosis may be confirmed by arthrography (Fig. 3.15) or by ultrasonography.

Tendon Rupture

Spontaneous tendon ruptures may occur secondary to erosion by pannus or bony spurs (Mannerfelt and Norman, 1969). In the hand, extensor tendon ruptures may cause sudden loss of finger extension. Tendon ruptures may be bilateral, particularly in the patellar tendon (see Fig. 3.5) and Achilles tendon.

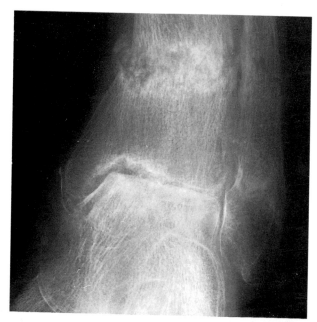

Figure 3.14 Insufficiency fracture in patient with rheumatoid arthritis. There is a fracture through the distal tibia with considerable bony sclerosis and irregularity. Note the asymmetric narrowing of the ankle joint and the area of linear density in the distal fibula representing an additional insufficiency fracture.

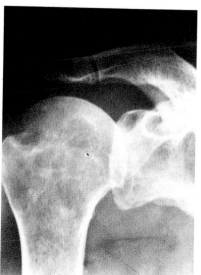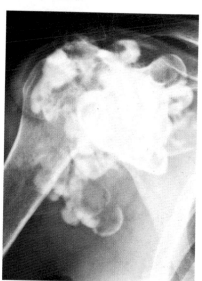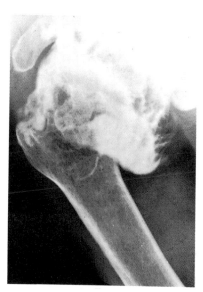

Figure 3.15 Rotator cuff tear. Plain film of the right shoulder (*left*) revealing multiple erosions in the region of the humeral head. Arthrogram (*middle*) demonstrating rotator cuff tear with contrast in the shoulder joint and the subacromial-subdeltoid bursa. There is marked enlargement and irregularity of the joint with filling defects secondary to synovial hypertrophy. Axillary view (*right*) demonstrating communication of contrast material with erosions.

Communicating Cysts

If there is an adjacent bursa, synovial fluid may dissect into the bursa or rupture into the soft tissues, decompressing the joint. This is most common around the knee. If fluid dissects posteriorly from the knee joint into the semimembranous gastrocnemius bursa, fluid flow is usually unidirectional from the joint into the cyst, with the narrow neck acting as a one-way valve. The bursa may enlarge, extending inferiorly into the calf (Fig. 3.16) or, less commonly, superiorly into the thigh. Occasionally, cysts may dissect or rupture, and the patient may present with calf swelling and pain, mimicking thrombophlebitis. Venography may be performed to exclude deep venous thrombosis. Occasionally, popliteal cysts and deep venous thrombosis may also occur simultaneously, secondary to pressure on the veins by the enlarged bursa or ruptured cystic contents (Patershank and Mitchell, 1977; Smurthwaite, 1976).

Rarely, dissection of joint fluid anteriorly from the knee into other bursa has been reported. When dissection occurs into the bursa deep to the medial collateral ligament, these patients typically present with pain and swelling on the anteromedial aspect of the medial tibial condyle (Palmer, 1972). Antefemoral cysts may occur when there is communication with the knee joint via the suprapatellar bursa (Seidl et al, 1979).

Enlargement of the subdeltoid bursa, which is usually continuous with the subacromial bursa, may occur alone but is usually associated with a rotator cuff tear. Radiographically, a soft tissue mass displaces the deltoid muscle laterally (Weston, 1969). Calcification within an enlarged subdeltoid bursa has also been reported in rheumatoid arthritis (Berger and Ziter, 1972).

Geodes

Erosion of the cartilage usually results in joint space narrowing. Occasionally, pannus can erode through a focal defect in the cartilage, creating subchondral cysts or geodes (Fig. 3.17). These geodes may occur around any joint but are more common in the weight-

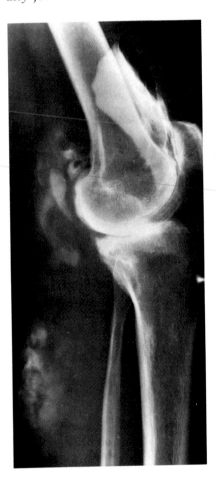

Figure 3.16 Knee arthrogram demonstrating large dissecting popliteal cyst in patient with rheumatoid arthritis.

bearing joints such as the knee or hip. They have been reported to become as large as 5 cm in diameter (Gohel et al, 1972; Magyar et al, 1974). Occasionally, geodes may be confused with a malignant tumor or pigmented villonodular synovitis (Gerster et al, 1982).

OTHER IMAGING MODALITIES

The advent of new imaging modalities may provide additional help in the evaluation of rheumatoid arthritis. In this section, the use and indications of these imaging modalities are briefly discussed.

Arthrography

Arthrography may be utilized for the evaluation of communicating or giant cysts in any joint or rotator cuff tears in the shoulder.

In the knee, arthrography is useful in both the diagnosis and treatment of a popliteal cyst (see Fig 3.16). Arthrography can determine the presence and size of the cyst, as well as whether it is intact or ruptured. Treatment by aspiration of the joint and instilling steroids either into the joint space or the cyst may also be performed.

The rotator cuff tendons separate the glenohumeral joint from the subacromial subdeltoid bursae. During arthrography, contrast passing from the glenohumeral joint into the

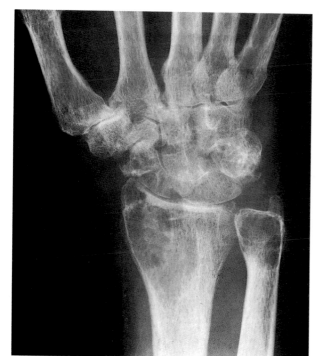

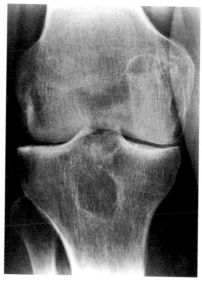

Figure 3.17 Large geodes (*left*) in the distal ulna and distal radius. Notice the extensive destruction of the intercarpal articulations. Another patient (*right*) with a large lucent lesion in proximal tibia representing geode. Note the narrowing of the knee joint.

subdeltoid or subacromial bursae indicates a tear of the rotator cuff (*see* Fig. 3.15). Nodular filling defects may be seen in the involved shoulder joint secondary to synovial hypertrophy (DeSmet et al, 1975). Lymphatic filling is a frequent but nonspecific finding.

Thermography

Thermography, is not popular in the United States, but has been used in Europe for the evaluation of inflammatory arthritis. Hyperemia or synovitis leads to temperature increases which may be detected early in the course of the disease (Colavita et al, 1983).

Ultrasonography

Ultrasound may provide a noninvasive alternative to arthrography in the diagnosis of rotator cuff tears or periarticular cysts. Although comparative studies have not been performed in patients with rheumatoid arthritis, ultrasonography has been shown to correlate well with arthrography in demonstrating rotator cuff tears (Mack et al, 1985; Middleton et al, 1985) and popliteal cysts (Carpenter et al, 1976) (Fig. 3.18).

Computerized Axial Tomography (CAT) Scans

CAT scans play a supplemental role to other imaging modalities in rheumatoid arthritis. CAT scans are helpful in the evaluation of the cervical spine, where they are superior to plain radiographs in demonstrating vertical (see Fig. 3.10) and posterior atlantoaxial subluxation.

In one study (Schwimmer et al, 1985), CAT scans were used to demonstrate synovial cysts associated with the knee. CAT scans were especially valuable for demonstrating cysts that occurred in unusual locations or that did not communicate with the joint, which precluded arthrographic diagnosis.

CAT scans have also been used to evaluate extraskeletal manifestations of rheumatoid arthritis, including rheumatoid lung disease

Figure 3.18 Large cystic lesion in popliteal region demonstrated on ultrasound.

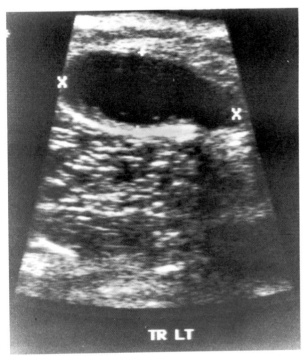

(Bergin and Muller, 1985), cricoarytenoid disease (Brazeau-Lamontagne et al, 1986), and hepatic deposition of gold during treatment of rheumatoid arthritis with gold salts (DeMaria et al, 1986).

Nuclear Medicine Scans

Nuclear medicine scans have been a valuable ancillary technique particularly in the evaluation of early avascular necrosis.

The earliest but often undetected abnormality in avascular necrosis is a cold defect on bone scan secondary to the acute vascular insult. With subsequent revascularization and healing, increased uptake is seen in the involved bone (Mettler and Guiberteau, 1986). Nuclear scintigraphy has largely been supplanted by magnetic resonance imaging when available, since the latter modality is considerably more sensitive in both early and late disease (Mitchell et al, 1987; Thickman et al, 1986).

One research team reported finding that radionuclide joint scanning was valuable for excluding inflammatory arthritis in patients with vague complaints of polyarthralgia (Shearman et al, 1982). Joint scanning may also detect the presence of inflammation in rheumatoid arthritis prior to radiographically evident erosions (Pitt et al, 1986).

Magnetic Resonance Imaging

Because of its superior contrast, magnetic resonance imaging (MRI) is quickly becoming the diagnostic study of choice for many soft tissue and bone lesions.

In the cervical spine, MRI has the advantage of imaging the spinal cord within the spinal canal. Cervical spine abnormalities have been demonstrated by MRI and myelography in four patients with rheumatoid arthritis (Masaryk et al, 1986). In one patient, MRI proved superior to myelography by visualizing the entire spinal cord, including the area distal to a high-grade stenosis. In another patient, MRI, with flexion and extension views, directly demonstrated impingement by the odontoid process on the cervicomedullary region.

In patients clinically suspected of having avascular necrosis, MRI detects changes in the femoral head before they appear on radiographs or nuclear medicine scans. Hence MRI is the most sensitive test for the early detection of avascular necrosis (Mitchell et al, 1986; Thickman et al, 1986).

Because of its excellent soft tissue resolution, MRI may be valuable in the evaluation of carpal tunnel syndrome associated with rheumatoid arthritis (Weiss et al, 1986). MRI can demonstrate soft tissue abnormalities in patients with normal radiographs and may be used in the evaluation of synovial cysts, geodes, or other soft tissue (Fig. 3.19) and osseous abnormalities.

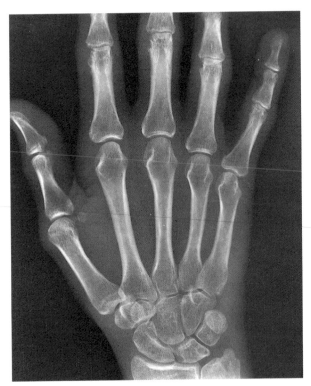

Figure 3.19 Plain film (*top, left*) of hand and wrist revealing moderate osteopenia and multiple subtle erosions. A 2000/80 MRI image (*bottom, left*) revealing area of increased intensity on the radial side of the wrist indicating inflammatory tissue. A 2000/80 spin echo image of same patient (*bottom, right*) in more anterior location indicating an area of increased intensity in the location of the radial ulna joint. Additional areas of high intensity are located in the region of the lunate and distal radioulnar joint.

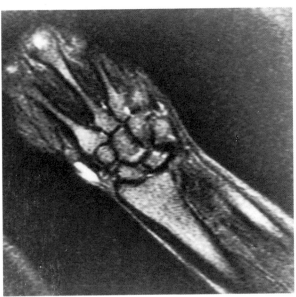
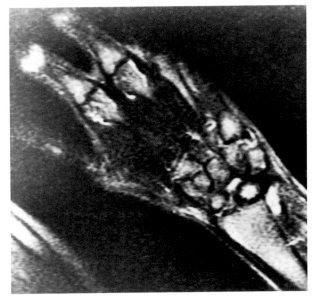

REFERENCES

Berger LS, Ziter FMH: Case reports: Calcification within enlarged subdeltoid bursae in rheumatoid arthritis. *Br J Radiol* 1972;45:530-531.

Bergin CJ, Muller NL: CT in the diagnosis of interstitial lung disease. *AJR* 1985;145:505-510.

Bland JH: Seronegative and seropositive rheumatoid arthritis: Clinical, radiological, and biochemical differences. *Ann Intern Med* 1963;60:88-94.

Bland JH, Davis PH, London MG, et al: Rheumatoid arthritis of cervical spine. *Arch Intern Med* 1963;112:892-898.

Brazeau-Lamontagne L, Charlin B, Levesque R, et al: Cricoarytenoiditis: CT assessment in rheumatoid arthritis. *Radiology* 1986;158:463-466.

Brower AC, NaPombejara C, Stechschulte DJ, et al: Rheumatoid nodulosis: Another cause of juxta-articular nodules. *Radiology* 1977;125:669-670.

Burry HC, Caughey D, Palmer DG: Benign rheumatoid nodules. *Aust NZ J Med* 1979;697-701.

Cabot A, Becker A: The cervical spine in rheumatoid arthritis. *Clin Orthop* 1978;131:130-140.

Carpenter JR, Hattery RB, Hunter GC: Ultrasound evaluation of the popliteal space: Comparison with arthrography and physical examination. *Mayo Clin Proc* 1976;51:498-503.

Colavita N, Orazi C, Fusco A: Role of telethermography and arthrography in rheumatoid wrist. *Diagn Imag* 1983;52:189-196.

Cruess RL: Rheumatoid arthritis of the shoulder. *Orthop Clin North Am* 1980;11:333-342.

Dalinka MK, Wunder JF: Unusual manifestations of rheumatoid arthritis. *Radiology* 1970;97:393-395.

DeCarvalho A, Graudal H: Radiographic progression of rheumatoid arthritis related to some clinical and laboratory parameters. *Acta Radiol Diagn* 1980;21:551-555.

DeHaas WHD, Griffioen F, Oosten-Elst P: Rheumatoid arthritis of the robust reaction type. *Ann Rheum Dis* 1974;33:81-85.

Del Paine JDW, Leek JC: Still's arthritis in adults: disease or syndrome. *J Rheumatol* 1983;10:758-762.

DeMaria M, DeSimone G, Laconi A, et al: Gold storage in the liver: Appearance on CT scans. *Radiology* 1986;159:355-356.

DeSmet AA, Ting YM, Weiss JJ: Shoulder arthrography in rheumatoid arthritis. *Radiology* 1975;116:601-605.

DeSilva RTD, Grennan DM, Palmer DG: Lymphatic obstruction in rheumatoid arthritis: a cause of upper limb oedema. *Ann Rheum Dis* 1980;39:260-265.

Dorfman HD, Norman A, Smith RJ: Bone erosion in relation to subcutaneous rheumatoid nodules. *Arthritis Rheum* 1970;13:69-73.

El-Khoury GY, Wener MH, Menezes AH, et al: Cranial settling in rheumatoid arthritis. *Diagn Radiol* 1980;137:637-642.

Esdaile JM, Tannenbaum H, Hawkins D: Adult Still's disease. *Am J Med* 1980;68:758-762.

Fleming A, Benn RT, Corbett M, et al: Early rheumatoid disease: II. Patterns of joint involvement. *Ann Rheum Dis* 1976;35:361-364.

Gelman MI, Ward JR: Septic arthritis: A complication of rheumatoid arthritis. *Radiology* 1977;122:17-23.

Gerster JC, Anani P, DeGoumoens P, et al: Lytic lesions of the femoral neck in rheumatoid arthritis simulating pigmented villonodular synovitis or malignancy. *Clin Rheum* 1982;1:30-34.

Ginsberg MH, Genant HK, T'sai FY, et al: Rheumatoid nodulosis: An unusual variant of rheumoid disease. *Arthritis Rheum* 1975;18:49-58.

Gohel V, Dalinka MK, Edeiken J: Giant rheumatoid pseudocyst: a case report. *Clini Orthop* 1972;88:151-153.

Good AE, Gayes JM, Kauffman CA, et al: Multiple pneumococcal pyoarthrosis complicating rheumatoid arthritis. *South Med J* 1978;71:502-504.

Halla JT, Fallahi S, Hardin JG: Small joint involvement: A systemic roentgenographic study in rheumatoid arthritis. *Ann Rheum Dis* 1986;45:327-330.

Karten I: Septic arthritis complicating rheumatoid arthritis. *Ann Intern Med* 1969;70:1147-1158.

Kelly MC, Hopkinson ND, Zaphiropoulos GC: Manubriosternal joint dislocation in rheumatoid arthritis: The role of thoracic kyphosis. *Ann Rheum Dis* 1986;45:345-348.

Kreel L, Urquhart W: Two unusual radiological features in rheumatoid arthritis. *Br J Radiol* 1963;36:715-718.

Mack LA, Matsen FA, Kilcoyne RF, et al: US evaluation of the rotator cuff tears. *Radiology* 1985;157:205-209.

Magvar E, Talerman A, Feher M, et al: Giant bone cysts in rheumatoid arthritis. *J Bone Joint Surg* 1974;56b:121-129.

Mannerfelt L, Norman O: Attrition ruptures of flexor tendons in rheumatoid arthritis caused by bony spurs in the carpal tunnel. *J Bone Joint Surg* 1969;51B:270-277.

Martel W, Bole GG: Pathologic fractures of the odontoid process in rheumatoid arthritis. *Ra-*

diology 1968;90:948–952.

Martis CS, Karakasis DT: Ankylosis of the tempo-romadibular joint caused by Still's disease. *Oral Surg Oral Med Oral Pathol* 1973;35:462–466.

Masaryk TJ, Modic MT, Geisinger MA, et al: Cervical myelopathy: A comparison of magnetic resonance and myelography. *J Comput Assist Tomogr* 1986;10:184–194.

Medsger TA Jr, Christy WC: Carpal arthritis with an-kylosis in late onset Still's arthritis. *Arthritis Rheum* 1977;19:232–242

Mettler FA, Guiberteau MJ: *Essentials of Nuclear Medicine* ed 2. Orlando, Florida, Grune & Stratton, 1986; pp 247–283.

Middleton WD, Edelstein G, Reinus WR, et al: Son-ographic detection of rotator cuff tears, *AJR* 1985;144:349–353.

Mitchell MD, Kundel HL, Steinberg ME, et al: Avas-cular necrosis of the hip: Comparison of MR, CT, and scintigraphy. *AJR* 1986;147:67–71.

Moldofsky PJ, Dalinka MK: Multiple loose bodies in rheumatoid arthritis. *Skeletal Radiol* 1979;4:219–222.

Monsees B, Murphy WA: Pressure erosions: A pat-tern of bone arthritis: resorption in rheumatoid arthritis. *Arthritis Rheum* 1985;28:820–824.

Monsees B, Destouet JM, Murphy WA, et al: Pressure erosions of bone in rheumatoid arthritis: A subject review. *Radiology* 1985;155:53–59.

Montgomery WW, Goodman ML: Rheumatoid cri-coarytenoid arthritis complicated by upper esophageal ulcerations. *Ann Otol Rhinol Laryngol* 1980;89:6–8.

Palmer DG: Anteromedial synovial cysts at the knee joint in rheumatoid disease. *Austr Radiol* 1972; 16:79–83.

Pastershank SP, Mitchell DM: Knee joint bursal ab-normalities in rheumatoid arthritis. *J Can Assoc Radiol* 1977;28:199–203.

Perrin RL, Poller WR, Perkins DG: Sternal destruction in rheumatoid arthritis. *Skeletal Radiol* 1977;2:95–97.

Pitt P, Berry H, Clarke M, et al: Metabolic activity of erosions in rheumatoid arthritis. *Ann Rheum Dis* 1986;45:235–238.

Rappoport AS, Sosman JL, Weissman B: Sponta-neous fractures of the olecranon process in rheu-matoid arthritis. *Radiology* 1976;119:83–84.

Resnick D: Pyoarthrosis complicating rheumatoid arthritis. *Radiology* 1975;114:581–586.

Resnick D: Rheumatoid arthritis of the wrist: Why the ulnar styloid? *Radiology* 1974;112:29–35.

Resnick D, Cone R: Pathological fractures in rheu-matoid arthritis: Sites and mechanisms. *Radio-graphic* 1984;4:549–562.

Resnick D, Gmelich JT: Bone fragmentation in the rheumatoid wrist: Radiographic and pathologic considerations. *Radiology* 1975;114:315–321.

Schneider R, Kaye JJ: Insufficiency and stress frac-tures of the long bones occurring in patients with rheumatoid arthritis. *Radiology* 1975;116:595–599.

Schwimmer M, Edelstein G, Heiken JP, et al: Synovial cysts of the knee: CT evaluation. *Radiology* 1985;154:175–177.

Sebes JI, Salazar JE: The manubriosternal joint in rheumatoid disease. *AJR* 1982;140:117–121.

Seidl G, Scherak O, Hofner W: Antefemoral dis-secting cysts in rheumatoid arthritis. *Radiology* 1979;133:343–347.

Shapiro RF, Resnick D, Castles JJ, et al: Fistulization of rheumatoid joints: Spectrum of identifiable syndromes. *Ann Rheum Dis* 1975;34:489–498.

Sharp JT, Lidsky MD. Collins LC, et al: Methods of scoring the progression of radiologic changes in rheumatoid arthritis: Correlation of radiologic, clinical, and laboratory abnormalities. *Arthritis Rheum* 1971;14:706–720.

Shearman J, Esdaile J, Hawkins D, et al: Predictive value of radionuclide joint scintigrams. *Arthritis Rheum* 1982;25:83–86.

Smurthwaite WA: Rupture of the knee joint in rheu-matoid arthritis: A reminder in differential diag-nosis. *Australas Radiol* 1976;20:95–97.

Snow C, Goldman JA, Casey HL, et al: Rheumatoid nodulosis: A continuum of extra-articular rheu-matoid disease. *South Med J* 1979;72:1572–1578.

Taylor RT, Huskisson EC, Whitehouse GH, et al: Spontaneous fractures of the pelvis in rheumatoid arthritis. *Br Med J* 1971;4:663–664.

Terkeltaub R, Esdaile J, Decary F, et al: A clinical study of older age rheumatoid arthritis with comparison to a younger onset group. *J Rheu-matol* 1983;10:418–424.

Thickman D, Axel L, Kressel HY, et al: Magnetic res-onance imaging of avascular necrosis of the fem-oral head. *Skel Radiol* 1986;15:133–140.

Weiss KL, Beltran J, Lubbers LM: High-field MR sur-face-coil imaging of the hand and wrist: Part II. Pathological correlations and clinical relevance. *Radiology* 1986;160:147–152.

Weston WJ: The enlarged subdeltoid bursa in rheu-matoid arthritis. *Br J Radiol* 1969;42:481–486.

Wisnieski JJ, Askari AD: Rheumatoid nodulosis: A

relatively benign rheumatoid variant. *Arch Intern Med* 1981;141:615–619.

Wu G, Whitehouse GH, Littler TR: Demonstration of lymphatic channels on wrist arthrography in rheumatoid disease with particular reference to associated lymphoedema. *Rheum Rehab* 1982;21:65–71.

Yaghmai I, Rooholamini SM, Faunce HF: Unilateral rheumatoid arthritis: Protective effect of neurological deficits. *AJR* 1977;128:299–301.

CHAPTER 4

PATHOLOGIC FINDINGS IN RHEUMATOID ARTHRITIS

H. RALPH SCHUMACHER Jr, MD

In rheumatoid arthritis morphologic changes can occur throughout the body and help to emphasize the systemic nature of this disease. This chapter focuses on the light and electron microscopic findings in joints and other structures. Recent immunohistologic studies which have some implications for pathogenesis of tissue changes are also discussed.

Findings in the joint fluid are never diagnostic of rheumatoid arthritis but since examination of joint fluid plays such a critical role in differential diagnosis of arthritis these findings are described in detail. Joint fluid aspiration and synovial fluid analysis provide the first morphologic information on most patients with rheumatoid disease.

SYNOVIAL FLUID EVALUATION

Indications

Joint aspiration and careful synovial fluid analysis should be done at least once in every patient with suspected rheumatoid arthritis or unexplained arthritis. Each year many patients are seen in consultation who have been treated for years for "rheumatoid arthritis"

but are found to have gouty arthritis or other diagnoses that are readily established by examination or culture of joint fluid. Thus, joint fluid study is important for excluding other causes of rheumatoid-like polyarthritis.

Joint fluid examination by itself can never be diagnostic of rheumatoid disease but the demonstration of an otherwise unexplained inflammatory fluid can meet one of the ARA criteria for diagnosis. Joint aspiration should also be performed whenever one or more joints are part of an exacerbation that is difficult to explain. Septic arthritis occurs more often in rheumatoid joints than in normal articulations and must be diagnosed promptly to prevent disastrous joint destruction. Recent studies have also shown that calcium pyrophosphate crystal deposition disease (CPPD) (Reginato et al, 1982), and oxalate crystal deposition (Schumacher et al, 1987) can complicate rheumatoid arthritis and can cause dramatic flares in single joints when rheumatoid disease is otherwise well controlled. The precise disease process in a given joint can only be decided with study of that joint that includes analysis of joint fluid. It is worth noting that gout seems to be a very rare complication and occurs with rheumatoid disease less often than would be expected by chance.

This procedure is to joint disease what urinalysis is to renal disease. Some diagnostic errors will be made if joint fluid is not aspirated and systematically analyzed. The routes for arthrocentesis of various joints, techniques used, and appropriate precautions have been well described (Hollander, 1985; Schumacher, 1985). Relative contraindications to arthrocentesis include only severe thrombocytopenia or other bleeding diatheses, and bacteremic infection if the joint itself is not considered as possibly infected. Superficial infection overlying the joint and preventing sterile access to the joint space is a contraindication unless the joint is also infected and in need of aspiration.

A systematic approach to joint fluid analysis should include gross examination of the fluid, a white blood cell count and differential, microscopic examination of a wet preparation for crystals and other particles, gram stain and cultures if infection is under consideration, and occasionally other special tests. A mucin clot test which was widely advised is now rarely recommended because it adds little or nothing to what can be determined from easier procedures. It is useful to consider which studies are most important in a given case and to plan priorities for the handling of small amounts of fluid.

Cultures

Prompt and careful culture of synovial fluid is very important if there is any suspicion of infection. Try to obtain laboratory help in planning cultures needed. If certain organisms are a possibility, specific media may be necessary. Most laboratories prefer prompt delivery of unadulterated specimens.

Gross Examination

Gross examination should be started at the bedside and findings can help plan which of the other studies are most pertinent.

The amount of effusion can serve as one measure of the severity of arthritis and can be used for comparison with previous arthrocenteses. Low volume does not mean absence of an important intra-articular process. Effusions may be difficult to aspirate because of thick fibrin, rice bodies, and other debris. Fluid may be loculated and not accessible by the route chosen.

Viscosity can be estimated by watching the synovial fluid as it is slowly expressed from the syringe and by manipulating several drops of fluid between the gloved thumb and index finger. Fluid of normal viscosity holds together and stretches to a string of one to two inches before separating. Low-viscosity fluid drips from a syringe like water. Very viscous fluid is seen in hypothyroid effusions and in ganglia. Viscosity is generally decreased in inflammation but also is low in edema fluid and tends to parallel the concentration of hyaluronate. In purulent effusions the massive numbers of white blood cells may make the fluid seem more viscous. The usual patterns of viscosity and other examination findings are given in Figure 4.1.

Perfectly normal joint fluid is clear and colorless. Noninflammatory fluids are yellow but still transparent. If print cannot be read easily through the fluid, the effusion is cloudy and this should suggest an inflammatory process (Fig. 4.2). The plastic of some syringes makes fluids appear falsely cloudy, so fluids should be examined in glass. Generally, the more cloudy fluids have more cells, but not all very cloudy or opaque fluids are due to increased cells. Microscopic examination is still needed to be certain that the opacity is not due to massive numbers of crystals, lipid droplets, fibrin, amyloid, or cartilage fragments. Sometimes chronically inflamed joints have effusions containing rice bodies, which might also be confused with pus on gross examination. Rice bodies are end results of synovial proliferation and degeneration; they contain collagen, cell debris, and fibrin (Fig. 4.3).

CLASSIFICATION OF SYNOVIAL EFFUSIONS

GROSS EXAMINATION	NORMAL	"NONINFLAMMATORY"	INFLAMMATORY	SEPTIC
Volume (mL) (knee)	<3.5	Often >3.5	Often >3.5	Often >3.5
Viscosity	High	High	Low	Variable
Color	Colorless to straw	Straw to yellow	Yellow	Variable
Clarity	Transparent	Transparent	Translucent	Opaque
Routine laboratory examination				
WBC (mm³)	<200	200 to 2000	2000 to 75,000	Often >100,000†
PMN leukocytes (%)	<25%	<25%	>50% often	>75%†
Culture	Negative	Negative	Negative	Often positive
Mucin clot	Firm	Firm	Friable	Friable
Glucose (AM fasting)	Nearly equal to blood	Nearly equal to blood	<50 mg% lower than blood	>50 mg% lower than blood

†WBC and %PMN leukocytes will be less if organism is less virulent or partially treated.

Figure 4.1 Classification of synovial effusions.

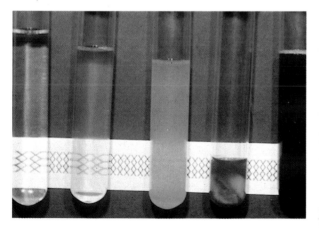

Figure 4.2 Normal, noninflammatory, inflammatory, purulent, and bloody fluids can be identified by gross examination.

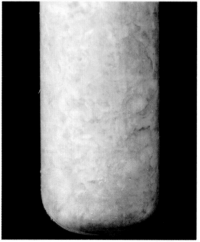

Figure 4.3 Rice bodies usually consisting of fibrin infiltrated necrotic villi are common in rheumatoid arthritis and some other joint effusions. A dense mass of such bodies is visible.

Ochronotic fluid may be speckled with dark particles ("ground pepper" sign) (Hunter et al, 1974). Black or gray debris from metal or plastic fragments after prosthetic arthroplasty can also discolor the fluid (Kitridou et al, 1969).

Rheumatoid and other chronic effusions occasionally have a greenish hue; pigmented villonodular synovitis can be grossly bloody or may produce an orange-brown color. Gouty or apatite-crystal laden fluids tend to be unusually white when they contain massive amounts of crystals. Streaks of blood can be the result of injury to a small vessel during the procedure. Causes of diffusely bloody fluid are listed in Figure 4.4. Partially-treated or low-grade infection can make the synovial fluid look like any other moderately inflammatory fluid that is not purulent. Slightly cloudy or clear fluids are common in systemic lupus erythematosus, rheumatic fever, polymyositis, and scleroderma and can be seen in the interim between attacks of gout and pseudogout.

White Blood Cell Count

Quantitation of the synovial fluid white blood cell (WBC) count is an important part of synovial fluid analysis (Ropes and Bauer, 1953), especially as it is the major basis for classification of an effusion as "septic", "inflammatory" (Fig. 4.5), or "noninflammatory" (Fig. 4.6). Note that many important systemic diseases such as hypertrophic pulmonary osteoarthropathy and sickle cell disease can be associated with noninflammatory effusions. Synovial fluid white blood cell counts along with volumes can be used as a rough measure of the intensity of inflammation in sequential samples.

The standard WBC counting chamber and techniques are used, except that ordinary WBC counting fluid should be replaced with normal or 0.3% saline. The 0.3% saline will lyse erythrocytes. The acid of ordinary WBC counting fluid clots synovial fluid and gives inaccurate WBC counts. One mL of the fluid to be counted should be placed in a heparinized tube and the tube shaken to mix the fluid thoroughly. The count must be done promptly, as there may be some spontaneous clotting and clumping of WBCs. Counts over 60,000/mm^3 should raise a suspicion of infection. However, remember that partially treated infections or low grade infections with gonococci, mycobacteria, and fungi often have lower WBC counts. Patients with rheumatoid disease, Reiter's syndrome, and crystal-induced arthritis may have counts over 100,000/mm^3.

CAUSES OF HEMARTHROSIS	
Trauma (with or without fractures)	Anticoagulant therapy
Pigmented villonodular synovitis	Myeloproliferative disease
Synovioma and other tumors	with thrombocytosis
Hemangioma	Thrombocytopenia
Charcot joint or other severe	Scurvy
joint destruction	Ruptured aneurysm
Hemophilia or other bleeding disorders	Arteriovenous fistula
Von Willebrand's disease	Idiopathic

Figure 4.4 Causes of hemarthrosis.

INFLAMMATORY JOINT EFFUSIONS*

Rheumatoid arthritis
Psoriatic arthritis
Reiter's syndrome
Ulcerative colitis
Regional enteritis
Post-ileal bypass arthritis
Ankylosing spondylitis
Juvenile rheumatoid arthritis
Rheumatic fever
Collagen-vascular disease
Systemic lupus erythematosus
Scleroderma
Polymyositis
Polychondritis
Polyarteritis
Polymyalgia rheumatica
Giant cell arteritis
Sjögren's syndrome
Wegener's granulomatosis
Goodpasture's syndrome
Henoch-Schönlein purpura
Familial Mediterranean fever
Whipple's disease
Behçet's syndrome
Lyme disease

Sarcoidosis
Multicentric reticulohistiocytosis
Erythema multiforme (Stevens-Johnson)
Postsalmonella, shigella, yersinia arthritis
Infectious arthritis
Parasitic
Viral (hepatitis, mumps, rubella, others)
Fungal
Mycoplasmal
Bacterial (staphylococcal, gonococcal,
tuberculous, others)
Treponemal
Carcinoid
Subacute bacterial endocarditis
Crystal-induced arthritis
Gout
Pseudogout
After intra-articular steroid injection
Hydroxyapatite arthritis
Hyperlipoproteinemias
Serum sickness
Agammaglobulinemia
Leukemia
Hypersensitivity angiitis
Palindromic rheumatism

*Leukocyte count greater than 2000/mm^3

Figure 4.5 Inflammatory joint effusions.

"NONINFLAMMATORY" JOINT EFFUSIONS*

Osteoarthritis
Traumatic arthritis
Acromegaly
Gaucher's disease
Hemochromatosis
Hyperparathyroidism
Ochronosis
Paget's disease

Mechanical derangement
Erythema nodosum
Villonodular synovitis,
tumors
Aseptic necrosis
Ehlers-Danlos syndrome
Sickle cell disease
Amyloidosis

Hypertrophic pulmonary
osteoarthropathy
Pancreatitis
Osteochondritis dissecans
Charcot's joints
Wilson's disease
Epiphyseal dysplasias

*Leukocyte count less than 2000/mm^3

Figure 4.6 Noninflammatory joint effusions.

Microscopic Studies

Probably the single most important step in synovial fluid analysis is prompt microscopic examination of a fresh drop of synovial fluid as a wet preparation. Even if only a single drop of fluid is obtained with aspiration, this can be examined for crystals and other constituents as a wet preparation and then the same fluid allowed to dry for staining with Gram's stain if required. Express one to two drops of unadulterated synovial fluid from the syringe onto a clean glass slide. Usually uncentrifuged fluids are examined, but examination of a pellet after centrifugation can help concentrate rare crystals or cells in a clear-appearing fluid. Cover the synovial fluid with a glass cover slip.

First examine each joint fluid with regular light microscopy. Red and white cells can be noted and their numbers estimated. Fragments of cartilage can be seen. Some white blood cells will be seen to contain cytoplasmic inclusions that have been felt to represent distended phagosomes and/or lipid droplets. Erythrocytes may be noted to be sickled in patients with sickle cell disease or trait, but this does not establish that the current effusion is due to sickle cell disease.

A variety of fibrillar materials can be seen in joint fluids. Some of these fibrils are fibrin, whereas others can be shown to be collagen from synovium or cartilage fragments (Cheung et al, 1980). Dark, irregularly shaped metal fragments can be seen in effusions of patients with implant arthroplasties (Kitridou et al, 1969). Polymer particles might also be seen. The rare shards of ochronotic cartilage are seen as yellow or ochre fragments with regular transmitted light microscopy (Schumacher and Holdsworth, 1977) (Fig. 4.7).

Large numbers of lipid droplets may be noted in traumatic arthritis (Graham and Goldman, 1978) (Weinberger and Schumacher, 1981), in inflammatory effusions of various types, including some otherwise unexplained effusions, (Reginato et al, 1985), and in pancreatic fat necrosis, or a few lipid droplets can simply result from the arthrocentesis. Fat droplets should rise to the top of a spun specimen. Oil red O will stain lipid red. The origin and full significance of lipid droplets are not yet clear. In trauma some lipid presumably comes from marrow and synovium. Marrow spicules may be found if fracture into the joint has occurred. Such spicules tend to adhere to glass and must be sought carefully.

Amorphous globular and irregular material, usually without birefringence, can be seen and can be due to amyloid masses (Gordon et al, 1973) in patients with primary amyloidosis, multiple myeloma, and Waldenstrom's macroglobulinemia. Congo red will stain this pink or red on the wet preparation (Fig. 4.8). Other globular or coin-like clumps can be seen from hydroxyapatite aggregates in joint and bursa fluids (Fig. 4.9). These clumps can be shown to contain calcium by staining with alizarin red S or von Kossa's stain (Paul et al, 1983). Apatite often appears to be phlogistic in bursae and joints.

Crystals can be noted with regular light microscopy and may be especially well seen with the illumination low or with the help of phase microscopy. Urate crystals are often acicular but may be blunt rods. Calcium pyrophosphate (CPPD) crystals can be rods or rhomboids. Other crystals also occasionally occur in joint fluids. Fluids must be examined promptly to avoid dissolution of CPPD crystals or appearance of artefactual crystals.

Compensated polarized light microscopy (Phelps et al, 1968) is used to help with further identification of crystals. Monosodium urate crystals have a yellow color when the crystal axis is parallel to the slow ray of the compensator. This is termed "negative birefringence." CPPD crystals have their slow ray in the long axis of the crystal, and thus they appear blue when parallel to the axis of slow vibration of the compensator (Fig. 4.10).

A variety of other birefringent materials will be seen on polarized light examinations of joint fluids. Depot corticosteroid preparations are crystalline (Kahn et al, 1970) and can remain in joints or adjacent connective tissue for long periods after local injections.

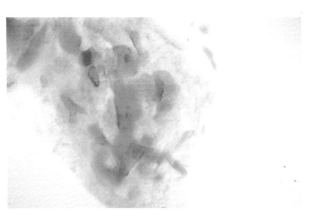

Figure 4.7 Among the particles that can occasionally be seen in joint fluids are ochronotic shards. The ochre fragments seen here are embedded in a villous synovial fragment found in the joint fluid.

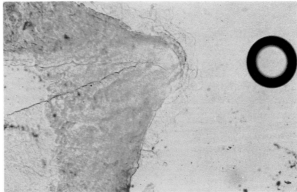

Figure 4.8 Amorphous material staining pink with Congo red is suggestive of amyloid. This is further confirmed by demonstrating apple-green birefringence with polarized light, or straight filaments by EM.

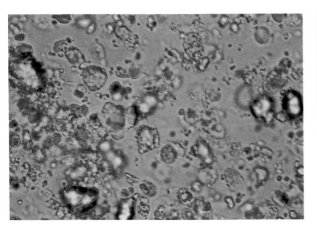

Figure 4.9 Shiny nonbirefringent clumps of apatite can complicate some rheumatoid joint effusions with secondary osteoarthritis. Here clumps are mixed with erythrocytes and leukocytes.

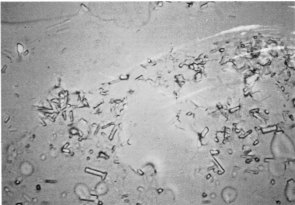

Figure 4.10 Calcium pyrophosphate crystals are positively birefringent rods or rhomboids, as seen with compensated polarized light.

These crystals can be phagocytized and occasionally induce a transient inflammation several hours after intra-articular injections. Corticosteroid crystals can appear as positively or negatively birefringent rods similar in size to urates or calcium pyrophosphate crystals, as granules, or as irregular debris (Fig. 4.11). Most other irregular birefringent material is artifact, such as dust from the slide or from the cover slip. Powder from rubber gloves is birefringent and generally shows a Maltese cross appearance.

Erroneous use of an oxalate or lithium heparin anticoagulant can introduce anticoagulant-derived crystals. Such crystals can be phagocytized by white blood cells in vitro and can thus be seen intracellularly. Oxalate and lithium heparin crystals are positively birefringent.

Cholesterol crystals can be seen in chronic joint or bursal effusions, especially in rheumatoid arthritis (Zucker et al, 1964). These crystals are usually plate-like with a notch in one corner (Fig. 4.12) and are larger than a cell. Crystals in cholesterol-laden effusions can occasionally also be negatively birefringent needles. Oxalate crystals recently described in joint effusions of patients with chronic renal failure may be pleomorphic but typically include some large bipyramidal forms (Hoffman et al, 1982) (Fig. 4.13).

Commercial polarizing microscopes are readily available and should generally be used. One can also obtain polarizing filters to be inserted in a regular light microscope. One filter is placed between the light source and condenser; another is placed above the objective or in the eyepiece. Filters are rotated until a black field is obtained. This produces the white birefringence that shows crystals more easily than ordinary light but cannot separate positive and negative birefringence. An effect similar to that obtained with a commerical compensated polarizing microscope can be achieved by applying two layers of cellophane tape to the top of a clean glass slide and placing this over the polarizing filter above the light source (Owen, 1971). The long axis of the slide then is substituted for the axis of slow vibration of the first order red compensator. Some variation has been noted with different tapes; newer tapes that appear semiopaque before use do not appear to work. Before using such a set-up, findings should be clinically compared on several crystals with the findings using a commercial compensator.

Dried Smears for Staining

Synovial smears are made using one to two drops of heparinized fluid on slides or coverslips in the same manner as with peripheral blood smears. If the white blood cell count is greater than approximately 5,000, a good smear can generally be made from the whole fluid. Fluids with lower counts often produce better smears if the fluid is centrifuged and the button is resuspended in a few drops of the supernatant before smearing. It should be allowed to air dry.

A Gram's stain is important if bacterial infection is being considered. Bacteria can be quickly classified into broad groups, but mucin artifacts can be confusing. The absence of bacteria on Gram's stain is much too common in infection and does not rule out a septic joint.

In most other cases the Wright's stain is more useful. Smears should be examined briefly under low magnifications to look for such findings as lupus erythematosus (LE) cells (Fig. 4.14). Although LE cells have so far been reported frequently in systemic lupus erythematosus (SLE) and only very rarely in rheumatoid arthritis, they need not be present in typical SLE.

The smear is next examined carefully under oil immersion. Cells can be separated into polymorphonuclear leukocytes, monocytes, small lymphocytes, and large mononuclear cells. The latter probably include some transformed lymphocytes, monocytes, and synovial lining cells. Although classification

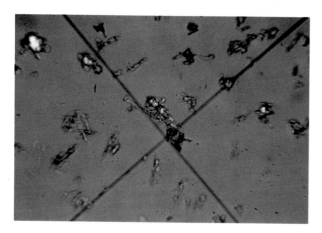

Figure 4.11 Irregular corticosteroid crystals are birefringent in polarized light.

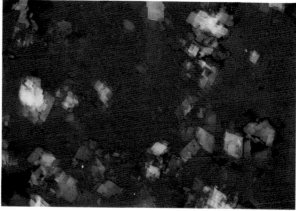

Figure 4.12 These birefringent cholesterol crystals were obtained from a chronically inflamed rheumatoid olecranon bursa.

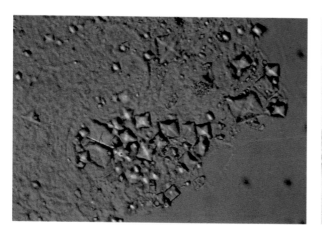

Figure 4.13 Oxalate crystals can be bipyramidal and are easily appreciated even with regular light microscopy.

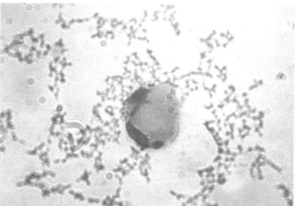

Figure 4.14 An LE Cell in a synovial fluid of a patient with polyarthritis due to SLE. (H&E).

of individual large mononuclear cells may be difficult, it may be worth attempting, since transformed lymphocytes are often seen in rheumatoid arthritis and are very rare in acute gout or pseudogout (Traycoff et al, 1976). Synovial lining cells typically are 20μ to 40μ in diameter, with an eccentric nucleus that occupies less than 50% of the cytoplasm. Some large monocyte-derived cells are similar in size, although they often have larger nuclei. These two large mononuclear cells can be distinguished with nonspecific esterase or Sudan black stains, since these stains are positive in monocytes and monocyte derived cells, but not in fibrocyte-like lining cells. Other large cells (15μ to 25μ in diameter) that have nuclei filling the majority of the cytoplasm are Sudan black negative and are transformed lymphocytes or lymphoblasts (Fig. 4.15). Both the lining cells and lymphoblasts may have prominent nucleoli. Mononuclear cells in joint fluid can now also be classifed by monoclonal antibodies (Duclos et al, 1982).

Determining the percentage of polymorphonuclear (PMN) cells is helpful in distinguishing some diseases (see Fig. 4.1). Among the inflammatory effusions, lower PMN cell counts have been seen in early rheumatoid arthritis, SLE, rheumatic fever, scleroderma, and chronic infections such as tuberculosis. Lining cells or large monocytes can be seen to have phagocytized polymorphonuclear leukocytes in a variety of diseases in which there are both exudation of neutrophils and lining cell proliferation. Such cells are common in Reiter's syndrome but are by no means diagnostic of this syndrome. (Fig. 4.16).

Eosinophils are uncommon in differential counts, but have been reported after arthrography with just air or contrast medium, and also in a variety of other causes of arthritis including hypersensitivity reactions and Lyme disease. Malignant cells can occasionally be identified in synovial fluid with Wright's or Papanicolaou's stains.

A Ziehl-Neelsen stain may be helpful in evaluation of possible tuberculosis, although cultures and synovial biopsy are often needed. Fat stains and alcian blue-PAS stains for proteoglycans (mucopolysaccharides) may show deposition of these materials in synovial macrophages. PAS-positive cells have been noted in Whipple's disease but are not unique to this disease. Other stains that may be useful include a Prussian blue stain that may show iron in synovial lining cells in pigmented villonodular synovitis or in hemochromatosis.

Glucose

Synovial fluid glucose can be measured by the standard Somogyi-Nelson true glucose method or the ortho-toluidine method and should be done simultaneously on fasting serum and synovial fluid for comparison (Ropes and Bauer, 1953) (Fig. 4.1). Synovial fluid glucose concentration is normally very slightly less than that of blood glucose. Equilibration between blood and synovial fluid after a meal is slow and unpredictable, so that fasting levels are most reliable. Effusions for glucose should be placed in a fluoride tube to stop glucose metabolism in vitro by the synovial fluid white bood cells, which would further lower the glucose level. Glucose measurements should not have a high priority, but a very low level of glucose in the synovial fluid suggests joint infections.

Complement

Total hemolytic complement is determined by the technique of Kabat and Mayer after storing at -70°C; C3 and C4 can be measured by immunoassay on any frozen fluid (Townes and Sowa, 1970). Synovial fluid complement is predominantly of value when compared with serum levels and with serum and synovial fluid protein determinations. In rheumatoid arthritis the serum complement is usually normal, while the synovial fluid level is often less than 30% of this. In SLE and hepatitis both serum and synovial fluid levels may be low. Synovial fluid complement levels in infectious arthritis, gout, and Reiter's syndrome may be high, but this is largely due to elevated serum levels. It is useful to measure serum and synovial fluid protein and globulin levels when evaluating complement, because synovial fluid complement may be very low in normal or noninflammatory fluids in which there is little escape of complement or other proteins into the joint space from the circulation.

Other Tests

Antinuclear factors, rheumatoid factor, immunoglobulins, and other substances involved in immune reactions can be measured in synovial fluid, but these assays have so far added little to the simple studies described here. Antinuclear factors, for example, are seen in synovial effusions in many conditions in which they are not identifiable in serum. Latex fixation tests for rheumatoid factor are occasionally positive in effusions when negative in the serum. However, the significance of such positive synovial fluids is not established. Several causes of false-positive tests for rheumatoid factor in synovial fluid have been described (Seward and Osterland, 1973). Immune complexes can be measured with a variety of techniques but are still largely investigational.

Other studies are not of much diagnostic value but may be of research interest. The pH of normal fluid is 7.4, and this is slightly lower in inflammation. Joint fluid pO_2 also falls in many inflammatory conditions. This tends to correlate with severity of leukocytosis and also with synovial fluid volume, which may lower pO_2 by affecting blood flow to the joint. Total protein normally averages only 1.7 g per dL, but rises with inflammation. Uric acid, electrolytes, and urea nitrogen tend to reflect the serum values. Fibrinogen and its products are normally absent, so that normal fluid does not clot upon standing. Bence Jones kappa light chains have been demonstrated in amyloid arthropathy secondary to multiple myeloma. For research lymphokines, fibronectin, proteinases, and prostaglandins can be assayed in joint fluid.

Gas chromatography on synovial fluid has been suggested as an aid in identifying bacterial products in culture-negative infections. Elevated synovial fluid lactic acid measurements have been found in untreated nongonococcal septic arthritis. Succinic acid levels are also elevated in septic arthritis and tend

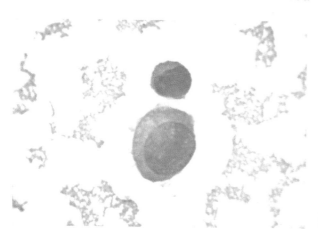

Figure 4.15 The larger cell in this figure is a transformed or activated lymphocyte.

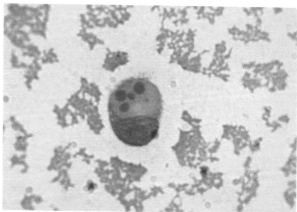

Figure 4.16 Some mononuclear cells in Reiter's syndrome have phagocytized necrotic neutrophils and have been termed "Reiter's cells." (H&E).

to persist even after treatment (Borenstein et al, 1982). Neither lactic nor succinic acid is specific for infection but may complement other tests for early diagnosis of infectious arthritis. Bacterial antigens can also be sought in synovial fluid by counter immunoelectrophoresis.

Occasionally crystals of urate or CPPD are so few or so small that they are detected only by electron microscopy (EM) (Schumacher et al, 1975, Honig et al, 1977). Urate crystals are dissolved out leaving a crystal-shaped cleft. CPPD crystals are dense chunks in electron microscopy. Individual apatite crystals can only be seen by EM (Fig. 4.17). Electron diffraction or electron probe analysis can be done on such crystals, but techniques for this are less standardized than those for x-ray diffraction. Infrared spectroscopy or electron microscopy can identify small amounts of crystals mixed with other predominant crystals.

RHEUMATOID SYNOVIAL FLUID

Joint fluid in rheumatoid arthritis is usually cloudy due to increased numbers of white blood cells. Counts generally range between 2,000 and 75,000 mm^3. Not all joints are involved or affected to the same degree in rheumatoid disease. Occasionally joints may have clear effusions in the noninflammatory range while others can have white blood cell counts over 100,000, which raise concern about infection. Rice bodies commonly occur. Viscosity tends to be low in actively inflamed joints.

Cytoplasmic inclusions due at least in part to distended phagocytic vacuoles (Fig. 4.18) are common in rheumatoid effusions. Immunoglobulins and complement can be identified in some vacuoles with immunofluorescent study (Hollander et al, 1965) (Fig. 4.19). These inclusions although of interest as

a sign of pathogenetic mechanisms are also seen in other joint exudates and are not specific for rheumatoid arthritis.

Large transformed lymphocytes as described above may be seen on Wright's stains of rheumatoid effusions and tend to help support this diagnosis although they are also not unique to rheumatoid arthritis.

CPPD, apatite, or lipid crystals can occasionally complicate chronic rheumatoid effusions and need not exclude the diagnosis of rheumatoid arthritis. Glucose levels are sometimes very low in rheumatoid disease but levels near zero should raise concern of infection. Low joint fluid complement levels may help favor rheumatoid disease over infection or Reiter's syndrome.

EVALUATION OF TISSUE PATHOLOGY

Indications For Biopsies

Most biopsies are done either to study the pathogenesis of a disease, to assist in the establishment of a diagnosis or the two functions may coexist. Either pathogenetic investigations or diagnostic procedures must be planned in advance. Investigations into pathogenesis usually do not require that the lesion studied be specific for the disease in question. The value of a biopsy for diagnosis is, however, determined by the specificity of the lesion to be examined. The degree of specificity required depends on the nature of the differential diagnosis in the particular case. For example, there is little chance that a joint biopsy for routine histology will be helpful in distinguishing between rheumatoid arthritis and psoriatic arthropathy; on the other hand, one is very likely to be able to distinguish rheumatoid arthritis from gout, tuberculosis, or pigmented villonodular synovitis by this procedure.

In patients with either proven rheumatoid

arthritis or under consideration for a diagnosis of rheumatoid disease there are several reasons for obtaining biopsies.

A biopsy may establish or exclude some diseases in the differential diagnosis. For example, infectious arthritis and crystal-induced arthritis may have pathognomonic lesions. Positive cultures or stains can sometimes be obtained from tissue in infectious disease when blood and synovial fluid cultures are negative. Some other less common joint diseases, such as hemochromatosis, ochronosis, and amyloidosis, also have virtually pathognomonic synovial or cartilage findings.

Positive support may be provided by a biopsy for a diagnosis of rheumatoid arthritis. Demonstrations of typical chronic prolifera-

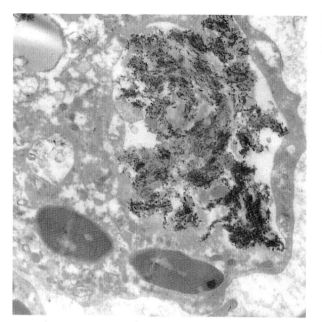

Figure 4.17 Tiny needle-like apatite crystals are seen only by electron microscopy. Crystals shown here are phagocytized by a synovial cell.

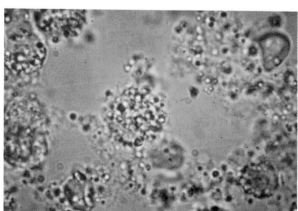

Figure 4.18 Cytoplasmic inclusions are seen in viable and degenerating synovial fluid cells.

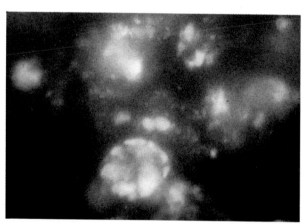

Figure 4.19 Immunofluorescence identifies immunoglobulin G in these rheumatoid joint fluid cells.

tive synovitis and rheumatoid nodules meet two of the ARA criteria for rheumatoid disease although neither one of these findings alone is specific.

A biopsy can also be used for pathologic study to confirm involvement of a specific organ system in rheumatoid arthritis. Perhaps most important is the confirmation and determination of the type of vasculitis which cannot usually be established in any other way.

By having the patient undergo a biopsy, it is possible to identify related diseases or coincidental complications of rheumatoid arthritis. Sjögren's syndrome is most definitively diagnosed by salivary gland biopsy, while lymph node biopsy can show the rare complication of lymphoma.

Synovial Membrane

Examination of the synovial membrane is a greatly underappreciated technique for diagnosis and investigation of joint diseases. Reasons for neglect of what should be an important part of evaluation of many patients with arthritis may include: Inexperience with biopsy techniques, the inconvenience to the physician and to the patient in getting a biopsy, superficial interpretations of little value provided by some pathologists without special expertise in joint disease, failure to pose specific questions to see if a biopsy would help and failure to consider which techniques, such as histochemistry, immunomorphology, and electron microscopy, might contribute to understanding the patient's condition.

Synovial membrane examination can be the only way to determine exactly what is happening in any given joint. One can make a definite diagnosis in some infectious, infiltrative, and deposition diseases (Schumacher and Kulka, 1972). In other situations biopsy can narrow diagnostic possibilities by demonstrating the presence or absence of an inflammatory process. Although a synovial biopsy is never diagnostic of rheumatoid arthritis, the characteristic findings can meet one of the criteria for diagnosis as established by the ARA (Ropes et al, 1959). As an example of potential utility, in a study of patients with a wide variety of diagnostic problems Schumacher and Kulka (1972) found that needle synovial biopsy was of assistance in diagnosis in about 35% of a group of patients with a variety of kinds of arthritis.

Obtaining Synovial Tissue

NEEDLE BIOPSY Probably the most popular current technique among rheumatologists for obtaining diagnostic synovial material is use of blind needle synovial biopsy. The original Polley-Bickel technique is increasingly replaced by use of the newer, smaller Parker-Pearson needles (Schumacher and Kulka, 1972) (Fig. 4.20). Such needle synovial biopsy can be performed in the hospital, clinic, or office with sterile precautions during the procedure and limitation of activity of the patient for the 24 hours after the biopsy.

The knee is by far the most frequently biopsied joint, but successful biopsies can also be obtained from shoulders, elbows, wrists, ankles, olecranon bursae, and occasionally even smaller joints if they are sufficiently swollen. The route of entry is generally that described for arthrocentesis. The procedure can be performed by a single operator with one assistant. Meperidine or diazepam is occasionally used for very anxious patients. Young children may even need general anesthesia. The biopsy area is widely prepared with soap, then iodine, and washed with alcohol. Using gloves, the operator places a transparent plastic adhesive drape with a two-inch hole over the biopsy site. The skin and subcutaneous tissue are infiltrated to the capsule with 1% lidocaine, using a 25-gauge needle. Caution is exercised to avoid instilling anesthetic into the joint space, which would distort the synovial fluid findings. Next, a 20- to 22-gauge needle is inserted through the anesthetized area into the joint space. Fluid is aspirated for analysis. Two to 4 mL of 1% lidocaine can be instilled into the joint space, but biopsy can also rarely be done without this if it is important to avoid any possible artifact that might be introduced by the local anesthetic. It is not necessary to distend the joint with fluid. As the needle is withdrawn another 1 mL of 1% lidocaine is infiltrated into the needle tract.

The biopsy trochar is next thrust decisively into the joint space through the anesthetized tissue. In the knee the trochar tip should be at the top of the retropatellar space and should move freely into the suprapatellar pouch. The biopsy needle is inserted through the outer needle. The side with the hooked notch is approximated against the synovium, and suction is applied with a 20 mL Luer-lock syringe. The needle is always directed away from the site of initial lidocaine infiltration to avoid possible artifacts in this area. Five to eight specimens (to minimize sampling error) from the various parts of the joint are taken by moving the tip of the needle without reinserting the outer needle (Lindblad and Hedforg, 1985). Suction is maintained with one hand on the syringe while the other retracts the inner needle through the outer with a slight twist. The outer needle remains in place. One must become familiar with the appearance of the specimens, so as not to mistake yellow-white fibrin or necrotic material for pink synovial tissue. Specimens may be transferred carefully by a 25-gauge needle from the needle to the fixative on a small piece of sterile paper.

Patients are instructed to rest biopsied joints until the following day, when they are permitted to resume usual activity, providing no increased pain or swelling has been noted. Hemarthrosis and infection are theoretical complications, but only two patients of more than 450 in one series had hemarthrosis that required aspiration the next day for pain relief. There are reports of needle tips breaking off in the joint (Bocanegra et al, 1980). Care must be taken before biopsy to check that the needle fits easily through the trochar and that the tip is not bent or weakened.

Other needles that have been used for synovial biopsy are those of Cope, Williamson, and Franklin and Silverman (Moon et al, 1980).

ARTHROSCOPY Most hospitals have orthopedists familiar with arthroscopy, and some rheumatologists are doing the procedure also. It has become an increasingly popular alternative for obtaining diagnostic biopsies. Arthroscopy has the advantage of direct visualization of the synovium which allows identification of discrete localized lesions which can be biopsied. The rest of the joint can be surveyed but such complete arthroscopy is done under general rather than local anesthesia in most centers. If a biopsy of only synovium from the anterior portion of the knee is needed, it can usually be done under local anesthesia. The procedure is

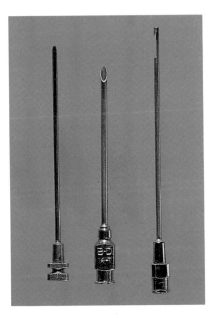

Figure 4.20 The three parts of the Parker-Pearson biopsy needle are shown.

generally limited to larger joints. If there is the possibility of focal granulomas, deeper lesions such as a vasculitis in larger capsular vessels, or other lesions that might have been missed on a closed needle biopsy, arthroscopic biopsy or open surgical biopsy must be considered.

OPEN SURGICAL SYNOVIAL BIOPSY
This procedure is indicated in many of the same situations as arthroscopic biopsy and is done when experienced arthroscopists are not available. Surgical biopsy is also very useful at small joints not suitable for needle biopsy. A small incision over a metacarpophalangeal joint is very effective and offers virtually no morbidity.

Open biopsy, even of a knee, can be done with a small incision; but if one wants the advantage of the full joint exploration, a large surgical incision and some more prolonged postoperative immobilization are obviously needed.

"FOUND" OR "FREE" BIOPSIES During evaluation of patients with arthritis, it is important not to forget to ask about useful synovial tissue that may have been obtained in the past. "Ganglions" that have been removed may in fact contain inflamed synovium and offer clues to rheumatoid or other types of inflammatory arthritis. If a specimen was submitted at the time of a past carpal tunnel release, this sample could provide the diagnosis of amyloidosis or support for an inflammatory or crystal deposition disease. Synovium removed at previous arthroscopies or surgery for suspected meniscus tears can reveal surprises when reexamined for careful diagnostic interpretation.

Synovial membrane fragments can occasionally be found floating in joint fluid after arthrocentesis (Fig. 4.21). These can be examined in a wet smear for crystals and can be collected by centrifugation and fixed for processing as with any biopsy.

Handling Synovial Tissue

The multiple small pieces of synovium from needle biopsy or the large specimens obtained at operation should be distributed among the several methods of handling, depending on the questions being asked. With large surgical specimens it can be important to identify the synovial surface before it is fixed and difficult to see. Only superficial tissue is desired for most electron microscopy (EM), since much effort can be wasted examining the large specimens with much capsular tissue.

Specimens for routine light microscopy are placed into neutral buffered formalin or Bouin's fixative. Some slides should be stained with hematoxylin and eosin and other tissue save for possible special stains. If gout is a consideration, a portion of the biopsy should be placed in absolute alcohol, since urates are water soluble. These specimens then should be processed without water and stained with the DeGolantha stain for urate, or sections can be examined with compensated polarized light. Frozen sections of unfixed biopsies can also be used for polarized light examination for urates (Fig. 4.22). If tissue is seen fresh, it is possible to tease out tophaceous material and confirm the diagnosis immediately with compensated polarized light.

Immunofluorescent study of synovium has not been of any convincing clinical value but is of research interest. One study (Bayliss et al, 1975) suggested that demonstration of synovial IgM deposition favored the diagnosis of rheumatoid arthritis. Specimens for immunofluorescence should be placed in saline until transferred to a cryostat chuck and quick frozen by immersion in liquid nitrogen. Immunoperoxidase studies can be done on paraffin-embedded tissue but are probably also better on frozen tissue.

Electron microscopy (EM) of synovium is also largely of research interest. For example,

EM can show electron-dense deposits (probably due to several different causes) in vessel walls in early rheumatoid arthritis (Schumacher, 1975b), in palindromic rheumatism (Schumacher, 1982), in subacute bacterial endocarditis, and also in the syndrome of hypertrophic pulmonary osteoarthropathy (Schumacher, 1976). Investigation into the components of the dense deposits in these diverse syndromes may give important clues to their pathogenesis. EM may also be a major diagnostic aid of immediate clinical value in identifying apatite or other small crystals, viruses, small amounts of amyloid with rod-like fibrils, bacilliform bodies of Whipple's disease, and Gaucher cell tubules.

Any specimen for EM should be placed immediately in a fixative such as 1% to 3% glutaraldehyde or half-strength Karnovsky's fixative (Karnovsky, 1965). Specimens should be minced into 0.5 mm by 0.5 mm pieces, fixed for up to four hours, and then switched into a buffer before further processing. Recent work suggests that immunoelectron microscopy (IEM) may be of great research and clinical value. Chlamydial antigen has recently been identified in synovium in early Reiter's syndrome (Schumacher, 1986). Bacterial cell wall peptidoglycan can be found in synovial macrophages with this technique in septic joints in which cultures have been negative (Schumacher, 1987). Fixation for IEM should be for only one hour in 1% glutaraldehyde as one method that minimizes denaturation of antigens. Crystals or other unexplained deposits seen by EM can be further analyzed by elemental analysis (Schumacher et al, 1983). Gold can be localized to synovial macrophages by this technique.

Synovial membrane can be grown in tissue culture to search for viruses or for other investigative purposes. Biopsies for tissue culture are placed promptly in culture medium and taken to the laboratory.

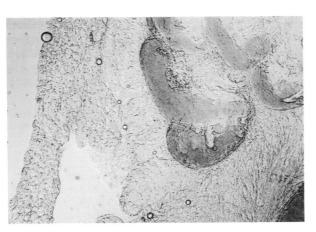

Figure 4.21 A synovial villus with its dilated vessels that was found floating in a joint effusion.

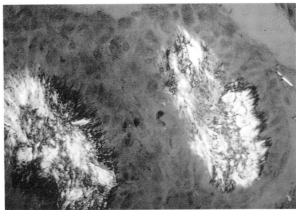

Figure 4.22 Birefringent urate crystals are nicely preserved in this gouty synovium prepared as a frozen section.

SYNOVIUM IN RHEUMATOID ARTHRITIS

Gross Examination

Synovial tissue in established disease as seen at arthroscopy or surgery is proliferated with large and numerous villi that tend to look more grainy and less smooth than normal tissue (Fig. 4.23). Vascular congestion can be evident or the surface can be covered with gray or yellow exudate. Brown staining can occur from extravasated erythrocytes and areas of necrosis. Villi may be long and thin or polyp-like with some processes or sheets extending over the cartilage. This invasive synovium is termed pannus. Gross involvement is often patchy with some areas appearing normal, especially in early disease. Burned-out disease may show only fibrous bands and scarring.

Microscopic Studies

LIGHT MICROSCOPY Active chronic disease as noted on hematoxylin and eosin stained tissue is characterized by many prominent villi seen in longitudinal or cross sections (Gardner, 1972). There is varying and focal deposition of fibrin on the synovial surface and in the interstitium (Fig. 4.24). Membranes with more fibrin and less inflammation have been suggested to be more typical of an anergic subset of patients (Malone et al, 1984). Neutrophils may occasionally be seen in the surface fibrinous exudate. Synovial lining cells are proliferated. Hypertrophic cells often extend their cytoplasmic processes toward the joint space. Nuclei of these cells are relatively pale with scattered chromatin. Hyperplasia of the lining layer increases from the normal one to two layers of cells to three to four and often more than 10 cells in depth (Fig. 4.25). Focal areas even in established disease show no such lining cell reaction and there may even be localized areas of necrosis.

Cells in mitosis and multinucleated giant cells can be seen in or just beneath the lining cell layer. The giant cells appear to be of monocyte or macrophage origin (Grimley and Sokoloff, 1966; Muirden, 1970) and have peripheral nuclei and abundant central basophilic or eosinophilic cytoplasm. Such cells must be recognized as part of the rheumatoid process and need not suggest other causes of giant cell formation such as tuberculous or fungal infection. Foreign body giant cells resulting from phagocytosis of bone and cartilage debris can also be seen in some chronic rheumatoid joints. Multinucleated plasma cells are also occasionally present (Muirden, 1970).

Evidence of erythrocyte extravasation is common and golden brown hemosiderin pigment from these cells is often seen in deep perivascular macrophages (Fig. 4.26). This iron deposition can lead to superoxide excess which has been suggested as a possible factor accentuating joint inflammation (Blake et al, 1984).

Clusters of perivascular lymphocytes and plasma cells are typical of rheumatoid joint

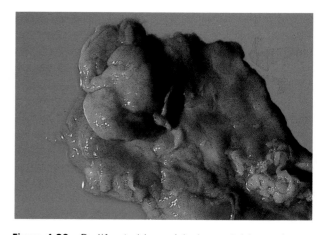

Figure 4.23 Proliferated brownish rheumatoid synovium removed at knee surgery.

involvement. Clumps can be massive, containing hundreds of cells. When lymphocytes are collected around germinal centers with larger pale cells with vesicular nuclei, they are termed "lymphoid follicles" (Cooper et al, 1981) (Fig. 4.27). These germinal centers are suggested to be virtually pathognomonic of rheumatoid arthritis but are infrequently encountered (Young et al, 1984). Similar lymphoid follicles have been described in synovial tissues adjacent to osteoid osteomas.

Neutrophils and eosinophils are infrequent in the synovium in chronic rheumatoid arthritis even though neutrophils are common in the joint space. Mast cells are detected only with Giemsa or other special stains but are prominent suggesting an important role for their vasoactive peptides (Crisp et al, 1984). Fibroblasts and histiocytes may be proliferated. Cellular changes are focal. There have been occasional observations that areas with lymphocytic infiltration have less lining

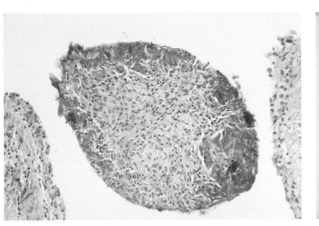

Figure 4.24 Pink fibrin coats a villus which is cut tangentially otherwise showing only proliferated lining cells. (H&E).

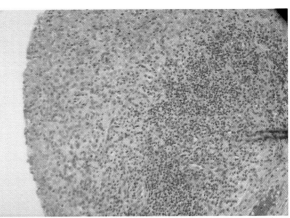

Figure 4.25 Rheumatoid synovium with massive proliferation of lining cells on the left and infiltration of lymphocytes on the right.

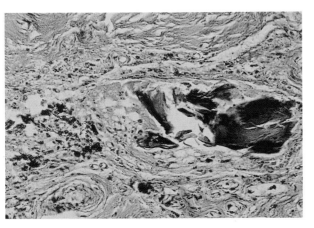

Figure 4.26 Golden brown iron is present in the deep synovial macrophages of synovium obtained at total hip surgery of this rheumatoid patient. Note bone fragments embedded in this tissue.

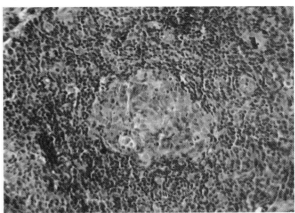

Figure 4.27 This rheumatoid synovium shows pale cells of a germinal center in this lymphoid follicle. (H&E).

cell proliferation (Muirden and Mills, 1971). The complex affects of lymphokines on the other cells could explain inhibition of proliferation in some situations.

Vascular congestion or endothelial proliferation have been described in chronic rheumatoid arthritis. Actual vasculitis has been described, but is rare. Focal ischemia has been felt to result from vascular occlusion. Such ischemia seems to be at least one factor in the formation of rice bodies. Rheumatoid nodules are rarely noted in synovium.

Synovium during the first several weeks of synovitis that eventually evolves into classic rheumatoid disease cannot be expected to show the changes seen in chronic arthritis. Plasma cells are very rare and lymphocytes are mainly perivascular and in small numbers. Vessels are often obliterated (Fig. 4.28) suggesting some role of a circulating material injuring small vessels (Schumacher, 1975). Also there is almost always some mild proliferation of lining cells.

IMMUNOHISTOPATHOLOGIC STUDIES

Histochemical studies in addition to confirming the presence of mast cells as noted above can also show increased activities of lysosomal enzymes. Collagenase, interleukins, gamma interferon, and different products of arachidonic acid can be identified in synovial cells. Immunofluorescent studies show complement and immunoglobulins in synovial surface cells as well as in deeper cells and vessel walls (Brandt et al, 1968). Rheumatoid factor can be identified in infiltrating plasma cells. Proteinases and protease inhibitors can be identified in lining and perivascular cells (Flory et al, 1982).

The infiltrating lymphocytes have been studied by monoclonal antibodies to surface markers using immunofluorescent and immunoperoxidase techniques. Most reports have shown a predominance of OKT_4 (helper) cells (Duke et al, 1984; Husby and Williams, 1985). Many express HLA-DR antigens and are in close proximity to activated B cells, mac-

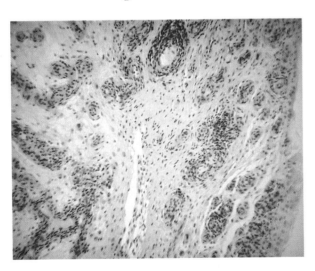

Figure 4.28 Early rheumatoid synovium shows intense mononuclear cell infiltration in venule walls and perivascular tissue with narrowing of lumens. There is slight lining cell proliferation at the *right*. (H&E).

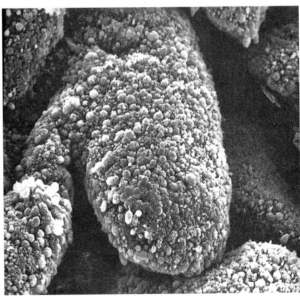

Figure 4.29 Hyperplastic synovial villi are seen here in the scanning EM. (Courtesy of Professor Alan Gaucher).

rophages, and dendritic cells. B-lymphocytes lie in the center of germinal centers. Small numbers of cells with natural killer (NK) activity can be stained in rheumatoid synovium (Young et al, 1984). Disease modifying drugs have been shown to be able to alter lymphocyte surface marker patterns (Walters et al, 1987). Fibronectin can be identified on the surface and in the interstitium by immunofluorescence or immunoperoxidase technique (Clemmensen et al, 1983) but seems to be no more common than in other inflammatory arthopathies.

ELECTRON MICROSCOPY (EM) Scanning EM can provide beautiful demonstrations of proliferated villi (Fig. 4.29). Information added by transmission EM includes further characterization of the proliferated lining cells. Both fibrocyte-like and monocyte-derived phagocytic cells (Mapp and Revell, 1987) are increased in size and numbers with the phagocytic cells most prominent in most studies (Fig. 4.30). Vacuoles of these cells contain a variety of types of material including finely granular material consistent in appearance with immune complexes, fibrin, ferritin

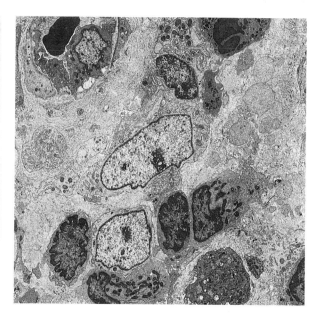

Figure 4.30 Proliferated phagocytic lining cells have many dense bodies and extend long processes toward the joint space in a patient with rheumatoid arthritis. One fibrocyte-like lining cell with prominent rough endoplasmic reticulum is seen on the left. (EM 10,000X).

Figure 4.31 The rheumatoid synovial venule at upper left has large endothelial cells. The basement membrane is multilaminated. Lymphocytes, other mononuclear cells, and a neutrophil lie in the adjacent tissue. (EM 7,000X).

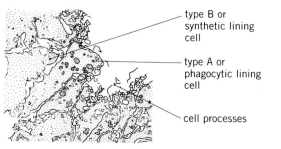

type B or synthetic lining cell

type A or phagocytic lining cell

cell processes

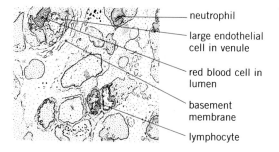

neutrophil

large endothelial cell in venule

red blood cell in lumen

basement membrane

lymphocyte

particles, cellular debris, and other unidentified particles that might include important antigens. Immunoglobulins and complement have been identified in vacuoles by immuno-electron microscopy (Cherian et al, 1984).

Vessels are best characterized by EM. Some endothelial cells are large (Fig. 4.31). These have been proposed to be at sites of emigration of lymphocytes (Freemont et al, 1983). Gaps can be seen between endothelial cells and can at times be seen to contain neutrophil processes. Basement membranes of venules are multilaminated (Matsubara and Ziff, 1987). Electron dense deposits in vessel walls (Fig. 4.32) and virus-like particles have been seen mainly in early cases (Schumacher, 1975), and more studies of such early lesions are needed. Synovial lymphocytes can be seen to be large activated cells with polyribosomes (Fig. 4.33). Distended cisternae of endoplasmic reticulum of plasma cells are clearly seen. Greater tissue damage has been related to iron deposits adjacent to phagocytic cells rather than when iron is in fibrocyte-like cells (Morris et al,

1986). Gold can be readily shown by EM in synovial macrophages in gold-treated patients (Figs. 4.34, 4.35).

CARTILAGE AND BONE IN RHEUMATOID ARTHRITIS

Cartilage or bone biopsies are infrequently studied in clinical investigation of rheumatoid disease but research on these structures is important in understanding several aspects of disease pathogenesis and may have implications for therapy. The surface of rheumatoid cartilage can be damaged in several ways (Fig. 4.36). It can be covered with a pannus which may consist primarily of proliferative and inflamed synovium or of a fibrous connective tissue (Fig. 4.37). Initially only a few surface chondrocytes are necrotic but even-

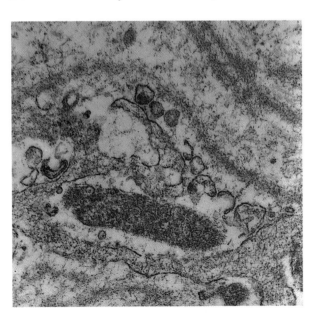

Figure 4.32 An early rheumatoid vessel wall with granular material and unidentified particles between layers of basement membrane. (EM).

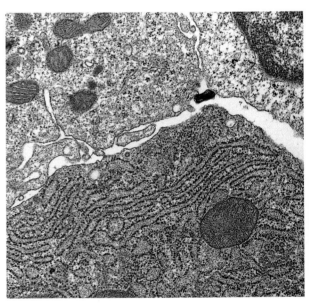

Figure 4.33 The lymphocyte above has many polyribosomes and lies close to a cell with layers of rough endoplasmic reticulum. (EM).

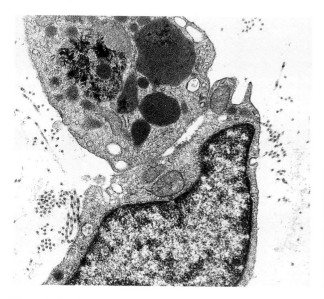

Figure 4.34 Dense curved metallic gold fragments are seen in a macrophage vacuole of a synovium in rheumatoid arthritis. (EM 40,000X).

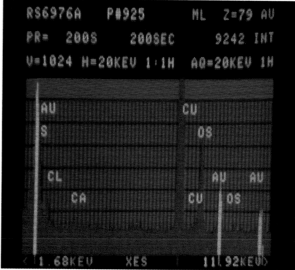

Figure 4.35 Energy dispersive elemental analysis confirms the presence of gold (yellow peaks) in a synovial macrophage. The copper is from the grid and the osmium from the fixation.

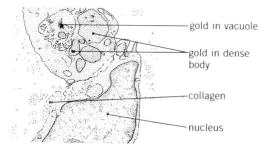

gold in vacuole

gold in dense body

collagen

nucleus

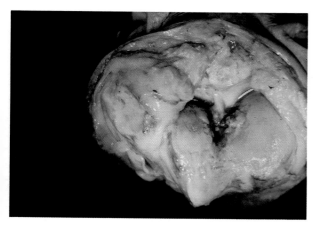

Figure 4.36 This rheumatoid knee after synovectomy shows areas of cartilage loss and disappearance of its normal lustre.

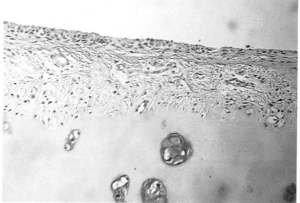

Figure 4.37 Pannus here is seen overlying cartilage with clusters of chondrocytes. There are a few inflammatory cells in this pannus.

tually cartilage in wide areas can be completely lost and pannus erodes through to bone (Fig. 4.38). Some cartilage loss also occurs in areas not covered by pannus. Mechanical factors, enzymes released from chondrocytes or synovium, free or adhering neutrophils at the cartilage-pannus surface (Mohr et al, 1981), and invasion of granulation tissue from subchondral bone have all been considered as possible factors. Most studies have emphasized an important role of fibrocyte-like cells and macrophages at the actual pannus-cartilage junction (Shiozawa et al, 1983).

Secondary osteoarthritis with osteophyte formation and bony sclerosis can occur in advanced disease. Of great potential pathogenetic interest is the immunofluorescent and EM demonstration by Cooke (1980) of granular deposits of IgG and C3 in about 90% of rheumatoid articular cartilages. Such deposits were mostly on the surface and suggested that the cartilage might be a repository for disease-perpetuating antigens or complexes.

Although often neglected in discussions of rheumatoid pathology, the involvement of subchondral bone can also be prominent and important. Granulation tissue that probably at least in part invades through vascular foramina from the synovium can be seen in the marrow space. This inflammatory tissue can destroy bone, leading to large cysts, and can accentuate joint destruction. Diffuse osteoporosis is also noted histologically.

DIFFERENTIAL DIAGNOSIS USING SYNOVIAL HISTOLOGIC FINDINGS

Normal

Normal synovial membrane consists of one or two layers of synovial lining cells overlying a richly vascular areolar or fibrous connective tissue. A biopsy containing several pieces of normal synovium does not absolutely exclude intra-articular disease, but should direct the search toward very focal disease or extrasynovial processes. Failure to identify a characteristic lesion does not exclude the di-

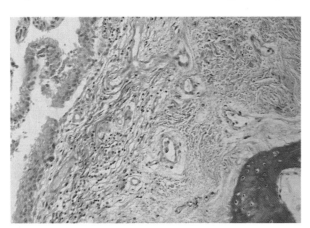

Figure 4.38 Pannus overlies a bone trabecula at the margin of this eroded joint. (H&E).

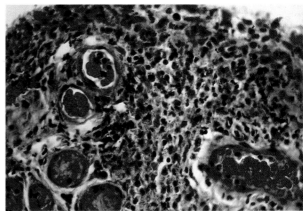

Figure 4.39 Reiter's syndrome synovium typically has dramatic vascular congestion and infiltration of neutrophils between the vessels and lining cells. (H&E)

agnosis of focal diagnosable diseases. For example, gouty, tuberculous, or ochronotic synovium can show only mild proliferation or changes indistinguishable from rheumatoid arthritis in tissue adjacent to a tophus, granuloma, or typical pigmented shard.

Seronegative Spondyloarthropathies

Psoriatic arthritis and ankylosing spondylitis can show synovial changes indistinguishable from rheumatoid arthritis. Early Reiter's syndrome has a typical superficial congestion and polymorphonuclear leukocyte infiltration (Fig. 4.39), which can, however, also be seen in some cases of early rheumatoid arthritis, Behcet's disease (Abdou et al, 1978), familial Mediterranean fever, and regional enteritis, as well as other conditions. Chronic Reiter's syndrome synovium is indistinguishable from that of rheumatoid arthritis. Synovium in Crohn's disease occasionally shows granulomas similar to those in the intestine. Synovium of peripheral joints can show dramatic plasma cell infiltration in ankylosing spondylitis.

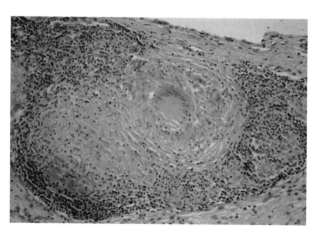

Figure 4.40 A Langhans giant cell is seen in a synovial granuloma in this patient with tuberculous arthritis. There are large numbers of surrounding lymphocytes. (H&E).

Collagen-Vascular Diseases

The synovial membrane in SLE typically shows less intense lining cell hyperplasia and less white blood cell infiltration than in rheumatoid arthritis (Labowitz et al, 1974) although inflammation may occasionally mimic rheumatoid arthritis. Synovial inflammation in polyarteritis is usually mild, and inflammatory cell infiltration of medium-sized vessel walls is only a rare finding. Early scleroderma (Schumacher, 1973) shows sparse lining cells, superficial fibrin, and chronic inflammatory cell infiltration. Similar findings of a paucity of lining cells can be seen also in some SLE, polymyositis, rheumatic fever, and some infections. In later scleroderma synovial fibrin and fibrosis predominate.

Infectious Arthritis

Infection is one of the sources of joint disease that can be definitively diagnosed by synovial biopsy. Sheets of neutrophils can be seen in acute bacterial arthritis. Bacteria can sometimes be demonstrated in synovium with a tissue Gram's stain. Cultures may be positive on synovial biopsy specimens even when they have been negative on blood and synovial fluid (Wofsky, 1980). In chronic or resolving infections, there are often large numbers of lymphocytes and plasma cells that could be confused with rheumatoid tissue.

Chronic infections such as tuberculosis and fungus disease can produce focal lesions that may be missed on limited biopsies. Mycobacterial granulomas in the superficial synovium do not always show caseation (Fig. 4.40). Ziehl-Neelsen and Kinyoun's stains can show acid-fast organisms. Staining for fungi should be attempted with Grocott and Gridley stains. Spirochaetes can be suggested with silver stain in the synovium in some patients with Lyme disease (Johnston et al, 1985). Immunoperoxidase techniques may be more definitive. Treponemes can also be sought in secondary syphilis with fluorescent and silver stains. Only a mild nonspecific synovitis has been seen in three cases of secondary syphilis. Sarcoidosis can involve the synovium with typical non-caseating granulomas, that could be confused with fungal disease.

Crystal-Induced Arthritis

Both gout and calcium pyrophosphate deposition disease ("pseudogout") often have tophus-like deposits in synovial membrane. Precautions for tissue handling to demonstrate water soluble urate tophi are described above (page 4.16). Calcium pyrophosphate or other calcium containing crystals are not as water soluble but can be dissolved by decalcification in specimens submitted along with bone. Thus, pseudogout synovium occasionally can have lucent areas where crystals were lost, as in gout. Usually only a fibrous capsule, a few histocytes, and giant cells surround the tophi. In acute crystal-induced arthritis there are areas of neutrophil infiltration, but in chronic disease large numbers of lymphocytes and plasma cells can be seen. Clumps of apatite crystals in synovium can appear as hematoxyphilic areas. The tiny crystals forming these clumps are identifiable only by EM. Oxalate crystals have also recently been found as pleomorphic birefringent bodies in synovium of one patient receiving chronic hemodialysis for renal failure (Schumacher et al, 1987). Calcium-containing crystals can be stained with Alizarin red S or Von Kossa stains for aid in identification.

Amyloidosis

In patients with primary amyloidosis, multiple myeloma, and Waldenstrom's disease amyloid can be deposited diffusely in the joint. This tissue appears pink on hematoxylin and eosin stain and red with Congo red. The Congo red-stained material has an apple-green birefringence when viewed with plain polarized light (Canoso et al, 1975). Most amyloid is found on the synovial surface and in the interstitium, but rarely in vessel walls. Recently amyloid deposits due to beta 2 microglobulin have been shown to cause some dialysis arthropathy. Such deposits are often interstitial.

Ochronosis

The synovial membrane in ochronosis is studded with brownish-pigmented shards from the friable cartilage (Schumacher and Holdsworth, 1977). Macrophages and giant cells adjacent to the cartilage fragments often contain pigment granules. Clusters of lymphocytes can also be seen (Fig. 4.41) and can also be found in areas of synovium in other patients with cartilage degeneration, such as in primary or secondary osteoarthritis. It should be noted that cartilage and bone fragments without the ochronotic pigment can also be seen embedded in the synovium in osteoarthritis, rheumatoid arthritis, Charcot joints, and other destructive arthropathies.

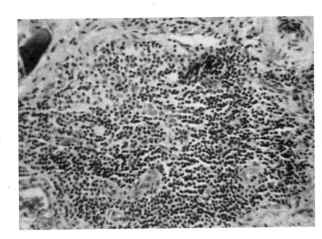

Figure 4.41 Brown ochronotic shards are embedded in this synovium but there is also a large potentially confusing lymphoid infiltrate. (H&E).

Hemochromatosis

Golden-brown hemosiderin pigment deposition in synovial lining cells and to a lesser degree in deeper phagocytes is characteristic of hemochromatosis (Schumacher, 1972) and other diseases with systemic iron overload. Iron in synovium from bleeding into the joint space or extravasation of erythrocytes into tissue as in hemophilia produces hemosiderin mainly in deep macrophages. Iron stains blue with Prussian blue for confirmation. Calcium pyrophosphate crystals can be seen in these synovia as well as in several other metabolic joint diseases.

Tumors

A variety of benign and malignant tumors or tumor-like conditions can involve the synovial membrane. Metastatic malignancies are occasionally identified in synovium (Goldenberg et al, 1975). Blast forms have been found infiltrating synovium in a few patients with leukemia or lymphoma and arthritis (Spilberg and Myer, 1972). Malignant synovioma is an extra-articular tumor that is very rarely seen in joint synovium. Osteochondromas developing in synovium can be seen as foci of osteometaplasia and chondrometaplasia in the synovial connective tissue. Pigmented villonodular synovitis, generally involving a single joint or tendon sheath, is characterized by giant cells, foamy cells, and hemosiderin deposits, predominantly in the deep synovium. There is villous or nodular proliferation with areas also showing some lymphocytes and plasma cells.

Other Diseases

Another condition that involves the synovial membrane is multicentric reticulohistiocytosis (Krey et al, 1974). Histological examination shows extensive infiltration of synovium with large foamy cells and/or multinucleated cells with eosinophilic "ground glass" cytoplasm.

Whipple's disease synovial membrane often shows just mild lining cell hyperplasia and scattered lymphocytes and neutrophils, but PAS-positive macrophages can be seen in some cases to suggest the diagnosis. Several reports suggest that EM can show the typical bacilliform bodies (Rubinow et al, 1976).

Despite large painful effusions, early hypertrophic osteoarthropathy (HPO) tissue tends to have virtually no inflammatory cell infiltration in synovium but does have marked vascular congestion (Schumacher, 1976). Electron-dense deposits in vessel walls can be seen in some biopsies by EM. In chronic HPO lymphocytic infiltration is reported.

Although basically "noninflammatory", varying degrees of lining cell proliferation and mononuclear infiltration can be seen in osteoarthritis. CPPD or apatite clumps are common.

Scurvy of the synovium shows edema, extravasation of erythrocytes, and large fibrocytes that have have been unable to release their collagen precursors because of the lack of vitamin C (Bevilacqua et al, 1976). Red cells extravasate because of poor collagenous support of the vessels.

A familial arthropathy with synovial coating with fibrin-like material and giant cells has been described in children (Athreya and Schumacher, 1978). Synovium in sickle cell disease can show obliterated vessels and occasionally some lymphocyte and plasma cell infiltration (Schumacher, 1975a). Sickled cells can be identified in the blocked vessels by EM.

Thorns or animal spines can occasionally penetrate into joints and be visible in biopsies as well as producing a chronic synovitis. Metallic or plastic particles in patients with joint arthroplasties can also occasionally be found in synovium. Lead fragments from a bullet have been found embedded in synovium.

Synovial fat necrosis and lipid laden macrophages can be associated with pancreatic disease (Smukler et al, 1979). Eosinophilic infiltration with fibrin deposition was found in a case later determined to have the hypereosinophilic syndrome (Brogadir et al, 1980).

BIOPSIES OF OTHER SITES IN RHEUMATOID ARTHRITIS

Subcutaneous Nodules

The most nearly diagnostic lesion of rheumatoid disease is the rheumatoid granuloma, typified in the subcutaneous nodule. The latter usually consists of a number of discrete granulomas, often in different stages of development, which are separated from each other by scar tissue containing scattered, small, vascular islands of lymphocytes, plasma cells, and histiocytes. The vessels in these aggregates, probably venules, generally have thick, nonmuscular walls and are lined by prominent endothelial cells.

The rheumatoid granuloma consists of a fairly large, amorphous, eosinophilic center surrounded by a zone of mononuclear cells, usually several cells deep. There is a tendency for large mononuclear cells immediately bordering the amorphous center to "palisade," that is, to be oriented with their long axes perpendicular to the rim of the necrotic area (Fig. 4.42). The outer portion of the nodule contains lymphocytes and histiocytes. Some histiocytes contain lipid droplets. Even in clinically old lesions, individual acute granulomas are often found, their centers sometimes containing neutrophils and fresh fibrin. Detailed studies of the necrotic centers of nodules show varying proportions of necrotic cellular debris, degenerated collagen, fibrin, fibronectin, lipids (Fig. 4.43), and proteoglycans. Vascular damage has been widely proposed as the primary event in the development of the subcutaneous nodule (Aherne et al, 1985; Rasker and Kuipers, 1983), but obvious vasculitis is only infrequently detectable even in apparently early biopsied lesions. Immunoglobins can be demonstrated in the necrotic center (Geiler, 1984). Immunohistologic studies of the surrounding cells identify the palisading cells as DR-expressing macrophages and the surrounding cells as helper and suppressor T lymphocytes (Duke et al, 1984). Further insight into the pathogenesis of this important lesion is needed and may reveal more about the most important factors in other extra-articular lesions too.

Rheumatoid granulomas can, of course, be seen in locations other than the subcutaneous nodule. The areas susceptible to biopsy in addition to the subcutaneous tissue include lung, pleura, pericardium, tendons, and rarely, synovium. The histologic appearance of lesions in the pleura and pericardium may be very suggestive of rheumatoid disease. However, the granulomatous reaction in these sections usually lies on the serous surface, where it is apt to be impossible to distinguish it with certainty from an organizing fibrinous exudate due to another cause. In the lung, silicotic nodules and infectious granulomas require care in differentiation. The lesions in tendons are often recognizable clinically. They are generally removed in the course of reparative surgical procedures, rather than for diagnostic purposes. Nevertheless, when they are seen, the diagnostic value of rheumatoid granulomas in tendons is as great as that of a subcutaneous nodule.

Although now infrequently seen, the subcutaneous nodule of rheumatic fever is very similar to the rheumatoid subcutaneous nodule. Characteristically, the rheumatic nodule as a whole and the granulomas within it are smaller than those of the rheumatoid lesion. The rheumatic granulomas are less well structured; the zones are not as clearly demarcated, and palisading is less evident. Both size and structure appear to be functions of the age of the lesions. If a rheumatic nodule has been present longer than the typical few weeks, or a biopsy is done on a rheumatoid nodule very early, the two lesions may be indistinguishable. The subcutaneous nodules that are found uncommonly in patients with SLE have a histologic appearance that shares some features of both rheumatic fever and rheumatoid arthritis, and can be indistinguishable from rheumatoid nodules. Subcutaneous nodules can also occur in some cases of palindromic rheumatism.

Granuloma annulare is another lesion that may be difficult to distinguish from a rheumatoid nodule. Usually it is intradermal, but it may also occur in subcutaneous tissue and, conversely, rheumatoid nodules sometimes involve the skin.

Peripheral Nerves

Mild chronic inflammatory cell infiltration of peripheral nerve areas and adjacent vessels seems to be surprisingly common in rheumatoid arthritis. Bauer and Clark (1948) found inflammation around peripheral nerves in 28 of 31 autopsies of rheumatoid patients. Any correlation of these findings with the mild symmetrical peripheral neuropathy of rheumatoid arthritis however is not clear. More dramatic neural changes are associated with either bland obliterative (Weller et al, 1970) or necrotizing arteritis (Peyronnard et al, 1982) of perineural vessels. These nerves can show varying degrees of demyelination and axonal degeneration. Both Wallerian degeneration of myelinated and unmyelinated fibers and segmental demyelination have been described and attributed to the effects of ischemia (Kim and Collins, 1981). Sural nerves are most often studied in patients with suspected vasculitis and mononeuritis multiplex involving the sural distribution (Fig.

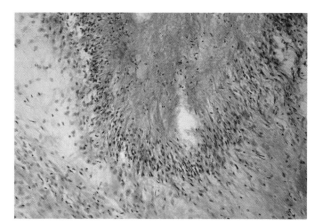

Figure 4.42 A classic rheumatoid nodule has central necrosis, pallisaded cells, and surrounding mononuclear cells. (H&E).

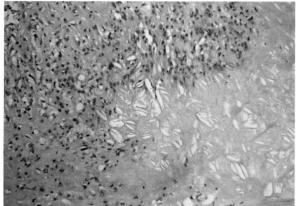

Figure 4.43 Clear clefts from dissolved lipids as shown here can be seen in some rheumatoid nodules.

4.44). Immunoglobulins and complement have been found in walls of epineural vessels and in the inner side of the perineural sheaths (Vanlis and Jennekens, 1977; Conn et al, 1972).

Compressive neuropathies in rheumatoid arthritis have not been studied histologically to see if there are any distinctive features. Amyloid neuropathy does not seem to develop in the secondary amyloidosis of rheumatoid arthritis (Kim and Collins, 1981).

Heart

Rheumatoid granulomas have been detected in the heart at autopsy in many reports. Valve leaflets, valve rings, myocardium, and epicardium have all been sites of such involvement. Although these lesions are localized and clearly different from the valvulitis of rheumatic fever, the valves are involved in the same descending order of frequency: mitral, aortic, tricuspid, and pulmonary. Valvular insufficiency can occur. Severe aortic insufficiency due to granulation tissue at the base of the valve, as can be observed in Reiter's syndrome, ankylosing spondylitis, po-

lychondritis, and Marfan's syndrome spondylitis, is not expected. Myocardial granulomas can cause conduction abnormalities or other abnormal EKG patterns.

Diffuse myocarditis can also occasionally occur but this has not been well correlated with clinical disease and may be due to other causes. Coronary arteritis can be seen most often in patients with arteritis elsewhere.

Pericardial tissue obtained at surgery for the rare complication of tamponade can show fibrin deposition, fibrous thickening, and infiltration with chronic inflammatory cells. Focal scarred fibrotic areas are also seen. Up to 40% of cases in autopsy studies show mild pericarditis, which is a much higher frequency than is ever clinically appreciated. Pallisaded histiocytes under fibrinous exudate and surrounded by lymphocytes can occasionally suggest a rheumatoid nodule-like lesion opening into the pericardial space (John et al, 1979).

Salivary Glands

Since Sjögren's syndrome is a common and potentially serious association with rheu-

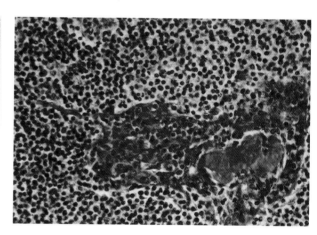

Figure 4.44 Inflammatory cell infiltration is seen in vessel wall in the sural perineurium of a patient with polyarteritis. An identical lesion can be seen in some patients with rheumatoid arthritis. (Courtesy of Arthritis Foundation.)

Figure 4.45 Classic salivary gland findings in Sjögren's syndrome include dense lymphoid infiltrates around metaplastic ducts.

matoid arthritis, definite diagnosis by salivary gland biopsy is occasionally called for. Biopsy of the parotid gland carries a risk of fistula formation so that a small minor salivary gland of the buccal lip mucosa (Greenspan et al, 1974), nasal mucosa, or lacrimal glands (Nasu et al, 1984) are more often studied. Some lip numbness often persists for many months at the biopsy site. Histologic findings tend to be less dramatic in rheumatoid patients with secondary Sjögren's syndrome than they are in primary Sjögren's syndrome (Greenspan et al, 1974). Inconsistent but characteristic changes can include metaplasia of salivary ducts forming "epimyoepithelial islands". Studies with immunohistochemistry demonstrate the presence of keratin from ducts and myoepithelial cells (Caselitz et al, 1986) but no smooth muscle antigen (Palmer et al, 1986). Type IV collagen containing basement membrane surrounds the islands. Lymphocytic infiltrates surround intralobular ducts and are an important feature (Fig. 4.45). Quantitation of severity of infiltration can be done by counting the number of aggregates that contain more than 50 lymphocytes. More than one such focus per 4 mm^2 of tissue is characteristic of Sjögren's syndrome (Greenspan et al, 1974). Plasma cells may be present. Infiltrating lymphocytes are predominantly helper-inducer T cells (Dalavanga et al, 1987). Other findings include acinar tissue atrophy. Interlobular fibrous septae are not destroyed. After years of disease there may be atrophy of acini with replacement by adipose tissue and loss of the inflammatory cell infiltration, making diagnosis more difficult. Cell infiltration and activation as identified by surface HLA-DR expression can be decreased by some therapies such as cyclosporin A (Dalavanga et al, 1987).

When complicating rheumatoid arthritis amyloid is occasionally demonstrable in gingival biopsies, as well as in viscera, subcutaneous fat, and rectal mucosa.

Pleuropulmonary

Rheumatoid nodules do occur in the lung but may be impossible to distinguish radiographically from infectious granulomas and tumors. Biopsy of a pulmonary parenchymal nodule is the most prudent course even in patients with widespread subcutaneous nodules. Large fibronecrotic parenchymal nodules occur in some patients such as anthracite miners. Granulomatous histology is often not evident; there are huge necrotic silica containing areas. Pulmonary fibrosis may be seen in about 2% of patients with rheumatoid arthritis.

Lung biopsies can be obtained by either the transbronchial route or by open surgical biopsies. Interstitial inflammation and fibrosis are common but show no unique features as they are similar to idiopathic lesions in other individuals. Immunoglobulins can be identified in alveolar septae and vessel walls (Cervantes-Perez et al, 1980).

Peribronchial inflammation may be seen more often in patients with Sjögren's syndrome.

Lymph Nodes

Lymph nodes are frequently enlarged in rheumatoid arthritis, but histopathologic study in uncomplicated disease reveals only nonspecific follicular hyperplasia. Prominent germinal centers can contain transformed lymphocytes.

In patients with associated Sjögren's syndrome there is an increased risk of lymphoma. This is about 20 times the level found in rheumatoid arthritis alone (Moutsopoulos et al, 1980). Lymphomas can be of the large transformed cell (histiocytic) type or, less often, of the small lymphocyte type. Lymph node specimens should always be evaluated by a pathologist experienced with this tissue as extreme follicular hyperplasia can be confused with malignancy. Immunopathologic stains can aid in this differentiation (Wilkens et al, 1980).

Immunocytologic studies have suggested that benign nodes in rheumatoid arthritis contain B lymphocytes that stain much more intensely for immunoglobulins than do the cells in malignant nodes (Wilkens et·al, 1980). Some lymphomas in rheumatoid patients with Sjögren's syndrome have been shown to be of T cell origin (Isenberg et al, 1987).

Muscle

Serially sectioned random muscle biopsies in patients with rheumatoid arthritis have revealed inflammatory infiltrates (Fig. 4.46) ("lymphorrhages") in the majority and a nonnecrotizing inflammation of small venules or arteries in about 10% of the patients (Sokoloff et al, 1951). The former lesion is nonspecific. The latter probably has some prognostic significance, but its infrequent occurrence limits the value of muscle biopsy as a diagnostic aid in most cases of rheumatoid disease. When a muscle biopsy is done in an area affected by peripheral neuritis, necrotizing arteritis is often found. Immunoglobulins can be identified in vessel walls (Oxenhandler et al, 1977). Except for disuse atrophy in areas immobilized as a re-

sult of joint disability, the muscle fibers themselves usually appear to be normal. Type II fiber atrophy demonstrated histochemically is another frequent but nonspecific finding (Kim and Collins, 1981). Muscle fiber degeneration and regeneration are not characteristic of rheumatoid arthritis and should suggest polymyositis.

Blood Vessels

A spectrum of pathologic changes in blood vessels is associated with varying clinical syndromes (see Chapter 14). Bland endothelial hyperplasia, perivascular lymphocytic collections, and leukocytoclastic vasculitis (Fig. 4.47) can occur. The most important finding is the rare necrotizing arteritis because of its associated poor prognosis. Vessels tend to be slightly smaller than those involved in periarteritis nodosa but show the same fibinoid necrosis of vessel walls. Aneurism formation seems to be less common in rheumatoid arthritis. Immunoglobulins and complement can be found in vessel walls in recent lesions (Conn et al, 1972) but are often not found in later lesions. Some other vessels seem to have similar immune deposits but no necrosis or cellular infiltration (Conn et al, 1976). The reasons for this are not clear.

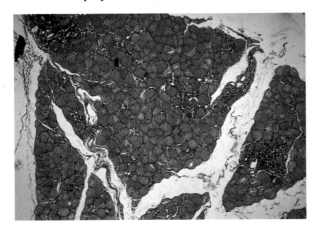

Figure 4.46 Lymphocytic inflitrates are seen in this rheumatoid muscle.

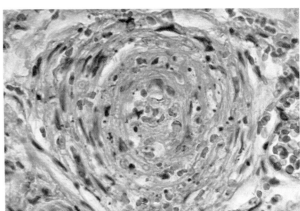

Figure 4.47 Leukocytoclastic vasculitis can occasionally be seen in rheumatoid disease.

REFERENCES

Abdou NI, Schumacher HR, Colman RW, et al: Behçet's disease: Possible role of secretory component deficiency, synovial inclusions and fibrinolytic abnormality in the various manifestations of the disease. *J Lab Clin Med* 1978;91:409–422.

Aherne MJ, Bacon PA, Blake DR, et al: Immunohistochemical findings in rheumatoid nodules. *Virchows Arch Path Anat* 1985;407:191–202.

Athreya B, Schumacher HR: Pathologic features of a recently recognized form of familial arthropathy. *Arthritis Rheum* 1978;21:429–437.

Bauer W, Clark WS: The systemic manifestations of rheumatoid arthritis. *Trans Assoc Am Physicians* 1948;61:339–350.

Bayliss CE, Dawkins RL, Cullity G, et al: Laboratory diagnosis of rheumatoid arthritis. *Ann Rheum Dis* 1975;34:395–402.

Bevilaqua FA, Hasselbacher P, and Schumacher HR: Scurvy and hemarthrosis. *JAMA* 1976;235:1874–1876.

Blake DR, Gallagher PJ, Potter AR, et al: The effect of iron on the progression of rheumatoid disease: A histologic assessment of patients with early rheumatoid synovitis. *Arthritis Rheum* 1984;27:495–501.

Bocanegra TS, McClelland JJ, Germain BF, et al: Intraarticular fragmentation of a new Parker-Pearson synovial biopsy needle. *J. Rheum* 1980;7:248–250.

Borenstein DG, Gibbs CA, Jacobs RP: Gas-liquid chromatographic analysis of synovial fluid. *Arthritis Rheum* 1982;25:947–953.

Brandt KD, Cathcart ES, Cohen AS: Studies of immune deposits in synovial membranes and corresponding synovial fluids. *J Lab Clin Med* 1968;72:631–647.

Brogadir SP, Golwein MI, Schumacher HR: A hypereosinophilic syndrome mimicking rheumatoid arthritis. *Am J Med* 1980;69:799–802.

Canoso JJ, and Cohen AS: Rheumatological aspects of amyloid disease. *Clin Rheum Dis* 1975;1:149–161.

Caselitz J, Osborn M, Wostrow J, et al: Immunohistochemical investigations on the epimyoepithelial islands in lymphoepithelial lesions: Use of monoclonal keratin antibodies. *Lab Invest* 1986;55:427–432.

Cervantes-Perez P, Toro-Perez A, Rodriquez-Jurado P: Pulmonary involvement in rheumatoid arthritis. *JAMA* 1980;243:1715–1719.

Cherian PV, Schumacher HR: Immunoelectron microscopic analysis of vessel walls in rheumatoid arthritis. *Arthritis Rheum* 1984;27:S34.

Cheung HS, Ryan LM, Kozin F, et al: Identification of collagen subtypes in synovial fluid sediments from arthritic patients. *Am J Med* 1980;68:73–79.

Clemmensen I, Holund B, Bach Anderson R: Fibrin and fibronectin in rheumatoid synovial membrane and rheumatoid synovial fluid. *Arthritis Rheum* 1983;26:479–485.

Cooke TDV: The interactions and local disease manifestations of immune complexes in articular collagenous tissues, in Maroudas A, Holborow EJ (eds): *Studies in Joint Disease* 1980;1:158–169.

Crisp AJ, Chapman CM, Kirkham SE, et al: Articular mastocytosis in rheumatoid arthritis. *Arthritis Rheum* 1984;27:845–851.

Conn DL, McDuffie FC, Dyck PJ: Immunopathologic study of sural nerves in rheumatoid arthritis. *Arthritis Rheum* 1972;15:135–143.

Conn DL, Schroeter AL, McDuffie FC: Cutaneous vessel immune deposits in rheumatoid arthritis. *Arthritis Rheum* 1976;19:15–20.

Cooper NS, Soren A, McEwen C, et al: Diagnostic specificity of synovial lesions. *Human Pathol* 1981;12:314–328.

Dalavanga YA, Detrick B, Hocks JJ et al: Effect of cyclosporin A on the immunopathological lesion of the labial minor salivary glands from patients with Sjögren's syndrome. *Ann Rheum Dis* 1987;46:89–92.

Duclos M, Zeidler H, Liman W, et al: Characterization of blood and synovial fluid lymphocytes from patients with rheumatoid arthritis and other joint diseases by monoclonal antibodies (OKT Series) and acid-naphthylesterase staining. *Rheum Internat* 1982;2:75–82.

Duke OL, Hobbs S, Panayi GS, et al: A combined immunohistological and histochemical analysis of lymphocyte and macrophage populations in the rheumatoid nodule. *Clin Exp Immunol* 1984;56:239–246.

Flory ED, Clarris BJ, Muirden KD: Deposits of β2M in the rheumatoid synovial membrane. *Ann Rheum Dis* 1982;41:520–526.

Freemont AJ, Jones CJP, Bromley M, et al: Changes in vascular endothelium related to lymphocyte collections in diseased synovia. *Arthritis Rheum* 1983;26:1427–1433.

Gardner DL: *The Pathology of Rheumatoid Arthritis*. Baltimore, Williams & Wilkins, 1972, 259 p.

Geiler G: Immunohistochemical examinations of

rheumatoid granulomas. *Histochem J* 1984;16:377–379.

Goldenberg DI, Kelley W, Gibbons RB. Metastatic adenocarcinoma of synovium presenting as an acute arthritis. *Arthritis Rheum* 1975;18:107–110.

Gordon OA, Pruzanski W, Ogryzlo MA: Synovial fluid examination in the diagnosis of amyloidosis. *Ann Rheum Dis* 1973;32:428–430.

Graham J, Goldman JA: Fat droplets and synovial fluid leukocytes in traumatic arthritis. *Arthritis Rheum* 1978;21:76–80.

Greenspan JS, Daniels TE, Talal N, et al: The histopathology of Sjögren's syndrome in labial salivary gland biopsies. *Oral Surgery* 1974;37:217–229.

Grimley M, Sokoloff L: Synovial giant cells in rheumatoid arthritis. *Am J Pathol* 1966;49:931–954.

Hoffman G, Schumacher HR, Paul H, et al: Calcium oxalate microcrystalline associated arthritis in end stage renal disease. *Ann Intern Med* 1982;97:36–42.

Hollander JL: Arthrocentesis technique and intrasynovial therapy, in McCarty DJ (ed): *Arthritis and Allied Conditions.* ed 10. Philadelphia, Lea & Febiger, 1985, pp 541–553.

Hollander JL, McCarty DJ, Rawson AJ: The "RA cell," "ragocyte," or "inclusion body cell." *Bull Rheum Dis* 1965;16:382–383.

Honig S, Gorevic P, Hoffstein S, et al: Crystal deposition disease diagnosis by electron microscopy. *Am J Med* 1977;63:161–164.

Hunter T, Gordon DA, Ogryzlo MA: The ground pepper sign of synovial fluid: A new diagnostic feature of ochronosis. *J Rheum* 1974;1:45–53.

Husby G, Williams RC: Immunohistochemical studies of interleukin 2 and interferon in rheumatoid arthritis. *Arthritis Rheum* 1985;28:174–181.

Isenberg DA, Griffiths MH, Rustin M, et al: T-cell lymphoma in a patient with long-standing rheumatoid arthritis and Sjögren's syndrome. *Arthritis Rheum* 1987;30:115–117.

John JT, Hough AJ, Sergent JS: Pericardial disease in rheumatoid arthritis. *Am J Med* 1979;66:385–390.

Johnston YE, Duray PH, Steere AC, et al: Lyme arthritis: Spirochaetes found in synovial microangiopathic lesions. *Am J Pathol* 1985;118:26–34.

Kahn CB, Hollander JL, Schumacher HR: Corticosteroid crystals in synovial fluid. *JAMA* 1970;211:807–809.

Karnovsky MJ: A formaldehyde-glutaraldehyde fixative of high osmolality for use in electron microscopy. *J Cell Biol* 1965;27:441A.

Kim RC, Collins GH: The neuropathology of rheumatoid disease. *Human Pathol* 1981;12:5–15.

Kitridou R, Schumacher HR, Sbarbaro JL, et al: Recurrent hemarthrosis after prosthetic knee arthoplasty: Identification of metal particles in the synovial fluid. *Arthritis Rheum* 1969;12:520–528.

Krey PR, Comerford FE, Cohen AS: Multicentric reticulohistiocytosis. *Arthritis Rheum* 1974;17:615–633.

Labowitz R, Schumacher HR: Articular manifestations of SLE. *Ann Intern Med* 1974:74:911–921.

Lindblad S, Hedforg E: Intra-articular variation in synovitis. *Arthritis Rheum* 1985;28:977–986.

Malone DG, Wahl SM, Tsokos M, et al: Immune function in severe, active rheumatoid arthritis. *J Clin Invest* 1984;74:1173–1185.

Mapp PI, Revell PA: Ultrastructural localization of muramidase in the human synovial membrane. *Ann Rheum Dis* 1987;46:30–37.

Matsubara T, Ziff M: Basement membrane thickening of post-capillary venules in rheumatoid synovium. *Arthritis Rheum* 1987;30:18–30.

Mohr W, Westerhellwig H, Wessinghage D: Polymorphonuclear granulocytes in rheumatic tissue destruction. III. An electron microscopic study of PMNs at the pannus-cartilage junction in rheumatoid arthritis. *Ann Rheum Dis* 1981;40:396–399.

Moon MS, Kim I, Kim J-M: Synovial biopsy by Franklin-Silverman needle. *Clin Orthrop* 1980;150:224–228.

Morris CJ, Blake DR, Wainwright AC, et al: Relationship between iron deposits and tissue damage in the synovium: An ultrastructural study. *Ann Rheum Dis* 1986;45:21–26.

Moutsopoulos HM, Chused TM, Mann DL, et al: Sjörgren's syndrome (sicca syndrome): Current issues. *Ann Intern Med* 1980;92:212–226.

Muirden KD: Giant cells, cartilage and bone fragments within rheumatoid synovial membrane: Clinicopathologic correlations. *Aust Ann Med* 1970;2:105–110.

Muirden KD, Mills KW: Do lymphocytes protect the rheumatoid joint? *Br Med J* 1971;4:219–221.

Nasu M, Matsubara O, Yamamoto TT: Post-mortem prevalence of lymphocytic infiltration of the lacrimal gland. *J Pathol* 1984;143:11–15.

Owen DS: A cheap and useful compensated polarizing microscope. *N Engl J Med* 1971;285:1152.

Oxenhandler R, Adelstein EH, Hart MN: Immunopathology of skeletal muscle. *Hum Pathol* 1977;8:321–328.

Palmer RM, Everson JW, Gusterson BA: "Epimyoepithelial" islands in lymphoepithelial lesions. *Virchows Arch Path Anat* 1986;408:603–609.

Paul H, Reginato AJ, Schumacher HR: Alizarin red S staining as a screening test to detect calcium compounds in synovial fluid. *Arthritis Rheum* 1983;26:191–200.

Peyronnard J-M, Charron L, Beaudet F, et al: Vasculitic neuropathy in rheumatoid disease and Sjögren's syndrome. *Neurology* 1982;32:839–845.

Phelps P, Steele AD, McCarty DJ: Compensated polarized light microscopy. *JAMA* 1968;203:508–512.

Rasker JJ, Kuipers FC: Are rheumatoid nodules caused by vasculitis? A study of 13 early cases. *Ann Rheum Dis* 1983;42:384–388.

Reginato AJ, Schumacher HR, Allan DA, et al: Acute monoarthritis associated with lipid liquid crystals. *Ann Rheum Dis* 1985;44:537–543.

Ropes MW, Bennett GA, Cobbs S, et al: 1958 revision of diagnostic criteria for rheumatoid arthritis. *Bull Rheum Dis* 1958;9:175–176.

Ropes MW, Bauer W: *Synovial Fluid Changes in Joint Disease*. Cambridge, Mass, Harvard University Press, 1953, 150 p.

Rubinow A, Canoso JJ, Goldenberg DL, et al: Arthritis in Whipple's disease. *Israel J Med Sci* 1981;17:445–450.

Schumacher HR: Ultrastructural characteristics of the synovial membrane in idiopathic hemochromatosis. *Ann Rheum Dis* 1972;31:465–473.

Schumacher HR: Joint involvement in progressive systemic sclerosis (scleroderma). *Am J Clin Pathol* 1973;60:593–600.

Schumacher HR: Rheumatological manifestations of sickle cell disease and other hereditary hemoglobinopathies. *Clin Rheum Dis* 1975a;1:37.

Schumacher HR: Synovial membrane and fluid morphologic alterations in early rheumatoid arthritis: Microvascular injury and virus-like particles. *Ann NY Acad Sci* 1975b;256:39–64.

Schumacher HR: The articular manifestations of hypertrophic pulmonary osteoarthropathy in bronchogenic carcinoma. *Arthritis Rheum* 1976;19:629–636.

Schumacher HR: Palindromic onset of rheumatoid arthritis: Clinical, synovial fluid and biopsy studies. *Arthritis Rheum* 1982;25:361–369.

Schumacher HR: Synovial fluid analysis, in Kelly WN et al (eds): *Textbook of Rheumatology* ed 2. Philadelphia, WB Saunders Co, 1985, pp 561–568.

Schumacher HR, Cherian PV, Reginato AR, et al: Intra-articular apatite crystal deposition. *Ann Rheum Dis* 1983;42:54–59.

Schumacher HR, Cherian PV, Sieck M, Clayburne G: Ultrastructural identification of chlamydial antigens in synovial membrane in acute Reiter's syndrome. *Arthritis Rheum* 1986;29(suppl):S31.

Schumacher HR, Cherian PV, Zeiger A, Wilder R: Immunological detection of peptidoglycan in synovium. *Arthritis Rheum* 1987;30(suppl):S106.

Schumacher HR, Holdsworth DE: Ochronotic arthropathy. I. Clinicopathologic studies. *Semin Arthritis Rheum* 1977;6:207–246.

Schumacher HR, Jimenez SA, Gibson T, et al: Acute gouty arthritis without urate crystals identified on initial examination of synovial fluid. *Arthritis Rheum* 1975;18:603–612.

Schumacher HR, Kulka JP: Needle biopsy of the synovial membrane: Experience with the Parker-Pearson technique. *N Engl J Med* 1972;286:416–419.

Schumacher HR, Reginato AJ, Pullman S: Synovial fluid oxalate deposition complicating rheumatoid arthritis with amyloidosis and renal failure: Demonstration of intracellular oxalate crystals. *J Rheumatol* 1987;14:361–366.

Seward CW, Osterland CK: The patterns of anti-immunoglobulin activities in serum, pleural and synovial fluids. *J Lab Clin Med* 1973;81:230–240.

Shiozawa S, Shiozawa K, Fujita T: Morphologic observations in the early phase of the cartilage-pannus junction. *Arthritis Rheum* 1983;26:472–478.

Smukler NM, Schumacher HR, Pascual I, et al: Synovial fat necrosis associated with ischemic pancreatic disease. *Arthritis Rheum* 1979;22:547–553.

Sokoloff L, Wilens SL, Bunim JJ: Arteritis in striated muscle in rheumatoid arthritis. *Am J Pathol* 1951;27:157–173.

Spilberg I, Meyer GI: The arthritis of leukemia. *Arthritis Rheum* 1972;15:630–635.

Townes AS, Sowa JM: Complement in synovial fluid. *Johns Hopkins Med J* 1970;127:23–37.

Traycoff RB, Pascual E, Schumacher HR: Mononuclear cells in human synovial fluid: Identification of lymphoblasts in rheumatoid arthritis. *Arthritis Rheum* 1976;19:743–748.

Van Lis JMJ, Jennekens FGI: Immunofluorescence studies in a case of rheumatoid neuropathy. *J Neurol Sci* 1977;33:313–321.

Walters MT, Smith JL, Moore K, et al: An investigation of the action of disease modifying antirheumatic drugs on the rheumatoid synovial membrane. *Ann Rheum Dis* 1987;46:7–16.

Weinberger A, Schumacher HR: Experimental joint trauma: Synovial response to blunt trauma and inflammatory response to intra-articular injection of fat. *J Rheumatol* 1981;8:380–389.

Weller RO, Bruckner FE, Chamberlain MA: Rheumatoid neuropathy: Histological and electrophysiological study. *J Neurol Neurosurg Psychiatry* 1970;33:592–604.

Wilkens FR, Roth GR, Husby G, et al: Immunocytological studies of lymph nodes in rheumatoid arthritis and malignant lymphomas. *Ann Rheum Dis* 1980;39:147–151.

Wofsky D: Culture-negative septic arthritis and bacterial endocarditis: Diagnosis by synovial biopsy. *Arthritis Rheum* 1980;23:605–607.

Young CL, Adamson TC, Vaughn JH, et al: Immunohistologic characterization of synovial membrane lymphocytes in rheumatoid arthritis. *Arthritis Rheum* 1984;27:32–39.

Zucker J, Uddin J, Gantner GE, et al: Cholesterol crystals in synovial fluid. *Ann Intern Med* 1964;60:436–446.

CHAPTER 5

PATHOGENESIS IN RHEUMATOID ARTHRITIS

DAVID E. YOCUM, MD

Although rheumatoid arthritis is classified as an autoimmune disorder, the only clear autoantibody seen in laboratory studies is rheumatoid factor. There is no direct evidence implicating a specific etiology of rheumatoid arthritis, but it is speculated that the initiating event is one or more foreign antigens invading a genetically susceptible host. After the initial inflammatory response occurs, a subsequent series of inflammatory events, vascular proliferation, cellular invasion and proliferation, and cytokine production occur. Which features are critical in the initiation and perpetuation of disease and which are epiphenomena is not yet known. Until the roles of various factors and the sequence of response is known, therapy is, of necessity, largely empiric.

The discussion of pathogenesis includes several important components: genetic background; etiologic agents; early inflammatory changes; chronic inflammatory changes; mediators of inflammation; and pathogenetic significance of extra-articular disease manifestations. Clinically, patients have pain, fatigue, and loss of function. The result is joint destruction. Appropriate management of this group of patients makes it necessary to understand these processes.

GENETIC BACKGROUND

Polygenetic factors appear to play a major role in familial development of rheumatoid arthritis. The risk of developing erosive arthritis has been shown to be increased two- to threefold in first-degree relatives of patients with rheumatoid arthritis (Lawrence et al, 1970). This risk is increased to six- to sevenfold if radiologic assessment is used. There is no increased risk in relatives of patients with seronegative rheumatoid arthritis more than in the general population (Lawrence et al, 1970). Monozygotic twins of seropositive patients with rheumatoid arthritis have a 33-fold increase in prevalence of rheumatoid arthritis (Lawrence, 1970).

Evidence demonstrates an association between class II HLA-DR region genes and presence of seronegative rheumatoid arthritis. Although the specificity of the HLA-DR4 allotype for rheumatoid arthritis is not as strong as that of HLA-B27 for ankylosing spondylitis, the association is very convincing (Fig. 5.1). The HLA-DR4 allele has been detected in 35% to 70% of rheumatoid arthritis patients as compared with 16% to 33% of normal whites (Stastny, 1978; Panayi et al, 1978; Dobloug et al, 1980). Other populations appear similarly affected. The most striking association between HLA-DR4 and rheumatoid arthritis is reported in a series of Felty's syndrome patients in whom 23 of 24 were HLA-DR4–positive (Dinant et al, 1980). At present, the relative risk of rheumatoid arthritis is approximately eightfold in HLA-DR4–positive individuals. In contrast, patients with rheumatoid arthritis expressing HLA-DR3 have an increased likelihood of developing proteinuria, rashes, and thrombocytopenia during gold therapy (Wooley et al, 1980; Bardin et al, 1982). As the HLA-DR genes are further separated, other correlations may appear.

The biological role of HLA-DR in the pathogenesis of rheumatoid arthritis is not known. HLA-DR genes correspond to the immune response genes in the mouse. These genes code for molecules that are expressed by B lymphocytes, activated T lymphocytes,

HLA-DR4 IN RHEUMATOID ARTHRITIS

Patients	% HLA-DR4 Positive	% Controls	References
White	60%*	29%	Dobloug et al, 1980; Karr et al, 1980; Panayi et al, 1978; Stastny, 1978 and 1980.
North American black	46%*	14%	Karr et al, 1980
Yakima Indians	7%**	4%	Willkens, 1982
Mexican	26%*	2.7%	Gorodezky et al, 1981
Jewish			
Ashkenazi	48%**	32%	Stastny, 1980
Non-Ashkenazi	27%**	23%	Stastny, 1980
Asian Indian	15%**	12%	Nichol and Woodrow, 1981
Japanese	71%*	46%	Maeda et al, 1981

*Significant difference between patients and controls
**Difference not significant

Figure 5.1   HLA-DR4 in rheumatoid arthritis.

and antigen-presenting cells. These molecules act as stimulators in the mixed lymphocyte reaction, as targets for cytotoxic T cells, and as controlling elements in antigen presentation (Albert and Gotze, 1977).

ETIOLOGIC AGENTS

Although various microbial infections may be followed by polyarthritis and multisystem disease in both animals and humans, none has been shown to cause rheumatoid arthritis. Several organisms have been implicated as the cause of rheumatoid arthritis (Fig. 5.2). Although infection of the synovium by a microbial agent could be the initiating event in rheumatoid arthritis, microbial antigens deposited in the synovium without infection must be considered. Bacterial cell wall components such as muramyl dipeptide, a component of peptidoglycan, are potent immune stimulants that are capable of prolonged inflammatory reactions with minimal antigen deposition (Schwab et al, 1967; Hadler and Granovetter, 1978). The relationship between streptococcal antigens and rheumatic fever, and other bacteria with the reactive arthritides are examples (Wannamaker et al, 1951).

Studies by Mansson and Olhagen demonstrating a high frequency of atypical *Clostridium perfringens* in fecal culture from rheumatoid patients would suggest that abnormal intestinal flora could be a source of such antigens (Mansson and Olhagen, 1974). Supporting this are studies of arthritis development in pigs in which the intestinal flora had been altered (Mansson et al, 1971). In other studies, mycoplasma and diphtheroids have been cultured from a number of rheumatoid synovial membranes and fluids (Stewart et al, 1969; Taylor-Robinson and Taylor, 1976). While provocative, these studies have not been substantiated by other researchers (Cassell and Cole, 1981).

As noted above, 18 viruses are capable of inducing arthritis in humans (Sauter and Utsinger, 1978). At least twice that number have been associated with arthralgias. Although

INFECTIOUS AGENTS ASSOCIATED WITH ARTHRITIS IN HUMANS

Bacteria	DNA Virus	RNA Virus
Streptoccoci	Hepatitis B	Rubella
Clostridia	Epstein-Barr	Parvovirus
Diphtheroids	Cytomegalovirus	Mumps
Mycoplasmas	Adenovirus	Measles
	Variola	Echo
	Vaccinia	Ross River
	Varicella	Chikungunya
	Herpes simplex	Sindbis
		Mayaro
		O'nyong Nyong

Figure 5.2 Infectious agents associated with arthritis in humans.

most of these are self-limited, there are reports of chronic arthropathy. At present, full evaluations to detect viral etiologies are costly and have led to many negative results. However, it is clear that viruses, with their many effects on the immune system, must be considered as possible etiologic agents. Arthritis associated with hepatitis B infections is well described (Inman, 1982). Of patients with hepatitis B infection 10% to 30% develop arthritis. Although surface antigen can be demonstrated in the synovium and synovial fluid (Schumacher and Gall, 1974), the virus has not been cultured.

The association of rubella virus with arthritis has been noted for nearly 30 years (Johnson and Hall, 1958). A number of patients with rubella arthritis have been noted to test positive for rheumatoid factor, whereas some patients develop classical rheumatoid arthritis. However, other patients have been followed for up to 10 years without developing rheumatoid arthritis (Fry et al, 1962). Rubella virus has been isolated from

the synovial fluid of patients with rheumatoid arthritis or chronic arthritis, and it has also been isolated from patients with chronic arthritis after rubella vaccine-related infections (Chantler et al, 1982; Ford et al, 1982; Grahame et al, 1983). Whether rubella virus actually causes rheumatoid arthritis or whether these findings only represent the rheumatoid arthritis patient's difficulty responding to the virus remains to be proven.

As with rubella, rheumatoid factor production is a feature of acute Epstein-Barr virus (EBV) infection (acute mononucleosis) (Chervenick, 1981). Following acute infection, EBV lies dormant in the host's B cells, probably controlled by interferon-mediated natural killer cells (Purtillo and Sakamoto, 1981; Svedmer and Jondal, 1975; Wallace et al, 1982). EBV can cause immune abnormalities as well as frank neoplasia (Old et al, 1966; Hanto et al, 1982). The virus is capable of cellular transformation and is frequently used to "immortalize" cells in culture (Miller, 1971). Lymphocytes from rheumatoid arthri-

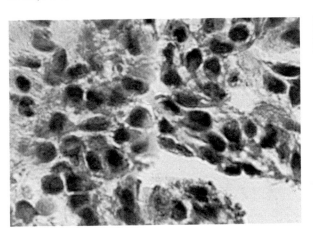

Figure 5.3 Synovial lining proliferation in early rheumatoid arthritis.

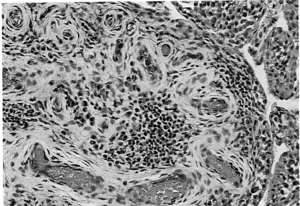

Figure 5.4 Hypertrophied rheumatoid synovium demonstrating a marked prominence of blood vessels around a small lymphoid nodule with narrowing or thrombosis of some vessels.

tis patients transform more readily with EBV, demonstrating an immune abnormality in dealing with this virus in this patient population (Bardwick et al, 1980). However, although arthritis can occur with EBV, EBV infection is not similar to rheumatoid arthritis and support for a causal relationship is lacking.

Recently, a parvovirus was cultured from the synovium of a patient with rheumatoid arthritis, suggesting an association with rheumatoid arthritis (Simpson et al, 1984). There are slow-growing viruses that can induce chronic disease in other tissues (Gajdusek, 1977). Such agents might infect and "transform" any one of the cell types present in the synovium and lead to chronic arthritis. Data from Fassbender suggest that such transformed synovial cells may exist in rheumatoid arthritis (Fassbender and Simmling-Annefeld, 1983). Clearly, cultured cells from rheumatoid synovium behave abnormally (Castor, 1971; Anastassiades et al, 1978). Whether this is a result of viral transformation or an indirect effect of humoral factors remains to be seen.

EARLY SYNOVIAL INFLAMMATION

The earliest event seen within the synovium of patients with rheumatoid arthritis is mild synovial lining layer proliferation (Fig. 5.3) and vascular changes with perivascular lymphocytes (Kulka et al, 1955; Schumacher, 1975; Schumacher and Kitridou, 1972). Synovial lining cells can be divided into three distinct subgroups (Burmester et al, 1981; Edwards et al, 1982). The first group, type A, appear to be macrophagelike in that the cells express monocyte antigens, are phagocytic

and have HLA-DR on their surface. The second group, type B, seen primarily in rheumatoid arthritis, appear dendritic and express abundant HLA-DR without expressing any of the other typical markers of monocytes, T cells, or B cells. The third cell group, type C, appear to be fibroblasts and lack HLA-DR or other typical differentiation surface antigens. Whether these cells are capable of invading the deep synovium and playing a role in tissue destruction is not known but seems very likely. When grown in culture rheumatoid synovial fibroblasts require less nutrients and grow more rapidly than normal synovial fibroblasts (Castor, 1971; Anastassiades et al, 1978). Early synovial cell changes have not been well studied.

The rheumatoid synovium is highly vascular (Fig. 5.4). Microvascular lesions lead to the obliteration of small blood vessels by inflammatory cells and organized thrombi. Electron microscopy demonstrates endothelial cell damage and gaps between endothelial cells. The increased number of blood vessels may be in response to hypoxia, which has been demonstrated in rheumatoid arthritis synovium, and/or in response to specific endothelial cell growth factors (Truehaft and McCarty, 1971; Polverini et al, 1977). The endothelial cell seems to play an important role in early synovial inflammation. Not only does it express HLA-DR antigens, but its morphology also changes to tall columnar endothelia (Freemont et al, 1983; Pober et al, 1983; Iguchi and Ziff, 1986). Such activated cells are more "adhesive" to macrophages and lymphocytes (Bevilacqua et al, 1985). The early, prominent vascular changes suggest that the etiologic agent might be carried to the synovium by the circulation.

Concomitantly with early cellular proliferation, various lymphokines and monokines (cytokines) are released from the synovial tissue. These biologically active nonimmunoglobulin substances are released from activated lymphocytes and monocyte–macrophages. These cytokines play a key role in the perpetuation of inflammation within the synovium.

CHRONIC RHEUMATOID ARTHRITIS INFLAMMATION

The chronic phases of rheumatoid arthritis are marked by proliferation of several cell types (Gardner, 1972; Zvaifler, 1985) (Fig. 5.5). The synovial lining becomes hyperplastic and the subsynovium becomes edematous and protrudes into the joint cavity, often forming villi. Focal and segmental vascular proliferation is seen, with areas of thrombosis and hemorrhage (Fig. 5.6). The synovium is frequently filled with mononuclear cells, a majority of which are T lymphocytes, often of the helper/inducer phenotype (Kurosaka and Ziff, 1983; Burmester et al, 1981) (Fig.

5.7). These cells as well as the monocytes display HLA-DR (Ia), a measure of cellular activation. Suppressor T lymphocytes, B lymphocytes, and plasma cells are also present (Konttinen et al, 1981; Ishikawa and Ziff, 1976). The contact between the T cells, macrophages, and B cells probably results in the activation of the B cells into plasma cells with resultant immunoglobulin production. The predominant immunoglobulins produced are IgG (30% to 60%) and IgM (10% to 30%). Most of the IgM and much of the IgG are rheumatoid factors. Approximately 20% of the IgG present in the synovial fluid is produced in the synovial membrane (Munthe and Natvig, 1972; Natvig and Munthe, 1975; Cecere et al, 1982). Immune complexes containing IgG, IgM, IgA, and C3 have been noted within the synovium of seropositive and seronegative patients. These complexes may be responsible for the perpetuation of the inflammatory reaction in rheumatoid arthritis.

At the sites of bone and cartilage erosion, the predominant cells are fibroblasts and macrophages (Bromley and Wooley, 1984) (Fig. 5.8). These cells release prostaglandins, collagenase, and other neutral proteases cap-

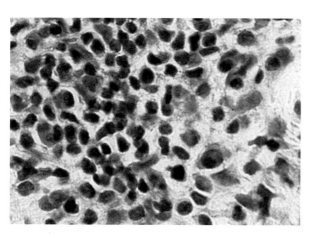
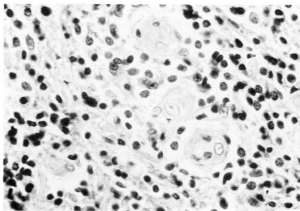

Figure 5.5 Multiple cell types invading and proliferating within rheumatoid synovium. (*Left*), A cluster of lymphocytes surrounded by monocytes, plasma cells, and polymorphonuclear leucocytes. (*Right*), Multinucleated giant cells surrounded by lymphocytes, monocytes, and polymorphonuclear leucocytes.

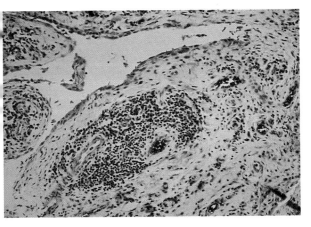

Figure 5.6 Lymphoid nodule surrounding blood vessels, one of which appears thrombosed. Note surrounding area which is highly vascular but relatively acellular.

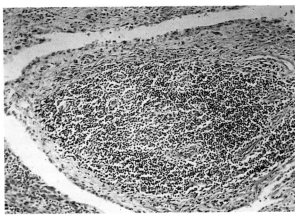

Figure 5.7 Intense cellular infiltration, primarily by lymphocytes.

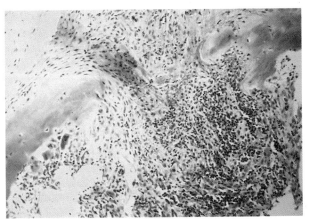

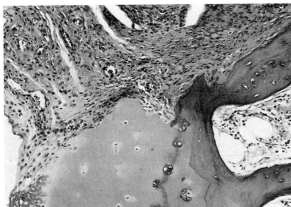

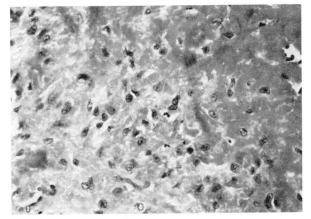

Figure 5.8 Cartilage and bone erosions. (*Top left*), Marginal erosion with invasion of both bone and cartilage. (*Top right*), Large cellular central erosion which has invaded both cartilage and bone. (*Bottom right*), Higher-power view of bony erosions. Note relative lack of mononuclear cells and predominance of fibroblast-like cells.

able of tissue destruction. The relationship between these cells and the other inflammatory cells is not clearly understood. However, the importance of other humoral factors in the stimulation of nonimmune cells is demonstrated by in vitro studies of cultured synovial cells. Upon removal from the joint these cells display stellate morphology and release collagenase and prostaglandin E_2 (PGE_2) (Dayer et al, 1976). However, after serial passage these cells lose their bizarre morphology and they produce less prostaglandin and collagenase. The addition of the monokine interleukin-1 (IL-1) and/or PGE_2 reproduces the morphologic changes. IL-1, but not PGE_2 predictably effect factor release (Baker et al, 1983).

Away from the site of erosions the pannus is composed of both dense, avascular, fibrous, acellular areas and vascular, very cellular areas (Malone et al, 1984; Kobayashi and Ziff, 1975) (Figs. 5.9 and 5.10). The former probably represent scarlike areas resulting from the intense inflammation. The latter are composed primarily of T lymphocytes that actively release lymphokines. These cellular areas may represent sites of antigen reactivation. The three areas of the pannus together suggest an ongoing cyclical reaction. Antigen deposition results in vascular proliferation and invasion of inflammatory cells, which release a series of cytokines that not only perpetuates the reaction but also activates fibroblasts, chondrocytes, and osteoblasts and degrades the surrounding tissue. Once the area has been destroyed, a fibrous scar is left

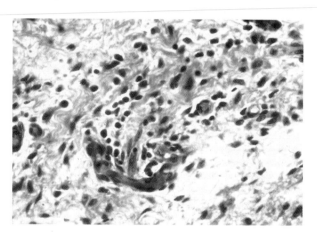

Figure 5.9 Acellular synovium showing decreased blood vessels, few lymphocytes, and predominance of amorphous fibrinoid material.

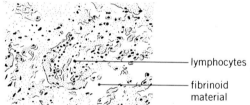

lymphocytes

fibrinoid material

behind. This series of reactions is well described in the stages of the inflammatory response. However, in rheumatoid arthritis these events continue to occur until the joint and surrounding tissue are destroyed. Whether this occurs in response to repeated challenges by antigen or whether the immune system is unable to turn itself off is not known.

Cells of rheumatoid synovial fluid differs from those of the synovial membrane. Polymorphonuclear leukocytes (PMNL) make up 75% to 85% of the total cells present (Zvaifler, 1985; Hollingsworth et al, 1967). Many of these cells have large cytoplasmic vacuoles containing immunoglobulins, rheumatoid factor, and complement components. These cells are frequently called ragocytes or rheumatoid arthritis cells and can be seen in nearly every form of inflammatory arthritis.

Synovial fluid also contains decreased levels of complement as compared with serum, demonstrating evidence of activation of both the classic and alternate complement pathways (Ward and Zvaifler, 1971). Also present are biologically active fragments of the complement sequence, anaphylatoxins, and chemotactic factors. The levels of these substances correlate with the presence of synovial fluid immune complexes. The complexes are composed of both IgM and IgG rheumatoid factor (Winchester, 1975). The IgG rheumatoid factors are able to self-associate, forming intermediate-size complexes that activate complement and enhance local inflammation.

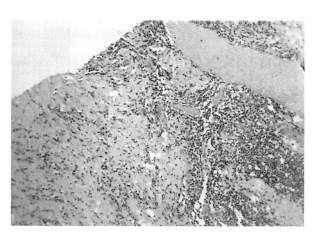 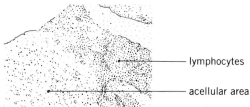

Figure 5.10 Section of synovium showing a very cellular lymphocyte-rich area with increased vasculature adjacent to an acellular area which is lacking in blood vessels and shows a marked decrease in the number of lymphocytes.

MEDIATORS OF INFLAMMATION

In rheumatoid arthritis the proliferation both of resident cells and of invading cells leads to chronic tissue destruction. Although this reaction can occur through cellular interaction, there are various soluble mediators whose actions during acute and chronic inflammation may be beneficial or deleterious. The relation between these effects and the exact role each mediator plays in the pathologic process is difficult to determine, but it is important to note the reactions in which these mediators are involved. Although it is probably overly simplistic to divide this complex disease into distinct phases, one can speculate about how mediators might contribute to different stages of the inflammatory process. Sources and interactions of mediators may vary depending on concentration, timing, and other factors.

Several factors may be involved in early synovitis of rheumatoid arthritis (Fig. 5.11). Vasoactive amines such as histamine, serotonin, and bradykinin are probably involved in early vascular permeability and pain. Histamine, which induces vascular contraction, intercellular gaps, and capillary permeability, is stored in tissue mast cells present even in normal synovium. Its release can be induced by several stimuli including immune complexes and complement fragments (Beaven, 1976). Serotonin, stored in platelets, increases vascular permeability (Essman, 1978). Bradykinin is a product of the clotting system and of fibrinolysis and is capable of enhancing vascular permeability (Movat, 1979).

MEDIATORS IN EARLY SYNOVITIS		
MEDIATORS	**PRIMARY CELL SOURCE**	**EFFECTS**
Vasoactive amines	Mast cells, basophils, platelets	Vasodilation, permeability, pain
Prostaglandins (PG)	Macrophages, synovial cells	Vasodilation, pain
Leukotrienes (LT)	Polymorphonuclear leukocytes (PMNL), macrophage	Chemotaxis, phagocytosis
Interleukin-1	Macrophage	Fever, chemotaxis, PG production
Platelet-activating factor	Basophils, PMNL, macrophages	PMNL adherence, platelet aggregation, LT production, vasoactive amine release
Complements C5a, C3b	Macrophages, serum	Chemotaxis, phagocytosis

Figure 5.11 Mediators in early synovitis.

The products of arachidonic acid metabolism are also important in the early phases of synovitis (Fig. 5.12). The association between rheumatoid arthritis and metabolites of cyclooxygenase, especially the prostaglandins, has been a major focus of research (Vane, 1971). The roles of prostaglandins of the E series are complex and sometimes contradictory. Prostaglandins enhance vascular permeability, probably by potentiating the effects of the vasoactive amines. On the other hand, PGs can suppress functions of T cells, B cells, natural killer cells, osteoclasts, and macrophages (Goodwin and Ceuppens, 1983). Many of these effects are reversed by nonsteroidal anti-inflammatory drugs. However, these effects are difficult to substantiate in vivo, especially in patients with rheumatoid arthritis. Lipoxygenase metabolites, especially the leukotrienes, are potent cellular chemoattractants (Ford-Hutchinson et al, 1980; Poubelle et al, 1984). The role of leukotrienes is yet to be elucidated in rheumatoid arthritis (Davidson et al, 1983). Other products of basophils, macrophages, PMNL, and platelets such as platelet-activating factor (PAF) and complement, play important roles in vascular activation, cellular recruitment, and release of further inflammatory mediators.

Interleukin-1 has been identified in synovial fluid and is probably an important mediator throughout the inflammatory process (Wood et al, 1983). Interleukin-1 plays a key role in T-cell activation and has been shown to stimulate fibroblasts, chondrocytes, and osteoclasts (Mizel, 1982; Mizel et al, 1981; Gowen et al, 1983). These target cells possess receptors for interleukin-1, the activation of which results in cellular proliferation and the release of collagenase and PGE_2.

During the proliferative stages of arthritis, mediators play key roles in the invasion and proliferation of various types of cells as well

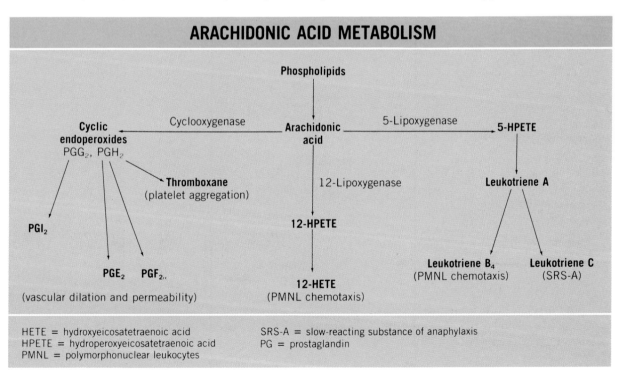

Figure 5.12 Arachidonic acid metabolism.

as vascularization of the synovium (Fig. 5.13). Interleukin-2 (IL-2) or T-cell growth factor results from the activation of T cells, which results in the release of a series of lymphokines with various cellular effects (Wilkins et al, 1983). Macrophage activating factor, macrophage inhibiting factor, and lymphocyte-derived chemotactic factor (LDCF) are probably responsible for the continued invasion of various inflammatory cells into the synovium (Stastny et al, 1975; Dayer and Demczuk, 1984). The release of LDCF correlates with the degree of cellular inflammation and peripheral anergy reported in some patients with rheumatoid arthritis (Malone et al, 1984).

The interferons (IFN) which are released by lymphocytes, monocytes, and fibroblasts, increase class I and class II antigen receptors,

Fc receptors, and enhance interleukin-1 production (Pober et al, 1983; Sztein et al, 1984). IFN have been detected in the sera and synovial fluid of patients with rheumatoid arthritis (Martin et al, 1981).

One can visualize how the release of all the above-mentioned mediators could result in the initiation and perpetuation of the inflammatory reaction. However, it cannot be assumed that the primary purpose of these factors is destructive (most have functions in normal homeostasis), and some may actually be important in attempting to regulate and/or inhibit the disease process.

Later, during the erosive stages of rheumatoid arthritis, osteoclast-activating factor released from lymphocytes results in bone resorption (Fig. 5.14). In addition, PGE_2 can activate osteoclasts, and epidermal growth

MEDIATORS IN ACUTE PROLIFERATIVE PHASE OF RHEUMATOID ARTHRITIS

MEDIATORS	PRIMARY CELL SOURCE	EFFECTS
Prostaglandin E_2	Macrophages	Increase T-cell suppressors
Interleukin-1	Macrophages	T-lymphocyte activation
Interleukin-2	T lymphocytes	T-lymphocyte proliferation
Colony-stimulating factor	T lymphocytes	Macrophage differentiation
Macrophage inhibitory factor	Lymphocytes	Inhibit macrophage movement
Lymphocyte-derived chemotactic factor	T lymphocytes	Macrophage chemotaxis
Lymphocyte inhibitory factor	Lymphocytes	Inhibit lymphocyte migration
Angiogenic factor	Macrophages	Endothelial cell proliferation
Interferons	Lymphocytes, macrophages, fibroblasts	Increase class I and II antigens, Fc receptors, and IL-1 production

Figure 5.13 Mediators in acute proliferative phase of rheumatoid arthritis.

factor (EGF) can induce bone resorption (Raisz et al, 1975; Yoneda and Mundy, 1979; Dayer and Demczuk, 1984).

Proteases such as collagenase, elastase, and cathepsin G result in further breakdown of collagen and proteoglycan (Dayer and Demczuk, 1984). Dayer and Demczuk (1984) have recently described a mononuclear cell factor (MCF) that may be IL-1, is released by synovial monocytes, and induces collagenese and PGE_2 release from other adherent synovial cells. Glucocorticoids and retinoids decrease PGE_2 and collagenase production by MCF-stimulated synovial cells, whereas nonsteroidal antiinflammatory drugs only suppressed PGE_2.

Growth factors may play important roles in both the destructive and repair stages of rheumatoid arthritis. Several of these mediators have recently been purified and identified as potent cellular activators. Alone, these substances can induce target-cell proliferation and enzyme–mediator release. In combination, growth factors such as epidermal growth factor (EGF) and transforming growth factor beta can induce transformation of normal synovial cells into tumorlike cells (Brinckerhoff, 1983). Such a process has been proposed by Fassbender in the pathogenesis of rheumatoid arthritis (Fassbender and Simmling-Annefeld, 1983).

Lymphotoxin, a mediator produced by lymphocytes, has been demonstrated in rheumatoid arthritis (Hazelton; 1984). This

MEDIATORS IN EROSIVE PHASE OF RHEUMATOID ARTHRITIS

MEDIATORS	PRIMARY CELL SOURCE	EFFECTS
Interleukin-1	Macrophages	Collagenase, PGE_2 production
Prostaglandin E_2	Macrophages	Osteoclast activation
Catabolite	Macrophages	Cartilage resorption
Osteoclast-activating factor	Lymphocytes	Bone resorption
Lymphotoxin	Lymphocytes	Lymphocyte, endothelial cell destruction
Tumor necrosis factor (TNF)	Macrophages	Collagenase and PG production, proliferation of synovial cells
Transforming growth factor beta	Lymphocytes, platelets	Fibroblast transformation
Epidermal growth factor	Fibroblasts	Bone resorption

Figure 5.14 Mediators in erosive phase of rheumatoid arthritis.

substance is responsible for destruction of lymphocytes and endothelium and results in cell necrosis and the release of cellular constituents within the synovium.

Within the same joint, both tissue destruction and tissue repair can be seen. However, the repair process is weak and the resultant product is primarily "scar" tissue. This is a reflection of the heterogeneous cell popula-

tion present. Many of the mediators that are believed to play a role in the erosive phase may also be important in repair (Fig. 5.15). While interleukin-1 induces collagen synthesis, PGE_2, EGF, and IFN decrease synthesis (Dayer and Demczuk, 1984). Fibroblast activating factor (FAF), a lymphocyte product, and platelet-derived growth factor induce fibroblast proliferation and collagen synthesis

MEDIATORS OF REPAIR AND FIBROSIS

MEDIATORS	PRIMARY CELL SOURCE	EFFECTS
Fibroblast-activating factor	Lymphocytes	Fibroblast proliferation, collagen synthesis
Interleukin-1	Macrophages	Collagen synthesis
Connective-tissue-activating peptide	Platelets	Cell proliferation, glycosaminoglycan synthesis
Platelet-derived growth factor	Platelets	Cell proliferation
Epidermal growth factor	Fibroblasts	Decreased collagen synthesis
Prostaglandin E_2	Macrophage synoviocytes	Decreased collagen synthesis
Interferons	Lymphocytes	Decreased collagen synthesis

Figure 5.15 Mediators of repair and fibrosis.

(Wahl et al, 1978; Russell et al, 1982). FAF has been shown to be produced by synovium and synovial fluid lymphocytes (Wahl et al, 1978). Finally connective-tissue-activating peptide, a platelet product, induces fibroblast proliferation and glycosaminoglycan synthesis (Castor et al, 1979).

The list of inflammatory mediators is long and complex, with new mediators being discovered regularly. The final effect of each depends upon multiple factors including their complicated interactions that are as yet to be understood. Although confusing, it is important to note that a better understanding of these factors will ultimately lead to better, more specific therapy.

EXTRA-ARTICULAR DISEASE

Although joint involvement is a hallmark of rheumatoid arthritis, the process is actually a systemic disease. Symptoms include fever, night sweats, weight loss, anorexia, fatigue, and myalgias, which may be due in part to interleukin-1. Arthritic patients frequently present with anemia, leukocytosis, thrombocytosis, elevated sedimentation rate, hypoalbuminemia, and hyperglobulinemia. Inflammatory lesions affect a wide variety of organs including the heart, lungs, central nervous system, vasculature, and the eyes. Although these lesions are usually asymp-

tomatic, they are present in a significant number of patients and may lead to clinically evident disease and death (see Chapter 14).

Although the occurrence of extra-articular manifestations is usually associated with more active articular disease, this is not always the case. With episcleritis and Felty's syndrome these manifestations may occur when the articular disease is relatively mild or in remission (Michels et al, 1984; Goldberg and Pinals, 1980). In general, extra-articular disease is seen in patients with persistently active, erosive arthritis in the presence of high titers of rheumatoid factor, circulating immune complexes, and low levels of serum complement. This suggests that the underlying pathogenesis of extra-articular disease is immunologically mediated. Although no primary antigen has been found, deposition of circulating immune complexes is considered the underlying cause of extra-articular disease (Hack et al, 1984). As in joint disease, the initial event in systemic rheumatoid involvement often is vessel damage, which is probably secondary to immune complex deposition followed by fibrinoid necrosis and imflammatory infiltration. Depending on the stage of the lesions, lymphocyte and monocyte infiltration may be seen or, if at a later stage, fibrosis. This suggests that the extra-articular inflammatory sites undergo changes similar to those seen in the joints. Immunofluorescent studies often demonstrate rheumatoid factor, IgG, IgM, and complement within the lesions.

SUMMARY

The pathogenesis of rheumatoid arthritis is complex and multifactorial (Fig. 5.16). The inflammatory cascade is initiated by an unknown agent(s) in genetically susceptible individuals, resulting in joint destruction and potential involvement of other nonarticular organs. The process can be, and frequently is, linked to a tumorlike process with abnormal tissue proliferation and mediator release. Indeed, the process is associated with increased morbidity and mortality. Only through better understanding of the cellular and humoral components can therapy be more specific.

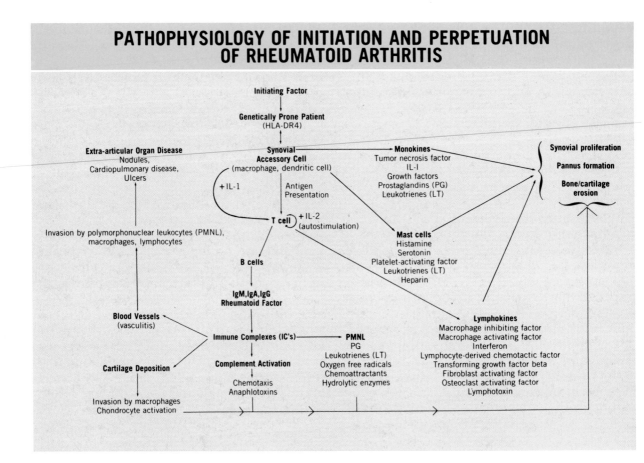

Figure 5.16 Pathophysiology of initiation and perpetuation of rheumatoid arthritis.

REFERENCES

Albert ED, Gotze D: The major histocompatibility system in man, in Gotze D (ed): *The Major Histocompatibility System in Man and Animals.* Berlin, Springer-Verlag, 1977, pp 7–58.

Anastassiades TP, Ley J, Wood A, et al: The growth kinetics of synovial fibroblast cells from inflammatory and noninflammatory arthropathies. *Arthritis Rheum* 1978;21:461–466.

Baker DG, Dayer J-M, Roelke M, Schumacher HR, Krane SM: Rheumatoid synovial cell changes induced by a mononuclear cell factor in culture. *Arthritis Rheum* 1983;26:8-14.

Bardin T, Dryll A, Debeyre N, et al: HLA system and side effects of gold salts and D-penicillamine treatment of rheumatoid arthritis. *Ann Rheum Dis* 1982;41:599–601.

Bardwick PA, Bluestein HG, Zvaifler NJ, et al: Altered regulation of Epstein-Barr virus induced lymphoblast proliferation in rheumatoid arthritis lymphoid cells. *Arthritis Rheum* 1980;23:626–632.

Beaven MA: Histamine. *N Engl J Med* 1976;294;30, 320–325.

Bevilacqua MP, Pober JS, Wheeler RS, et al: Interleukin-1 acts on cultured human vascular endothelium to increase adhesion of polymorphonuclear leukocytes, monocytes and related leukocyte cell lines. *J Clin Invest* 1985;76:2003–2011.

Brinckerhoff CE: Morphologic and mitogenic responses of rabbit synovial fibroblasts to transforming growth factor beta require transforming growth factor alpha or epidermal growth factor. *Arthritis Rheum* 1983;26:1370–1378.

Bromley M, Woolley DE: Histopathology of the rheumatoid lesion. *Arthritis Rheum* 1984;27:857–863.

Burmester GR, Yu DTY, Irani AM, et al: Ia+ T cells in synovial fluid and tissues of patients with rheumatoid arthritis. *Arthritis Rheum* 1981;24:1370–1376.

Cassell GH, Cole BC: Mycoplasmas as agents of human disease. *N Engl J Med* 1981;304:80–89.

Castor CW: Connective tissue activation: II. Abnormalities of cultured rheumatoid synovial cells. *Arthritis Rheum* 1971;14:55–66.

Castor CE, Ritchie JC, Williams CH, et al: Connective tissue activation: XIV. Composition and actions of human platelet autacoid mediator. *Arthritis Rheum* 1979;22:260–272.

Cecere F, Lessard J, McDuffey S, et al: Evidence for the local production and utilization of immune reactants in rheumatoid arthritis. *Arthritis Rheum* 1982;25:1307–1313.

Chantler JK, Ford DK, Tingle AJ: Persistent rubella infection and rubella-associated arthritis. *Lancet* 1982;1:1323–1325.

Chervenick PA: Infectious mononucleosis. *DM,* 1971;1:1–29.

Davidson EM, Rae SA, Smith MJH: Leukotriene B4, a mediator of inflammation present in synovial fluid in rheumatoid arthritis. *Ann Rheum Dis* 1983;42:677–679.

Dayer JM, Demczuk S: Cytokines and other mediators in rheumatoid arthritis. *Springer Semin Immunopathol* 1984;7:387–413.

Dayer JM, Krane SM, Russell RG: Production of collagenase and prostaglandins by isolated adherent rheumatoid synovial cells. *Proc Natl Acad Sci USA* 1976;73:945–949.

Dinant HJ, Muller WH, Vandenberg-Loonen EM, et al: HLA-DRw4 in Felty's syndrome. *Arthritis Rheum* 1980;23:1336.

Dobloug JH, Forre O, Kass E, et al: HLA antigens and rheumatoid arthritis. *Arthritis Rheum* 1980;23:209–313.

Edwards JC, Sedgwock AD, Willoughby DA: Membrane properties and esterase activity of synovial lining cells: further evidence for a mononuclear phagocyte subpopulation. *Ann Rheum Dis* 1982;41:282–286.

Essman WB (ed): Serotonin in health and disease in *Jamaica Spectrum Publications:* New York, SP Medical & Science Books, 1978

Fassbender HG, Simmling-Annefeld M: The potential aggressiveness of synovial tissue in rheumatoid arthritis. *J Pathol* 1983;139:399–406.

Ford DK, DaRoza DM, Reid GD, et al: Synovial mononuclear cell responses to rubella antigen in rheumatoid arthritis and unexplained persistent knee arthritis. *J Rheumatol* 1982;99:420–423.

Ford-Hutchinson AW, Bray MA, Doig MV, Shipley ME, Smith MJH: Leukotriene B, a potent chemokinetic and aggregating substance released from polymorphonuclear leukocytes. *Nature* 1980;286:264–265.

Freemont AJ, Jones CJP, Bromley M, et al: Changes in vascular endothelium related to lymphocyte collections in diseased synovia. *Arthritis Rheum* 1983;26:1427–1433.

Fry J, Dillane JB, Fry L: Rubella. *Br Med J* 1962;2:833–834.

Gajdusek DC: Unconventional viruses and the origin and disappearance of kuru. *Science* 1977;197:943–960.

Gardner DL: *The Pathology of Rheumatoid Arthritis.* London, Edward Arnold, 1972.

Goldberg J, Pinals RS: Felty syndrome. *Semin Arthritis Rheum* 1980;10:52–65.

Goodwin JS, Ceuppens J: Regulation of the immune response by prostaglandins. *J Clin Immunol* 1983;3:295–315.

Gorodezky C, Lavelle C, Castro-Escobar LE, et al: HLA antigens in Mexican patients with adult rheumatoid arthritis. *Arthritis Rheum* 1981;24:976–977.

Gowen M, Wood DD, Ihrie EJ, et al: An interleukin-1-like factor stimulates bone resorption in vitro. *Nature* 1983;306:378–380.

Grahame R, Armstrong N, Simmons JM, et al: Chronic arthritis associated with the presence of intrasyno vial rubella virus. *Ann Rheum Dis* 1983;42:2–13.

Hack CE, Eerenberg-Belmer AJM, Lim UG, et al: Lack of activation of C1 despite circulating immune complexes detected by two C1q methods, in patients with rheumatoid arthritis. *Arthritis Rheum* 1984;27:40–48.

Hadler NM, Granovetter DA: Phlogistic properties of bacterial debris. *Semin Arthritis Rheum* 1978;8:1–16.

Hanto DW, Frizzera G, Gajl-Peczalski KJ, et al: Epstein-Barr virus-induced B-cell lymphoma after renal transplantation. *N Engl J Med* 1982;306:913–918.

Harris ED: Pathogenesis of rheumatoid arthritis. *Am J Med* 1986;80:4–10.

Hazelton RA: A study of lymphocytotoxins in the sera of families of patients with rheumatoid disease. *Arthritis Rheum* 1984;27:233–236.

Hollingsworth JW, Siege ER, Creasey WA: Granulocyte survival in synovial exudate of patients with rheumatoid arthritis and other inflammatory joint diseases. *Yale J Biol Med* 1967;39:289–296.

Iguchi T, Ziff M: Electron microscopic study of rheumatoid synovial vasculature: intimate relationship between tall endothelium and lymphoid aggregation. *J Clin Invest* 1986;77:355–361.

Inman RD: Rheumatoid manifestations of hepatitis B virus infection. *Semin Arthritis Rheum* 1982;11:406–420.

Ishikawa H, Ziff M: Electron microscopic observation of immunoreactive cells in the rheumatoid synovial membrane. *Arthritis Rheum* 1976;19:1–14.

Johnson RE, Hall AP: Rubella arthritis: report of cases studied by latex tests. *N Engl J Med* 1958;258:743.

Karr RW, Rody GE, Lee T, et al: Association of HLA-DRw4 with rheumatoid arthritis in black and white patients. *Arthritis Rheum* 1980;23:1241–1245.

Kobayashi I, Ziff M: Electron microscopic studies of cartilage-pannus junction in rheumatoid arthritis. *Arthritis Rheum* 1975;18:475–483.

Konttinen YT, Reitamo S, Ranki A, et al: The characterization of the immunocompetent cells of rheumatoid synovium from tissue sections and eluates. *Arthritis Rheum* 1981;24:71–79.

Kulka JP, Bocking D, Ropes MW: Early joint lesions of rheumatoid arthritis. *Arthritis Pathol* 1955;59:129–150.

Kurosaka M, Ziff M: Immunoelectron microscopic study of distribution of T cell subsets and HLA-DR expressing cells in rheumatoid synovium. *Arthritis Rheum* 1983;26(suppl 4)553.

Lawrence JS: Rheumatoid arthritis—nature or nurture? *Ann Rheum Dis* 1970;29:357–379.

Lawrence JS, Laine VAI, DeGraaf R: Epidemiology of RA in northern Europe. *Proc Soc Med* 1970;29:357–379.

Maeda H, Juji T, Mitsue H, et al: HLA-DR4 and rheumatoid arthritis in Japanese people. *Ann Rheum Dis* 1981;40:299–302.

Malone DG, Wahl SM, Tsokos M, et al: Immune function in severe, active rheumatoid arthritis: a relationship between peripheral blood mononuclear cell proliferation to soluble antigens and synovial tissue immunohistologic characteristics. *J Clin Invest* 1984;74:1173–1185.

Mansson I, Norberg R, Olhagen B, et al: Arthritis in pigs induced by dietary factors. *Clin Exp Immunol* 1971;9:677–693.

Mansson I, Olhagen B: Fecal *Clostridium perfringens* and rheumatoid arthritis. *J Infect Dis* 1974;130:444–447.

Martin DA, Treadwell TL, Michalski JP, et al: Analysis of interferon levels in synovial fluids and sera in rheumatoid disease, abstracted. *Arthritis Rheum* 1981;24:S93.

Michels ML, Cobo LM, Caldwell DS, et al: Rheumatoid arthritis and sterile corneal ulceration. *Arthritis Rheum* 1984;27:606–614.

Miller G: Human lymphoblastoid cell lines and Epstein-Barr virus: a review of their interrelationships and their relevance to the etiology of leukoproliferative states in man. *Yale J Biol Med* 1971;43:358–384.

Mizel SB: Regulations of immune and inflammatory responses by interleukin-1. *Clin Immunol Newslett* 1982;3:123.

Mizel SB, Dayer JM, Krane SM, et al: Stimulation of rheumatoid synovial cell collagenase and prostaglandin production by partially purified lymphocyte-activating factor (interleukin-1). *Proc Natl Acad Sci USA* 1981;78:2474–2477.

Movat HZ: The acute inflammatory reaction, in Movat HZ (ed): *Inflammation, Immunity and Hypersensitivity: Molecular and Cellular Mechanisms.* New York, Harper & Row; 1979, p 1.

Munthe E, Natvig JB: Immunoglobulin classes, subclasses and complexes of IgG rheumatoid factor in rheumatoid plasma cells. *Clin Exp Immunol* 1972;12:55–70.

Natvig JB, Munthe E: Self-associating IgG rheumatoid factor represents a major response of plasma cells in rheumatoid inflammatory tissue. *Ann NY Acad Sci USA* 1975;256:88–95.

Nichol FE, Woodrow JC: HLA-DR antigens in Indian patients with rheumatoid arthritis. *Lancet* 1981; 1:220–221.

Old LJ, Boyse EA, Oettegen HF: Precipitating antibody in human serum to an antigen present in cultured Burkitt's lymphoma cells. *Proc Natl Acad Sci USA* 1966;56:1699–1704.

Panayi GS, Wooley P, Batchelor JR: Genetic basis of rheumatoid disease: HLA antigens, disease manifestations and toxic reactions to drugs. *Br Med J* 1978;1326–1328.

Pober JS, Gimbrone MA, Cotran RS, et al: Ia expression by vascular endothelium is inducible by activated T cells and by human interferon. *J Exp Med* 1983;157:1339–1353.

Polverini PJ, Cotran RS, Gimbrone MA Jr, et al: Activated macrophages induce vascular proliferation. *Nature* 1977;269:804–805.

Poubelle P, Beaulieu AD, Borgeat P: Synthesis of leukotrienes (LTs) by synovial polymorphonuclear leukocytes (PMNL) and macrophages from patients with rheumatoid arthritis (RA). *Arthritis Rheum* 1984;27:S72.

Purtillo DT, Sakamoto K: Epstein-Barr virus and human disease: immune response determines the clinical and pathologic expression. *Hum Pathol* 1981;12:677–679.

Raisz LG, Luben RA, Mundy GR, et al: Effect of os-

teoclast activating factor from human leukocytes on bone metabolism. *J Clin Invest* 1975;56:408–413.

Rothschild BM, Masi AT: Pathogenesis of rheumatoid arthritis: a vascular hypothesis. *Semin Arthritis Rheum* 1982;12:11–31.

Russell R, Raines E, Bowen-Pope D: Growth factors from platelets, monocytes, and endothelium: their role in cell proliferation. *Ann NY Acad Sci* 1982;397:18–24.

Sauter SVH, Utsinger PD: Viral arthritis. *Clin Rheum Dis* 1978;4:255.

Schumacher HR: Synovial membrane and fluid morphology alterations in early rheumatoid arthritis: microvascular injury and virus-like particles. *Ann NY Acad Sci* 1975;256:39.

Schumacher HR and Gall EP: Arthritis in acute hepatitis and chronic active hepatitis. *Am J Med* 1974;57:655.

Schumacher HR, Kitridou RC: Synovitis of recent onset: a clinicopathologic study during the first month of disease. *Arthritis Rheum* 1972;15:465–485.

Schwab JH, Cromartie WJ, Ohanian SH, et al: Association of experimental chronic arthritis and the persistence of group A streptococcal cell walls in articular tissues. *J Bacteriol* 1967;94:1728–1735.

Simpson RW, McGinty L, Simon L, et al: Association of parvoviruses with rheumatoid arthritis of humans. *Science* 1984;223:1425–1428.

Stastny P: Association of the B-cell alloantigen DRw4 with rheumatoid arthritis. *N Engl J Med* 1978; 298:869–871.

Stastny P, Rosenthal M, Andresis M, et al: Lymphokines in the rheumatoid joint. *Arthritis Rheum* 1975;18:237.

Stastny P: Rheumatoid arthritis, in Terasaki P (ed): *Histocompatibility.* Los Angeles, University of California Press, 1980, pp. 681–686.

Stewart SM, Alexander WRM, Duthie JJR: Isolation of diphtheroid bacilli from synovial membrane and fluid in rheumatoid arthritis. *Ann Rheum Dis* 1969;28:477.

Svedmer E, Jondal J: Cytotoxic effector cells specific for B cell lines transformed by Epstein-Barr virus are present in patients with infectious mononucleosis. *Proc Natl Acad Sci USA* 1975;72:1622.

Sztein MB, Steeg PS, Johnson HM, Oppenheim JJ: Regulation of human peripheral blood monocyte DR antigen expression in vitro by lymphocytes and recombinant interferons. *J Clin Invest*

1984;73:556–565.

Taylor-Robinson D, Taylor G: Do mycoplasmas cause rheumatic disease? in Dumonde DC (ed): *Infection and Immunology in the Rheumatoid Diseases*. Oxford, Blackwell Scientific Publications, 1976, pp. 177–186.

Truehaft P, McCarty D: Synovial fluid pH, lactate, oxygen and carbon dioxide partial pressure in various joint disease. *Arthritis Rheum* 1971;14:475–484.

Vane J: Prostaglandins as mediators of inflammation. *Adv Prostaglandin Thromboxane Res* 1971;14:475–484.

Wahl SM, Wahl LM, McCarthy JB: Lymphocyte-mediated activation of fibroblast proliferation and collagen production. *J Immunol* 1978;121:942–946.

Wallace LE, Rickinson AB, Rowe M, et al: Epstein-Barr virus-specific cytotoxic T-cell clones restricted through a single HLA antigen. *Nature* 1982;297:413–415.

Wannamaker LW, Rammelkamp CH, Denny FW, et al: Prophylaxis of acute rheumatoid fever by treatment of the preceding streptococcal infection with various amounts of depo-penicillin. *Am J Med* 1951;10:673.

Ward PA, Zvaifler NJ: Complement-derived leukotactic factors in inflammatory synovial fluids of humans. *J Clin Invest* 1971;50:606.

Wilkins JA, Warrington RJ, Sigurdson SL: The demonstration of an interleukin-2-like activity in the synovial fluids of rheumatoid arthritis patients. *J Rheumatol* 1983;10:109.

Willkens RF, Hansen JA, Malmagren JA, et al: HLA antigens in Yakima indians with rheumatoid arthritis. *Arthritis Rheum* 1982;25:1435–1438.

Winchester RJ: Characterization of Ig complexes in patients with rheumatoid arthritis. *Ann NY Acad Sci* 1975;156:73.

Wood DD, Ihrie EJ, Dinarello CA, et al: Isolation of an interleukin-1-like factor from human joint effusions. *Arthritis Rheum* 1983;26:975–983.

Wooley PH, Griffin J, Panayi GS, et al: HLA-DR antigens and toxic reactions to sodium aurothiomalate and D-penicillamine in patients with rheumatoid arthritis. *N Engl J Med* 1980;303:300–303.

Yoneda T, Mundy GR: Monocytes regulate ostoclast activating factor production by releasing prostaglandins. *J Exp Med* 1979; 150:338–350.

Zvaifler NJ: Overview of Etiology and Pathogenesis, in Utsinger Zvaifler NJ, Ehrlich GE (eds): *Rheumatoid Arthritis*. Philadelphia, JB Lippincott, 1985, pp 151–158.

2

RHEUMATOID INVOLVEMENT OF SPECIFIC ANATOMIC SITES

Rheumatoid arthritis has features at the various anatomic regions that deserve emphasis because of their value in differential diagnosis and because of their implications for understanding pathogenesis or therapy. The following chapters emphasize these. Some findings that may be sources of confusion, such as diseases with findings that mimic rheumatoid arthritis, are stressed. Potential complications of progressive rheumatoid arthritis at each site are also selected for emphasis. Note that not all features that are important are articular.

CHAPTER 6

THE HAND AND WRIST

H. RALPH SCHUMACHER, Jr, MD

The hands, along with the feet, are the most commonly affected sites in rheumatoid arthritis. There is prominent but not complete symmetry (Halla et al, 1983). The dominant hand is frequently both more involved and more inflamed (Owsianik, 1980) (Fig. 6.1). Symptoms most often arise directly from the inflamed joints. However pain felt in joints can also be referred from flexor tendon sheaths. Compression of the median nerve by inflamed tissues at the wrists typically produces distal pain and dysesthesia (the carpal tunnel syndrome).

JOINT INVOLVEMENT

Rheumatoid inflammation can involve any joint, but is most readily and commonly detected at the metacarpophalangeal (MCP) and proximal interphalangeal (PIP) joints where a soft swelling can be noted obscuring the normally palpable joint line (Fig. 6.2). Only rarely does rheumatoid inflammation produce a hot red joint. One must detect the more subtle swelling of rheumatoid arthritis to suggest the diagnosis in the common case of indolent onset. Persistent swelling and pain tends to gradually lead to irreversible limited motion although some patients retain motion and function despite widespread destructive disease. The earliest objective evidence of wrist involvement may be limitation of motion; this is often easier to detect than mild wrist swelling. Soft tissue swelling is prominent around the ulnar styloid due both to ulnocarpal synovitis and to inflammation in the sheath of the extensor carpi ulnaris (Fig. 6.3).

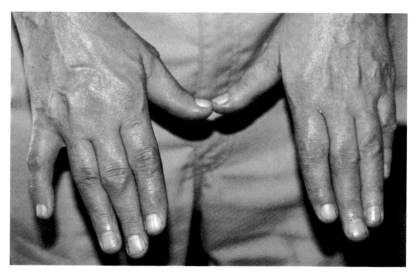

Figure 6.1 The hands of a man with chronic arthritis show more marked swelling of MCP and PIP joints of the dominant right hand.

Destruction of supporting ligaments produces a prominent ballotable ulnar styloid.

Synovitis has been felt to be more persistent at wrist and MCP joints than at PIP joints (Kay, 1971). The MCP joints of the thumb, second, and third fingers are involved most often. Distal interphalangeal (DIP) joints can be affected with tenderness (McCarty and

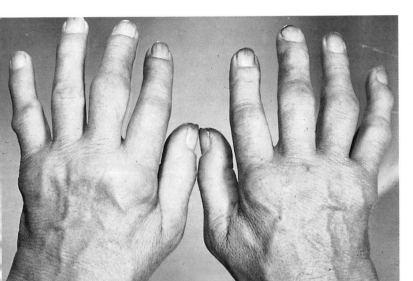

Figure 6.2 Moderately advanced soft tissue swelling at the MCP joints obliterates the normally palpable joint space.

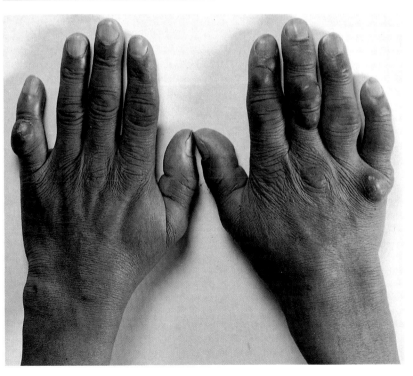

Figure 6.3 Synovial soft tissue swelling is seen at the ulnar styloid of the left hand. There is more diffuse swelling of the radiocarpal joint on the right. Firm rheumatoid nodules are adjacent to and overlying some PIP and MCP joints of both hands.

Gatter, 1966) or, less often, with full-blown synovitis. Jacob et al (1986) found some radiographic evidence of DIP joint erosions in 37% of patients with rheumatoid arthritis compared to 14% of age-matched controls.

Objective measurement of finger joint swelling is an important part of documentation before and during treatment. Jewelers' rings or the arthrocircameter (Fig. 6.4) can measure fairly accurately the circumference of the interphalangeal joints (Heyman, 1974). A measure of total hand swelling can also be made by recording the volume displacement after immersion of the hand in water (Sternberg et al, 1980).

It is important to consider hand function as well as signs of joint disease. Although hand function deterioration can be shown to correlate with the extent of deformity in advanced cases, there is also detectable loss of function even before deformity is apparent (Moutevilis and Schumacher, 1972). Function can be measured by questioning the patient about difficulties he or she has and by observing the performance of important or frequent tasks. The Jebsen hand function test is a standardized functional assessment used by many occupational therapists.

TENOSYNOVITIS

Fifty-five percent of 100 patients with rheumatoid arthritis had flexor tenosynovitis in a study done by Gray and Gottlieb (1977). Second to fourth tendons are most often involved. Difficulty extending fingers after flexion ("triggering") can occur but flexion can also be limited. The carpal tunnel syndrome, due to compression of the median nerve at the volar aspect of the wrist, is more common in patients with flexor tenosynovitis than in those without it (Fig. 6.5). Other tendinitis is also more common in these same patients.

Flexor tenosynovitis can be palpated anywhere along the various tendon sheaths but is most readily detected at the palmar side of the MCP joints as a nodular thickening. Subtle thickening can be felt and pain elicited by palpating this site during finger flexion and extension. Mild tendinitis can be difficult to confirm on physical examination. The most common tendons to rupture in rheumatoid arthritis are the abductors of the thumb and the extensor carpi ulnaris of the fourth to fifth fingers. Rupture of the latter is usually due to a combination of synovitis in the tendon

Figure 6.4 The arthrocircameter can be used for measurement of PIP joint circumference in millimeters.

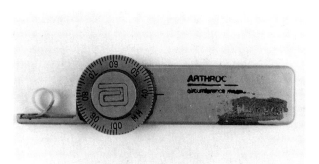

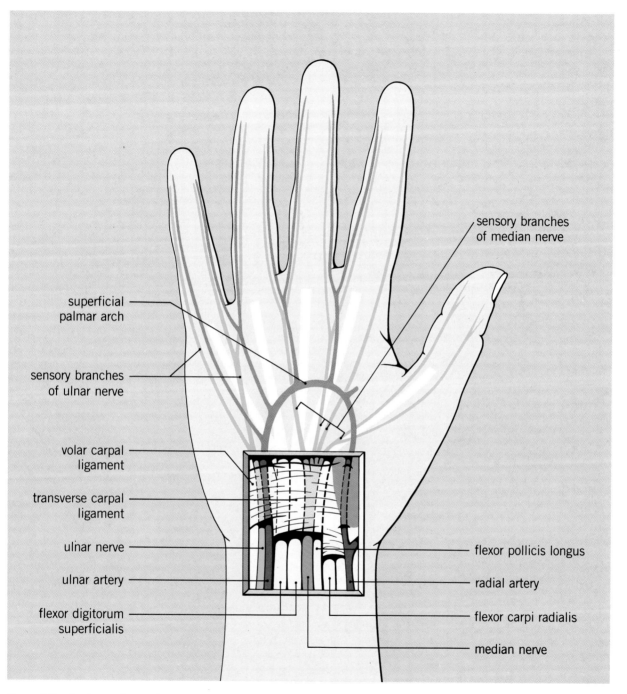

Figure 6.5 Anatomy of carpal tunnel. The highlighted area is the site where the median nerve passes beneath the transverse carpal ligament. Inflammation in the tendon sheaths, such as that found with rheumatoid arthritis, produces swelling of the surrounding tissues, compressing the median nerve and resulting in the condition known as the carpal tunnel syndrome. Surrounding structures are also noted.

sheaths and mechanical irritation from an eroded and subluxed distal ulna (Fig. 6.6).

Tenosynovitis of extensor tendons around the wrist is occasionally massive, leading to quite diffuse swelling. This is usually less painful or limiting than flexor tendon sheath involvement (Fig. 6.7). More diffuse swelling may rarely be due to lymphatic obstruction in rheumatoid arthritis but should also suggest consideration of other diagnoses, as discussed below.

DEFORMITIES

Ulnar drift at the MCP joints is a characteristic finding in rheumatoid arthritis (Fig. 6.8); its cause is not completely established. Both muscle-tendon forces and joint damage are probably involved. Flexor forces normally tend to exert greater force toward ulnar de-

viation at the MCP joints (Smith et al, 1966). Early radial deviation at the wrist may lead to compensatory ulnar deviation distally (Resnick, 1976a). Distention of MCP joints can also be shown to produce ulnar drift (Clark et al, 1978) and to favor flexion positioning.

In advanced cases extensor tendons will be noted to have slipped off the metacarpal heads on the ulnar side. These extensor tendon findings appear to be a result of the synovitis and deformity rather than a cause of deformity.

The most common deformity at the thumb consists of flexion deformity and/or instability at the MCP joint with hyperextension at the interphalangeal (IP) joint (Fig. 6.9). Either extreme deformity or instability of the thumb can be a major factor in loss of function.

The PIP joint positioning may become altered into either a swan neck or boutonnière

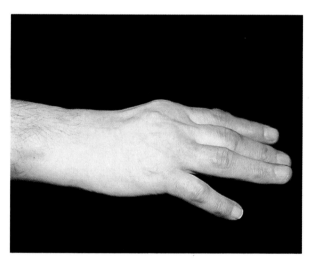

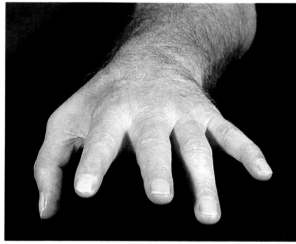

Figure 6.6 Rupture of fifth finger extensor tendons in a patient with rheumatoid arthritis wrist synovitis is shown on the *left*. A ruptured abductor pollicus longus tendon is shown on the *right*.

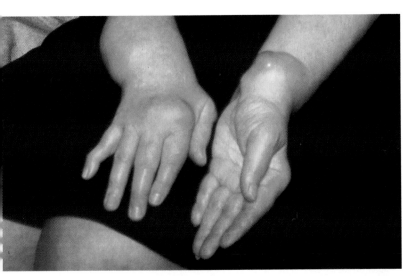

Figure 6.7 Massive synovial cysts are present in tendon sheaths around wrists.

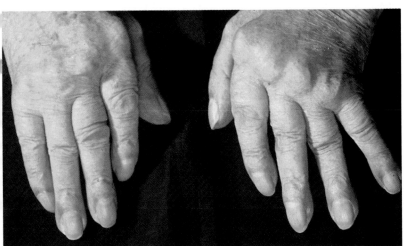

Figure 6.8 Ulnar drift at the MCP joints is seen more dramatically in the left hand. There is also volar subluxation of the phalanges.

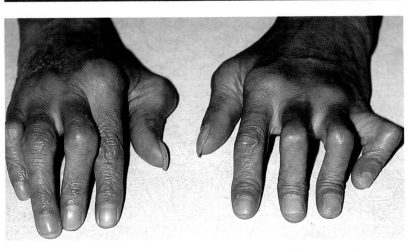

Figure 6.9 Flexion deformity and synovial swelling are demonstrated at the right thumb MCP joint with hyperextension at the IP joint. Note also other PIP joint flexion contractures and right second MCP joint swelling.

deformity (Fig. 6.10). Factors involved in swan neck deformities include increased activity of intrinsic muscles at the PIP joints, excessive pull of the extrinsic extensor tendons, and weakening of the joint structures by synovitis (Dreyfuss and Schnitzer, 1983). Boutonnière deformity consists of a flexed position at the PIP joint and hyperextension at the DIP joint. This deformity is said to resemble the position used to secure a carnation in the lapel; hence the French term, boutonnière, or button hole (Forrester et al, 1978). PIP joint swelling weakens the lateral bands that connect the central and lateral slips of the extensor tendons. The lateral slips slide in a palmar direction, the central slip lengthens, and the extensor forces become flexors. Attempts at extension of the DIP joint

actually flex the PIP joint. Boutonnière deformities are initially reversible but become fixed with time. Occasionally joint erosion and instability result in medial or lateral deviation, producing other, less common deformities (Fig. 6.11).

OTHER FEATURES

Skin and other extra-articular features of the hand are also important in rheumatoid arthritis. Muscle atrophy is prominent in advanced cases (Fig. 6.12). Atrophy, most prominent at the thenar eminence, is a typical late result of carpal tunnel syndrome complicating the rheumatoid arthritis. Palmar erythema may be seen (Fig. 6.13) and is felt

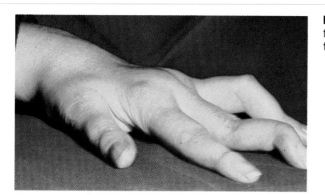

Figure 6.10 This hand has a boutonnière deformity of the fourth finger and a swan neck deformity of the third finger.

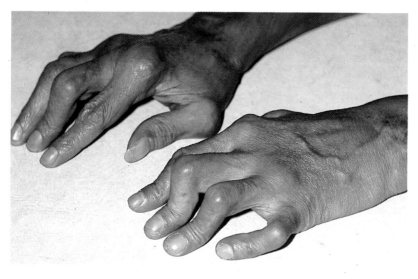

Figure 6.11 These digits show boutonnière deformities. Note radial deviation at the unstable left fifth PIP joint.

o be due to the vasomotor changes in rheumatoid arthritis. Neuropathy involving the hands may include a distal diffuse neuropathy and mononeuritis multiplex related to vasculitis as well as the carpal tunnel syndrome and other compression neuropathies. Small, dark, occasionally tender infarcts can develop in the nailfolds (Fig. 6.14) or elsewhere. These are usually benign but they are due to a low-grade rheumatoid vasculitis. Rheumatoid nodules can occur anywhere on the hands but are often at sites of repetitive irritation such as on the volar aspects of the fingers (Fig. 6.15). These must be distinguished from

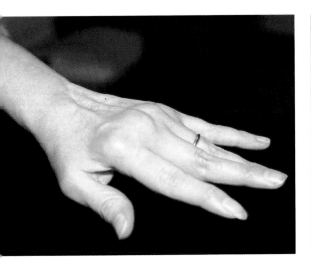

Figure 6.12 Dorsal muscle atrophy is demonstrated in a patient with previous extensor tendon ruptures.

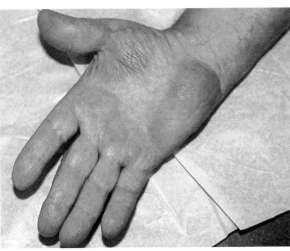

Figure 6.13 Palmar erythema is dramatic in this rheumatoid hand.

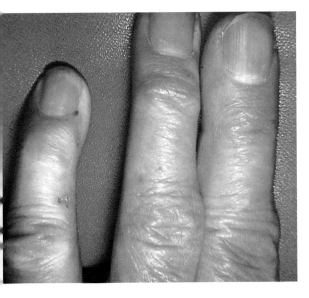

Figure 6.14 This hand reveals a nail fold infact and other small vasculitic lesions.

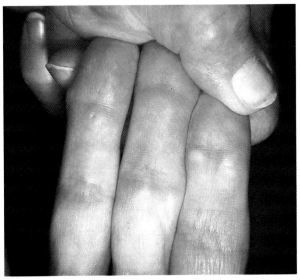

Figure 6.15 Firm rheumatoid nodules have appeared on the volar aspects of these fingers.

less symmetrical synovial protrusions (Fig. 6.16) in rheumatoid arthritis that are softer than the typically firm rheumatoid nodules.

DIFFERENTIAL DIAGNOSIS

As noted above, rheumatoid arthritis is largely a diagnosis of exclusion. Other joint diseases that mimic rheumatoid arthritis have some features that aid in their differentiation from rheumatoid arthritis (Dorwart and Schumacher, 1974) (Fig. 6.17). Psoriatic arthritis often produces less diffuse joint involvement but is especially destructive and more likely than rheumatoid arthritis to produce "arthritis mutilans," with resorption of large amounts of bone and pencil and cup deformities. Distal IP joint destruction also

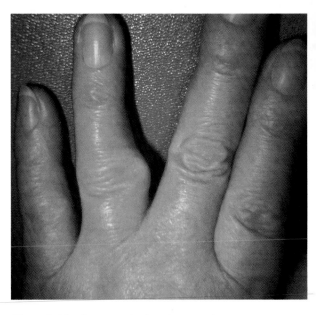

Figure 6.16 Asymmetrical, soft, synovial outpouching is seen at the fourth PIP joint.

DIFFERENTIAL DIAGNOSIS OF HAND PROBLEMS

Diseases are classified by prominent features that might cause confusion with rheumatoid arthritis.

Polyarticular Joint Swelling

Psoriatic arthritis

Reiter's syndrome

Osteoarthritis

Hemochromatosis

Gout

Calcium pyrophosphate deposition disease (pseudogout)

Thiemann's disease

Finger Deformities

Parkinson's disease

Ehlers-Danlos syndrome

Systemic lupus erythematosus

Jaccoud's postrheumatic fever arthropathy

Wilson's disease

Dupuytren's contracture

Camptodactyly

Mucopolysaccharidoses

Other Hand Swelling

Scleroderma

Mixed connective tissue disease

Sickle-cell disease (only in young children)

Drug addiction

Thyroid acropachy

Shoulder-hand syndrome

Hypertrophic pulmonary osteoarthropathy

Acromegaly

Tendinitis and Fasciitis

Malignancies

Diabetes

Amyloidosis

Isoniazid and other drug reactions

Hypothyroidism

Pregnancy

Trauma

Nodules

Calcinosis

Gout

Knuckle pads

Ganglia

Multicentric reticulohistiocytosis

Giant cell tumors

Xanthomas

Hypereosinophilic syndrome

Fibromas

Sarcoidosis

Figure 6.17   Differential diagnosis of hand problems.

suggests psoriatic arthritis (Fig. 6.18). Prominent periostitis resulting in diffuse swelling of the digit beyond the joints favors this diagnosis or Reiter's syndrome.

Swan neck deformities can be seen with Parkinsonism, Ehlers-Danlos syndrome, Jaccoud's postrheumatic fever arthropathy, and systemic lupus erythematosus (SLE) (Labowitz and Schumacher, 1971) (Fig. 6.19). In the latter two conditions erosion is usually absent, with initial laxity and later fixed deformities resulting purely from the soft tissue disease. A rare example of a similar deformity occurred secondary to tendon ruptures at sites of subperiosteal bone resorption in one case of hyperparathyroidism (Fig. 6.20). The choreoathetotic hand posturing in Wilson's disease results in a reversible boutonnière deformity.

Osteoarthritis typically involves the DIP and PIP joints with predominantly a bony enlargement. Inflammation can occur at these joints and, especially when the PIP joints are initially involved, can be confused with rheumatoid arthritis (Fig. 6.21). MCP joint involvement is relatively uncommon in osteoarthritis. When bony enlargement with or without some inflammation is more common at MCP joints than more distally it should suggest the possibility of metabolic disease (as noted below) or rheumatoid arthritis. Some manual laborers also develop potentially confusing osteoarthritic changes at MCP joints.

Gout typically produces a knobby and less symmetrical swelling than does rheumatoid arthritis (Fig. 6.22). White or yellow discoloration suggests that a tophus is bulging from the joint.

Palmar fasciitis and an inflammatory arthritis that mimics the findings of rheumatoid arthritis can be seen associated with ovarian

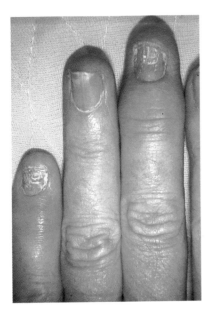

Figure 6.18 Psoriatic arthritis is shown especially involving the third DIP joint. Note also the psoriatic nail disease in the same digit.

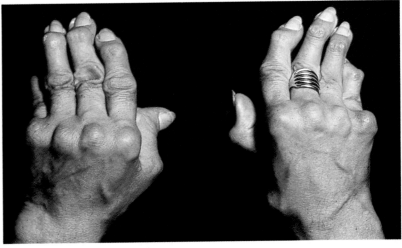

Figure 6.19 Extreme joint deformities as shown here can occur in systemic lupus erythematosus (SLE). Radiographs showed no erosive arthritis.

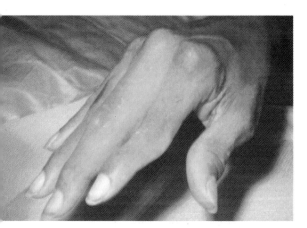

Figure 6.20 This swan neck deformity of the second finger is a rare result of tendon ruptures in hyperparathyroidism.

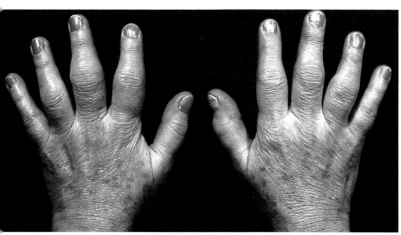

Figure 6.21 Osteoarthritis in this case is seen most prominently at the PIP joints. Palpation revealed swelling to be predominantly bony.

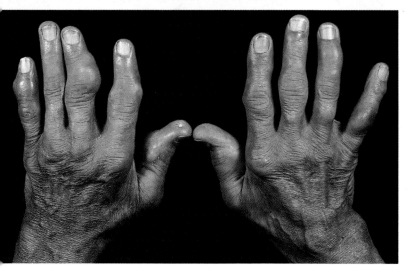

Figure 6.22 Gouty tophi are usually asymmetric and firm. Note the pale color where the tophi bulge under the skin.

neoplasms and other malignancies (Pfinsgraff et al, 1984). Metastatic tumors can also be seen in the hands (Fig. 6.23). They are usually at a single site. Initial radiographs may be inconclusive.

Dupuytren's contractures cause thickening in the superficially palpable palmar fascia. Fingers are drawn into flexion without actual joint involvement. Camptodactyly is often a developmental problem giving flexion deformities of fifth fingers that should be distinguished from residuals of synovitis. In a few cases this has been associated with an unusual syndrome of knee and other joint synovial proliferation in children (Athreya and Schumacher, 1978). Fibrosis with contractures and/or flexor tendon involvement occurs in diabetes, amyloidosis, after isoniazid therapy, and late in shoulder-hand syn-drome. Hand tenosynovitis is also seen with occupational trauma, hypothyroidism, and pregnancy.

MCP joint involvement (second to fourth especially) can be prominent in hemochromatosis (Fig. 6.24) (Schumacher, 1964), calcium pyrophosphate deposition disease and some patients with unexplained MCP disease (Williams et al, 1985). All these conditions have a firmer, more indurated swelling than is typical of rheumatoid arthritis and show changes like osteoarthritis or chondrocalcinosis on radiograph.

Ganglia are localized, usually nontender, noninflammatory swellings that can appear on the dorsum of the wrist. Occasionally an indistinguishable mass will contain tissue showing chronic synovitis and will actually be an early manifestation of rheumatoid ar-

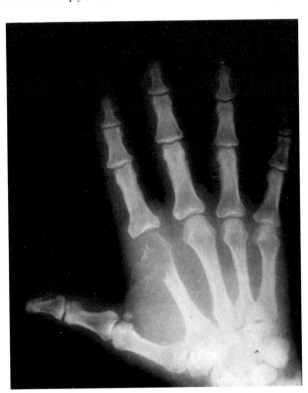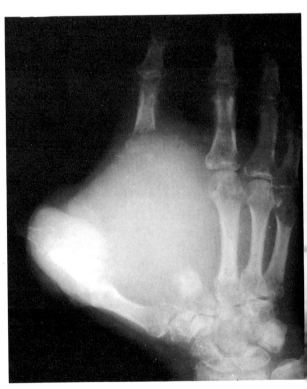

Figure 6.23 This early lytic lesion at the right second MCP joint, shown on the *left*, is due to metastatic adenocarcinoma. This patient had pain but no swelling at this site. On the *right*, massive destruction from the tumor is present several months later.

thritis or other inflammatory diseases. Most dorsal wrist swelling in rheumatoid arthritis is more diffuse.

PIP joint swelling in young people can be due to Thiemann's disease; it is usually a hard swelling. This epiphysitis is identified by beaking at the epiphyses visible on radiographs.

A diffusely puffy hand can occur in drug addiction, early scleroderma or mixed connective tissue disease, sickle cell disease in very young children (Fig. 6.25), shoulder-hand syndrome, or active acromegaly.

Finger nodules can be due to calcinosis in the collagen diseases, hypereosinophilic syndrome, fibromas (Chaquat et al, 1980), xantho-

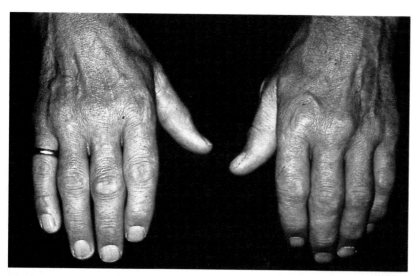

Figure 6.24 Firm swelling at the MCP and PIP joints is seen in a patient with the arthropathy of hemochromatosis.

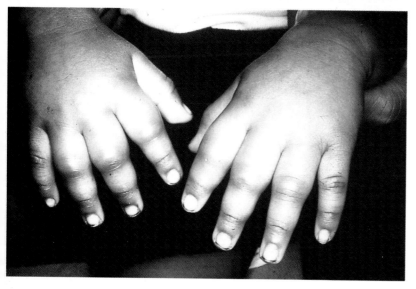

Figure 6.25 Diffuse painful hand swelling in a young child with sickle cell disease is typical of the hand-foot syndrome.

mas, tophi, multicentric reticulohistiocytosis (Fig. 6.26), sarcoidosis, or metastatic tumors. Giant cell tumors can complicate rheumatoid arthritis and can be confused with rheumatoid or other nodules (Reginato et al, 1974).

Fingers are stiff in chronic scleroderma largely due to the tight skin although joint fibrosis also occurs. In mucopolysaccharidoses claw hands are also due to connective tissue changes (Fig. 6.27). Knuckle pads are purely extra-articular structures over the dorsum of joints that could be confused with rheumatoid arthritis on a cursory examination (Fig. 6.28). More diffuse swelling around one or several digits occurs in thyroid acropachy. This com-

plication of Grave's disease can occur before or after treatment of the hyperthyroidism. Hypertrophic pulmonary osteoarthropathy may in severe cases result in swelling along the shafts of fingers in addition to the typical clubbing (Fig. 6.29).

With any unusual joint or hand problem always look for other systemic clues to support the diagnosis of rheumatoid arthritis or clues to the other diseases mentioned above. Remember that rheumatoid arthritis is a diagnosis of exclusion. Some of the diseases potentially confused with rheumatoid arthritis have specific or more effective therapy and should not be missed.

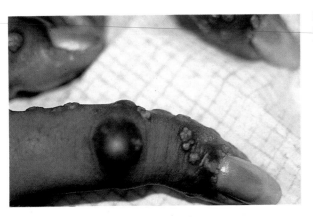

Figure 6.26 This nodule over the third MCP joint was shown on histologic examination to be due to multicentric reticulohistiocytosis.

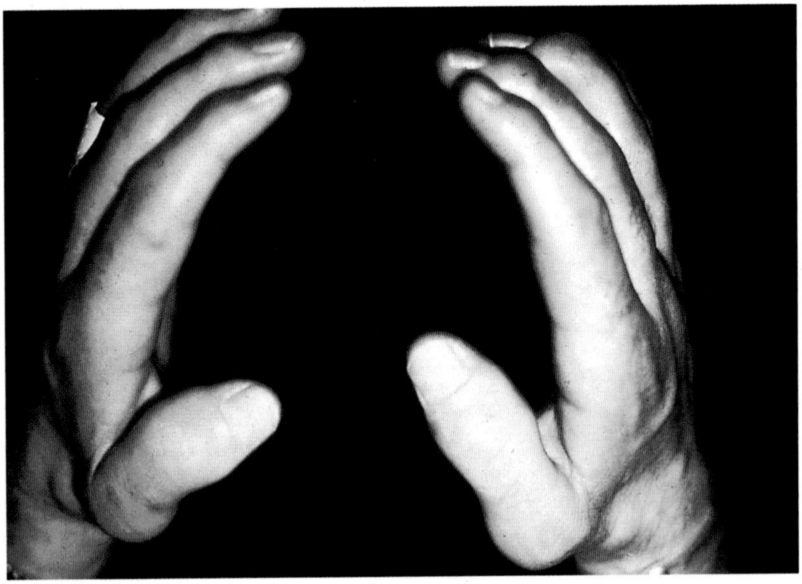

Figure 6.27 These stiff fingers with periarticular swellings are characteristic of Hurler's syndrome.

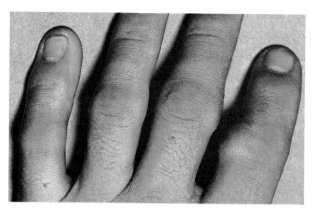

Figure 6.28 Fibrous knuckle pads do not involve the joints but can be confused with joint disease.

Figure 6.29 This radiograph from a patient with congenital hypertrophic osteoarthropathy shows periosteal thickening at the second to fourth proximal phalanges that can produce diffuse digital swelling. There is also periosteal reaction at the distal ulna and radius, and clubbing of the fingertips.

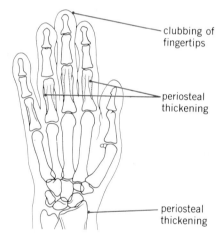

clubbing of fingertips

periosteal thickening

periosteal thickening

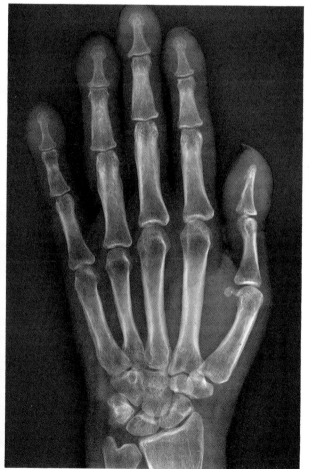

RADIOGRAPHIC FINDINGS

Demineralization is an early bony change in rheumatoid arthritis with periarticular accentuation around inflamed PIP and MCP joints and at the wrists. Such demineralization is not specific, but its distribution is consistent with the pattern of soft tissue swelling and synovial disease. Not all rheumatoid patients develop erosions but they are characteristic in chronic cases. Early erosions occur at the radiovolar aspect of the metacarpal heads at their junction with the shafts and/or at either side at the joint margin at the proximal ends of the proximal phalanges (Bywaters, 1960). These marginal erosions occur where the synovium contacts bone at the margin of the cartilage. Second and third MCP joints, wrist, and third and fourth PIP joints were the earliest involved in one series (Fletcher and Rowley, 1952). Erosions usually are detected only after the disease has persisted for 3 to 6 months.

Small defects in the bony cortex can also be associated with a very localized periosteal reaction. As defects become deeper a punched out appearance is seen (Fig. 6.30). Other early erosions in the hands occur at the first MCP joint beneath the sesamoid, at the ulnar styloid (Fig. 6.31) and in the intercarpal joints. Erosion of the radiocarpal joint can also be seen but is less common. Later a large scalloped erosion can occur on the radial side of the radioulnar joint (Fig. 6.32).

Calcium pyrophosphate deposition disease is a potential cause of confusion as it produces wrist and MCP joint involvement. Typically, however, erosions are not seen; joint space narrowing, bony sclerosis, and subchondral cysts predominate suggesting this diagnosis even without visible chondrocalcinosis. Gouty erosions are often sharper than those in rheumatoid arthritis and have an overhanging edge; less joint space narrowing is seen and the disease is less symmetrical.

Pseudocysts can be noted in subchondral bone in rheumatoid arthritis from invasion of granulation tissue from the marrow (Fig. 6.33). Narrowing of the cartilage space is also common in rheumatoid arthritis. Early loss of cartilage occurs independent of erosions

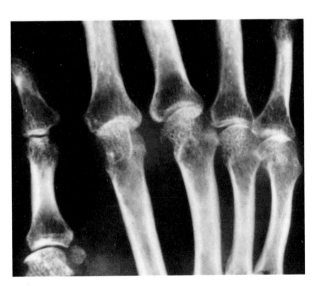 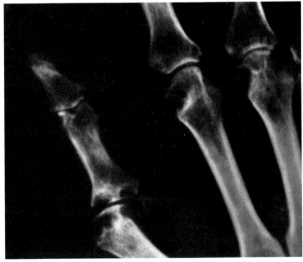

Figure 6.30 Erosions typical of rheumatoid arthritis are shown on the *left*, at the radial sides of the metacarpals at the MCP joints. More advanced MCP joint erosions (*right*) undermine the subchondral bone.

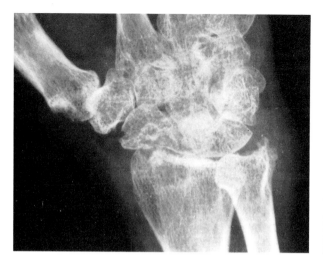

Figure 6.31 This radiograph shows jagged erosion of the ulnar styloid. There are also carpal cystic changes and narrowing between the carpal bones.

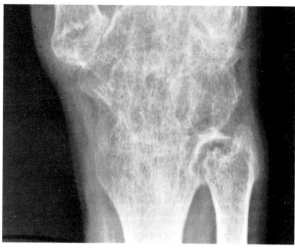

Figure 6.32 Rheumatoid arthritis resulted in this scalloped erosion of the radioulnar joint. Note also the bony carpal fusion.

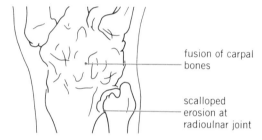

fusion of carpal bones

scalloped erosion at radioulnar joint

Figure 6.33 Bone pseudocysts are seen in the distal end of the fifth metacarpal.

(Resnick, 1976b). Note that flexion contractures can make joint space narrowing difficult to assess on AP radiographs. As erosions, cyst formation, and cartilage loss increase, the entire joint structure can be destroyed, sometimes leading to striking fragmentation of bone (Resnick and Gmelich, 1975). Typical subluxations such as described above result relatively early from the soft tissue disease. Bizarre subluxations can occur from the joint destruction. Pencil and cup deformities can be seen (Fig. 6.34). The destructive process can also eventually result in fibrous or bony joint fusion in 5% to 10% of cases.

It is of interest to note that hand radiographic features in many patients with seronegative rheumatoid arthritis do differ from classical seropositive rheumatoid arthritis. In one study of patients with seronegative rheumatoid arthritis there was more juxta-articular osteosclerosis, less erosion, more new bone formation, more fusion, less symmetry and more prominent carpal involvement (Burns and Calin, 1983). Osteoarthritic radiographs also show more periarticular sclerosis and osteophyte formation along with early joint space narrowing. Some erosions can occur but they are more often at the joint space than at the margins. In late rheumatoid arthritis secondary osteoarthritic changes can occur and the two diseases can coexist.

IMPLICATIONS FOR THERAPY

Hand joints are among the easiest to examine to assess both need for and effect of therapy. Persistent synovial swelling, even with acceptable levels of pain, in general means that more effective drug and other therapy should be considered. Education in joint conservation techniques can help the patients perform their daily activities in a manner that will reduce the stress and thus the pain and inflammation of involved joints. Avoiding excessive force in flexion and ulnar deviation may help slow the rate of deformity. Simple proximal interphalangeal (PIP) splints can help align fingers with correctible deformities (Fig. 6.35). Compliance with complicated splinting techniques is poor and there is no proof such finger splints can prevent digital deformities. Range of motion exercises can minimize stiffness and muscle atrophy. Splinting can prevent fusion from developing in nonfunctional positions. Wrist splints in slight extension allow better grips, decrease pain during activity, control carpal tunnel symptoms and, if fusion is to develop, assure fusion in a position of function (Fig. 6.36). Flexor tenosynovitis, which is often underappreciated, can be a major factor in PIP joint stiffness. Aggressive local treatment of the tenosynovitis (for example, with corticosteroid injections or physical medicine) may decrease stiffness (Millis et al, 1976). Since hand function can deteriorate quickly and is so critical for many activities, team care of the hands should begin early. Many assistive devices are available for specific functional problems.

Hand surgery has been most valuable when used to stabilize the thumb to allow pinching. Metacarpal phalangeal subluxations can be realigned surgically. This may also improve the grip but motion usually remains limited. Repair of ruptured tendons and wrist fusions in a position of function are also often effective.

It is intriguing that the dominant hand is usually, but not always, more severely involved. There must be a delicate balance between rest (joint protection) and exercise to minimize inflammation and maintain hand function. This may differ from patient to patient. More objective studies on the effects of joint conservation, splinting and exercise programs are needed.

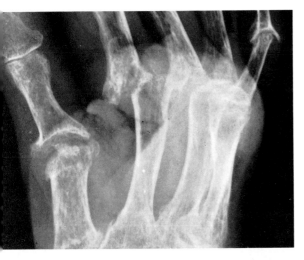

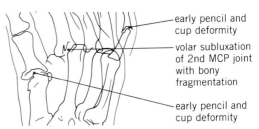

Figure 6.34 Pencil and cup deformities are forming at the first MCP joint and fifth PIP joint.

- early pencil and cup deformity
- volar subluxation of 2nd MCP joint with bony fragmentation
- early pencil and cup deformity

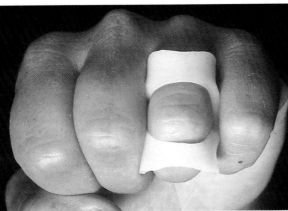

Figure 6.35 This proximal interphalangeal joint splint is used to prevent hyperextension in swan neck deformity.

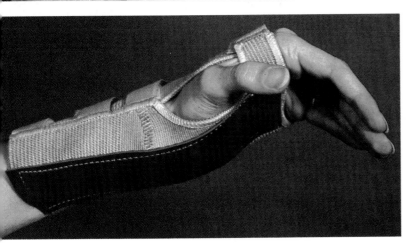

Figure 6.36 This lightweight wrist splint holds the wrist slightly extended in the position of function.

REFERENCES

Athreya B, Schumacher HR: Pathologic features of a recently recognized form of familial arthropathy. *Arthritis Rheum* 1978;21:429–437.

Burns TM, Calin A: The hand radiograph as a diagnostic discriminant between seropositive and seronegative rheumatoid arthritis. A controlled study. *Ann Rheum Dis* 1983;42:605–612.

Bywaters EGL: The early radiological signs of rheumatoid arthritis. *Bull Rheum Dis* 1960;11:231–234.

Chaquat Y, Aron-Bruentiere R, Faures B, et al: A new entity. The fibroblastic rheumatism. *Rev Rheum Mal Osteoartic* 1980;47:345–351.

Clark IP, James DF, Colwill JC: Intraarticular pressure as a factor in initiating ulnar drift. *J Bone Joint Surg* (Am) 1978;60A:325–327.

Dorwart BB, Schumacher HR: Hand deformities resembling rheumatoid arthritis. *Semin Arthritis Rheum* 1974;4:53–71.

Dreyfuss JN, Schnitzer TJ: Pathogenesis and differential diagnosis of the swan neck deformity. *Semin Arthritis Rheum* 1983;13:200–211.

Fletcher DE, Rowley KA: The radiographic features of rheumatoid arthritis. *Br J Radiol* 1952;25:282–295.

Forrester DM, Brown JC, Nesson JW: *The Radiology of Joint Disease*. Philadelphia, W B Saunders Co, 1978, pp 42–43.

Gray RG, Gottlieb NL: Hand flexor tenosynovitis in rheumatoid arthritis. *Arthritis Rheum* 1977; 20:1003–1007.

Halla JT, Fallahi S, Hardin JG: Small joint involvement: a systematic roentgenographic study in rheumatoid arthritis. *Ann Rheum Dis* 1986;45:327–330.

Heyman ER: Variability of proximal interphalangeal joint size measurements in normal adults. *Arthritis Rheum* 1974;17:79–84.

Jacob J, Sartoris D, Kursunoglu S, et al: Distal interphalangeal joint involvement in rheumatoid arthritis. *Arthritis Rheum* 1986;29:10–15.

Kay AGL: Natural history of synovial hypertrophy in the rheumatoid hand. *Ann Rheum Dis* 1971;30:98–102.

Labowitz R, Schumacher HR: The articular manifestations of systemic lupus erythematosus. *Ann Intern Med* 1971; 74:911–921.

McCarty DJ, Gatter RA: A study of distal interphalangeal joint tenderness in rheumatoid arthritis. *Arthritis Rheum* 1966;9:325–336.

Millis MB, Millender LH, Nalebuff EA: Stiffness of the proximal interphalangeal joints in rheumatoid arthritis. *J Bone Joint Surg* (Am) 1976;58A:801–80. (Abst).

Moutevilis K, Schumacher HR: Hand function and rheumatoid arthritis. *Arthritis Rheum* 1972;25:519 (Abst).

Owsianik WDJ, Kundi A, Whitehead JN, et al: Radiological articular involvement in the dominant hand in rheumatoid arthritis. *Ann Rheum Dis* 1980;39:508–510.

Pfinsgraff J, Buckingham RB, Keister SR, et al: Palmar fasciitis and arthritis associated with malignant neoplasms. *Clin Res* 1984;32:722A.

Reginato AJ, Schumacher HR, Martinez VA, Torres J: Giant cell tumor associated with rheumatoid arthritis. *Ann Rheum Dis* 1974;33:333–341.

Resnick D: Interrelationship between radiocarpal and metacarpophalangeal joint deformities in rheumatoid arthritis. *J Canad Assoc Radiol* 1976;27:29–36.

Resnick D: Rheumatoid arthritis of the wrist: The compartmental approach. *Med Radiogr Photogr* 1976;52:50–88.

Resnick, D, Gmelich JT: Bone fragmentation in the rheumatoid wrist: Radiographic and pathologic considerations. *Radiology* 1975;114:315–321.

Schumacher HR: Hemochromatosis and arthritis. *Arthritis Rheum* 1964;7:41–50.

Smith LM, Juvinall RC, Bender LF, et al: Flexor forces and rheumatoid metacarpophalangeal deformity. *JAMA* 1966;198:150–154.

Sternberg VI, Tveter K, Maxwell J: Accurate measurements of the extent of hand swelling in patients with rheumatoid arthritis. *Arthritis Rheum* 1980;12:1411–1412.

Williams MV, Hoyt TS, Cope R, et al: Unusual metacarpophalangeal arthropathy. *Arthritis Rheum* 1985;28(Suppl):593.

CHAPTER 7

THE ELBOW

SUZANNE ALGEO, MD, GINGER CONSTANTINE, MD AND
H. RALPH SCHUMACHER JR, MD

The elbow is comprised of the humeroulnar, humeroradial, and proximal radioulnar joints (Fig. 7.1). The humeroulnar and humeroradial joints are critical in elbow flexion and extension, while the humeroradial and radioulnar joints control forearm pronation and supination. These articulations inhibit significant lateral mobility (Vollertsen and Hunder, 1985).

While elbow synovitis and pain affect the majority of patients with rheumatoid arthritis at some time, only 15% to 20% of patients develop severe, potentially disabling involvement. The most severely affected elbows are seen in the 10% of the rheumatoid population who have advanced disease involving the shoulders and hands. The elbow, unlike the hand, does not exhibit increased incidence or severity of disease in the dominant limb (Amis et al, 1982).

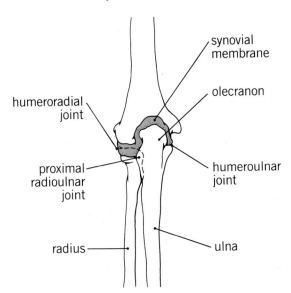
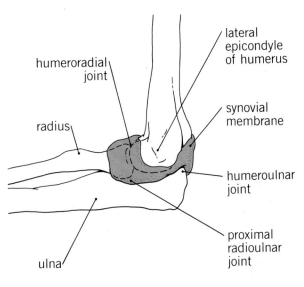

Figure 7.1 The posterior aspect of the elbow joint shows the radius and the ulna in extension. The distribution of synovial membrane is marked in dark blue (*left*). Lateral view of the elbow is also shown (*right*).

JOINT INVOLVEMENT

Flexion contractures due to inflamed synovium or effusions are commonly found in rheumatoid arthritis (Fig. 7.2). The mean flexion deformity is approximately 20°, with the majority of patients retaining 120° of flexion (Amis et al, 1982). Most daily activities can be accomplished with a flexion arc of only 100° (Morrey et al, 1981) compared with the normal range of elbow motion of 140°. Elbow limitation is not an early complaint for most patients. In fact, careful screening for an elbow contracture and effusion can provide a clue to polyarticular disease that the patient has not recognized. Effusions are generally detected by the presence of a fluctuant, ovoid swelling from the distended capsule noted on the posterolateral aspect of the elbow and limited by the lateral joint ligament (Fig. 7.3) (Palmer, 1969). Synovial thickening may also be detected as a fullness palpated in this lateral paraolecranon groove (Fig. 7.4).

In addition to flexion and extension deformities, there can be limitation of motion between the capitellum of the humerus and the radial head that inhibits pronation and supination (Shaffer et al, 1985). The normal humeroradial joint permits forearm rotation to about 70° of pronation and 85° of supination (Morrey et al, 1981). With advancing disease and limitation of motion, the shoulder compensates for loss of elbow pronation by abduction. Loss of supination is less easily compensated. While 40° of pronation suffices

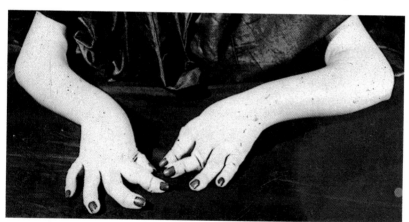

Figure 7.2 Severe flexion deformities at the elbows result from chronically inflamed synovium. (Courtesy of Joseph Hollander, MD).

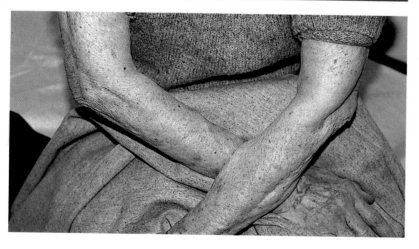

Figure 7.3 Synovial effusion or hypertrophy can easily be palpated in the paraolecranon grooves. Here only the right elbow has an effusion.

for most activities of daily living, 60° of supination are required. The majority of patients with rheumatoid arthritis fortunately retain a large degree of forearm rotation.

Elbow instability is an uncommon late complication of rheumatoid arthritis. Collateral stability is maintained in 80% of patients. When ligamentous laxity occurs, lateral instability causes more difficulty than medial instability with activities of daily living (Amis et al, 1982) (Fig 7.5).

Synovial rupture at the elbow is a rare occurrence in rheumatoid arthritis. Synovial dissection or rupture should be suspected

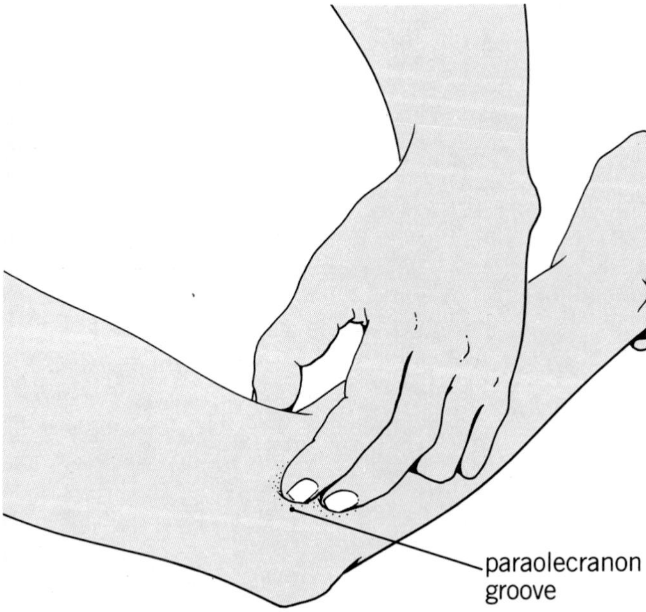

Figure 7.4 The lateral paraolecranon groove is palpated as shown.

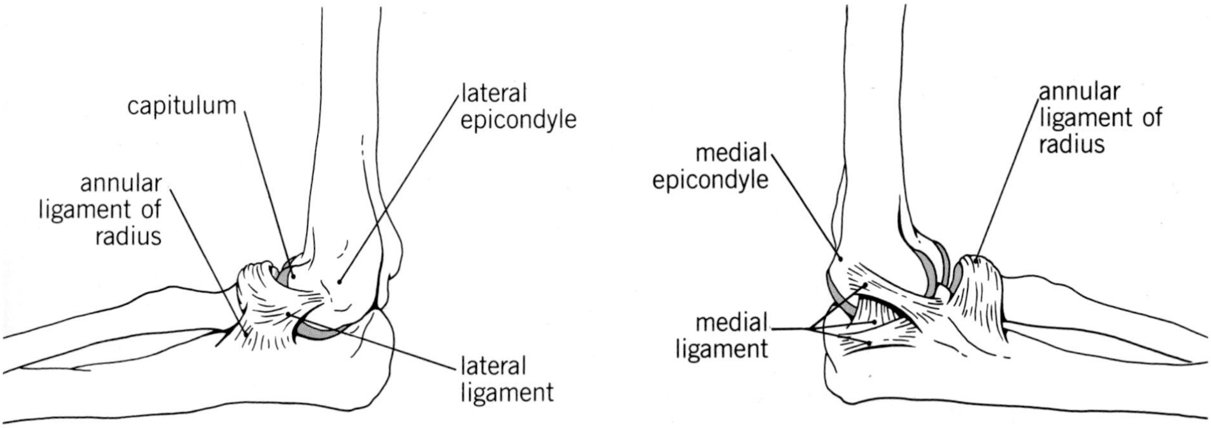

paraolecranon groove

capitulum

annular ligament of radius

lateral epicondyle

lateral ligament

medial epicondyle

medial ligament

annular ligament of radius

Figure 7.5 The elbow capsule is supported by the lateral (radial) and medial (ulnar) collateral ligaments. Lateral ligament weakness can lead to instability and increased disability.

when forearm swelling extends anteriorly from the elbow (Fig. 7.6). This can be accompanied by pitting edema and erythema. It is easily confirmed by arthrography (Pirani and Lange-Mechlen, 1982).

Another unusual complication in rheumatoid arthritis is fracture of the olecranon process (Fig. 7.7). The contracting triceps may provide sufficient force to shear the olecranon process against the distal end of the humerus. If the olecranon process is weakened by erosions or cyst formation, a spontaneous fracture may result (Rappoport et al, 1976).

PERIARTICULAR INVOLVEMENT

The olecranon bursa is commonly involved in rheumatoid arthritis with a fluctuant swelling secondary to effusion (Fig. 7.8). The distended bursa is usually of minimal concern except that patients may complain of pain on local pressure, or express anxiety about its appearance or significance. Because it can become secondarily infected, it is im-

portant to be aware of any acute change in the swelling (Fig. 7.9). Dramatic red bursal swelling can occasionally occur in rheumatoid arthritis (Fig. 7.10), and this sign should always raise the concern of infection. Rarely, a distended olecranon bursa may dissect down the dorsum of the forearm leading to signficant edematous swelling (Palmer, 1969). On occasion, the bursa may communicate with the elbow joint (Resnick, 1981). Antecubital cystic swelling can compress the interosseus nerve and can cause forearm edema (Gerber and Dixon, 1974) possibly by compressing veins in the fossa. Goode (1968) detected anterior synovial cysts in 6 of 140 patients with rheumatoid arthritis. Cysts were detected in all stages of disease in one study (Pirani and Lange-Mechlen, 1982). A ball valve communication may exist between the anterior synovial cyst and the elbow. Rice bodies and synovial villous extensions allow fluid to escape into the cyst, while preventing it from returning into the joint. On rare occasions the cysts may rupture (Ehrlich and Guttman, 1973).

Subcutaneous nodules are most commonly detected over the extensor surface of the

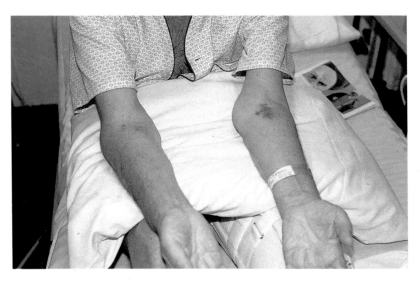

Figure 7.6 Antecubital forearm swelling appears in severe destructive elbow synovitis.

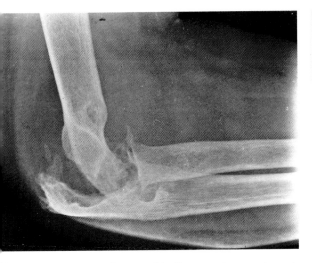

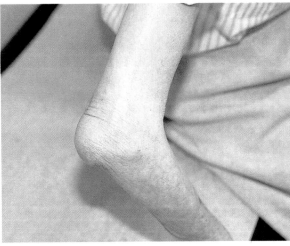

Figure 7.7   A severe rheumatoid elbow erosion can be seen with a small fracture fragment above the olecranon process.

Figure 7.8   A distended olecranon bursa is a common abnormality in rheumatoid arthritis.

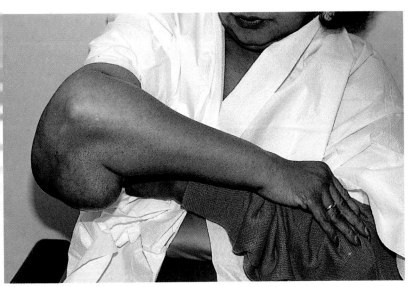

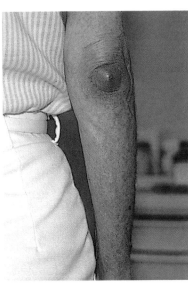

Figure 7.9   This recurrent, massively swollen olecranon bursa became secondarily infected with *Staphylococcus aureus* in this patient with rheumatoid arthritis.

Figure 7.10   The dramatic red swelling of the olecranon bursa seen here was due to acute rheumatoid inflammation. Such tense swelling and erythema required joint aspiration to exclude infection or superimposed crystal deposition disease.

proximal ulna (Fig. 7.11). The firm nodules may be freely movable or fixed to the periosteum. Nodules can also be palpated within enlarged olecranon bursae (Fig. 7.12). Nodules must be differentiated from epitrochlear lymph nodes which can be enlarged in rheumatoid arthritis or in any elbow or hand inflammatory process. The subcutaneous tissues and skin overlying the elbow may be involved with cutaneous vasculitis (Fig. 7.13).

NERVE ENTRAPMENT

Symptoms of ulnar nerve entrapment may develop in the setting of elbow synovitis or antecubital cysts, and can be confirmed by EMG (Ehrlich, 1972). The ulnar nerve may be compressed as it descends beneath the fascial tunnel roof connecting the two heads of the flexor carpi ulnaris muscles. The two heads are attached at the medial epicondyle and the

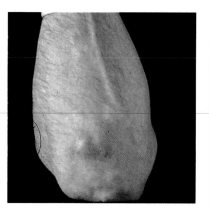

Figure 7.11 Subcutaneous nodules such as these are commonly detected over the extensor surface of the proximal ulna.

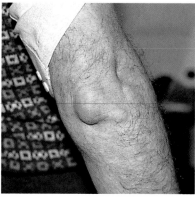

Figure 7.12 Distended olecranon bursal effusion can be irregular because of nodules in the bursal wall.

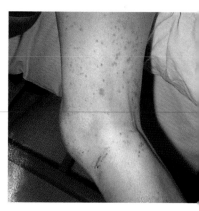

Figure 7.13 Cutaneous vasculitis secondary to rheumatoid arthritis is shown extending over the elbow and arm.

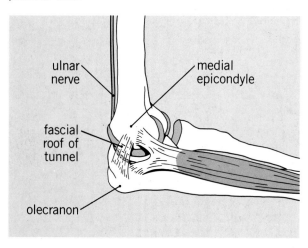

Figure 7.14 In the cubital tunnel syndrome, the ulnar nerve may be compressed as it passes beneath the aponeurosis connecting the two heads of the flexor carpi ulnaris muscle, which attach at the medial epicondyle and olecranon.

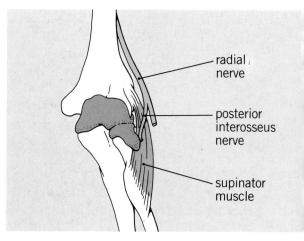

Figure 7.15 The posterior interosseous nerve may be compressed by inflamed synovium as it penetrates the supinator muscle.

medial aspect of the olecranon. This compression of the ulnar nerve beneath the aponeurosis is termed the cubital tunnel syndrome (Balagtas-Balmaseda et al, 1983) (Fig. 7.14). This produces numbness of the fourth and fifth fingers, and the ulnar aspect of the palm, and may produce a claw hand deformity with hyperextension at the MCP joints and flexion at the interphalangeal joints.

The posterior interosseous nerve, a branch of the radial nerve, may rarely be compressed in rheumatoid arthritis. The nerve is entrapped by inflamed synovium as it penetrates the supinator muscle (Chang et al, 1972) (Fig. 7.15). Fullness and tenderness in the antecubital fossa are detected on examination with loss of extensor tendon function to the fingers and the thumb. The posterior interosseous nerve syndrome must be distinguished from acute tendon rupture in the hand (Millender and Nalebuff, 1973). Ulnar or posterior interosseous nerve entrapment at the elbow must be differentiated from cervical radiculopathy and metabolic neuropathies (Upton and McComas, 1973).

DIFFERENTIAL DIAGNOSIS

Most diseases that involve other joints can also involve the elbow, and few of these have any unique features. Single joint involvement suggests the possibility of metastatic tumor or various types of infectious arthritis. Tuberculous arthritis and fungal arthritis have an indolent onset that can be confused with rheumatoid disease, and are distinguishable by laboratory findings (Fig. 7.16).

Crystal-induced arthritis is common at the elbow. Gout often involves the olecranon bursa as well as the elbow joint (Fig. 7.17). Tophaceous material in the bursa can easily be confused with a rheumatoid nodule by palpation. Yellow or white deposits can occasionally be seen under the skin and suggest crystal deposition rather than rheumatoid disease (Fig. 7.18). Diagnosis is only established by aspiration and search for crystals with compensated polarized light.

Calcium pyrophosphate deposition disease (CPPD) can be suggested on radiograph by the

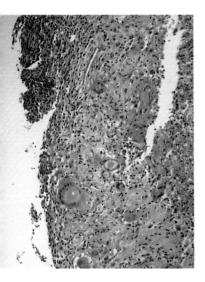

Figure 7.16 Elbow synovium reveals multiple granulomas of tuberculosis (H&E).

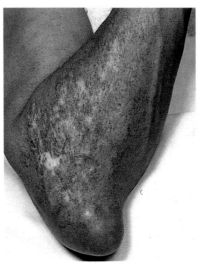

Figure 7.17 Unusually large chronic olecranon swellings may develop in gouty arthritis.

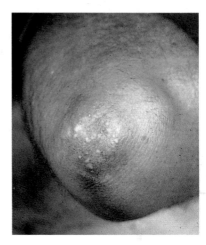

Figure 7.18 Yellowish gouty tophi are visible in the olecranon bursa.

linear calcification of articular cartilage (chondrocalcinosis) typical of this disease (Fig. 7.19). Any of the crystal-associated diseases can produce extreme joint destruction. Apatite crystal deposition is most notorious for producing severe destruction in some cases. In this disease, calcifications are typically noted in soft tissues rather than in articular cartilage. Calcification is not always visible on radiographs. CPPD or apatite crystals (Fig. 7.20) can be dispersed throughout the joint fluid in destroyed joints so that definitive diagnosis requires synovial fluid ex-amination. Even if showing calcification the radiograph is not definitive since tophi and granulomas can also calcify. Apatite crystal clumps are not birefringent but produce shiny chunks in the synovial fluid that should suggest this diagnosis.

Systemic lupus erythematosus and other collagen diseases most often produce mild transient arthritis but are occasionally complicated by apatite deposition or gout with acute apatite or urate crystal arthritis, even in young people (Fig. 7.21).

The various seronegative spondyloarthrop-

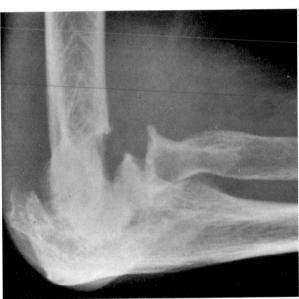

Figure 7.20 Hydroxyapatite deposition disease may lead to severe destructive arthritis.

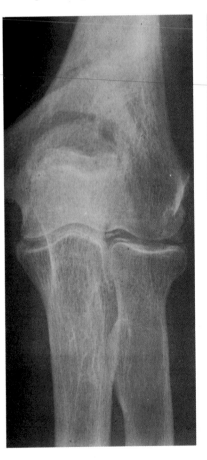

Figure 7.19 Anteroposterior view of the elbow reveals linear calcium pyrophosphate deposition in the articular cartilage between the distal humerus and proximal radius and ulna.

athies can begin with single joint involvement at the elbow or with oligoarthritis including the elbow. A prominent periosteal reaction seen on radiographs can favor this diagnosis. A more diffuse periosteal reaction of the long bones adjacent to the elbow can be seen in hypertrophic pulmonary osteoarthropathy. Osteoarthritis of the elbow is fairly uncommon and is most frequently the result of occupational trauma such as the use of compressed air tools. Tenderness only at the lateral or medial epicondyle without elbow joint swelling is usually due to a mechanically induced epicondylitis rather than to rheumatoid arthritis.

RADIOGRAPHIC FINDINGS

Of radiographic changes found secondary to capsular dilatation, olecranon bursal swelling (Fig. 7.22), as well as rheumatoid nodules

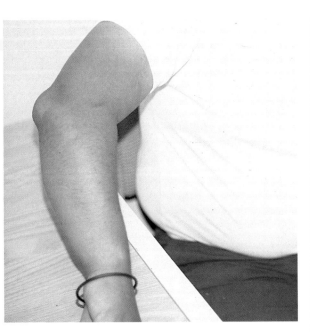

Figure 7.21   Acute gouty bursitis developed around an olecranontophus in a young man with systemic lupus erythematosus on chronic prednisone therapy.

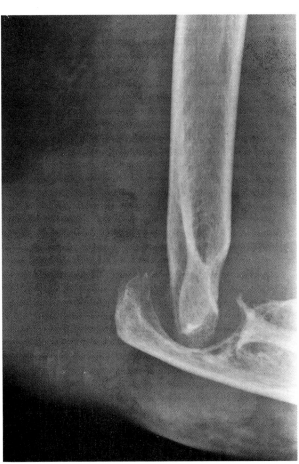

Figure 7.22   A large olecranon bursal swelling is seen in a patient with recurrent bursal effusions and destructive rheumatoid arthritis.

(Fig. 7.23) are the most frequent soft tissue abnormalities. Effusions or synovial hypertrophy are identified by noting fat pad displacement around the radial, coronoid, and olecranon fossae (Weissman and Sosman, 1975) (Fig. 7.24). An anteroposterior view of the rheumatoid elbow may show findings of an effusion, synovitis, joint space narrowing (Fig. 7.25), and joint deformity (Fig. 7.26). Lateral views of the elbow are most useful in revealing the extent of osteophyte formation (Edwards et al, 1983) (Fig. 7.27). As the dis-

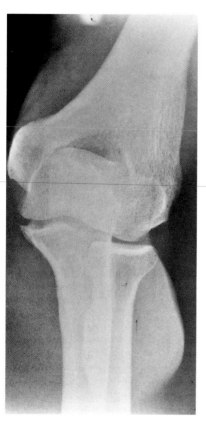

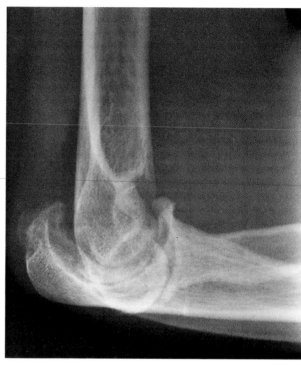

Figure 7.24 In this radiograph, fat pad displacement is evident at the distal humerus.

Figure 7.23 Soft tissue abnormalities may be detected on radiograph as depicted here with a large subcutaneous rheumatoid nodule evident over the proximal radius and significant swelling noted over the olecranon bursa.

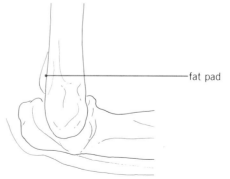

fat pad

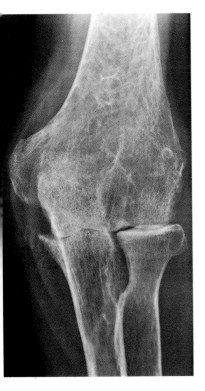

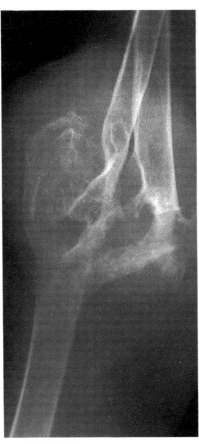

Figure 7.26 This anteroposterior view of the elbow reveals marked erosive disease with complete destruction of the elbow joint. Significant adjacent soft tissue swelling is also visible.

Figure 7.25 Uniform joint space narrowing is evident on this anteroposterior view.

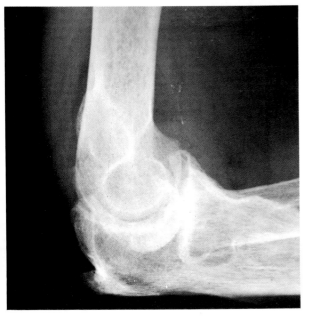

Figure 7.27 A large posterior spur is seen on this lateral elbow radiograph.

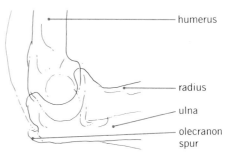

humerus

radius

ulna

olecranon
spur

ease progresses, demineralization is seen periarticularly. There is uniform joint space narrowing and erosions. This may eventually lead to extreme deformity (Fig. 7.28) and subluxation (Fig. 7.29). Deterioration seen radiographically does not correlate well with disability as function may be retained even with severe damage (Amis et al, 1982).

Arthrographic findings are similar in most rheumatoid joints. Irregularity of the synovial lining with multiple fixed filling defects and enlargement of the joint capsule are typical of rheumatoid arthritis (Hug et al, 1977). Arthrography may be useful in confirming the presence and extent of a cyst (Weissman et al, 1981).

IMPLICATIONS FOR THERAPY

Acutely inflamed painful joints frequently benefit from splinting in positions of least intra-articular pressure (Seeger et al, 1984). For the elbow, this is achieved with flexion of 30° to 75°. During acute inflammation, splinting may reduce damage to the joint capsule and provide pain relief. Intra-articular corticosteroid injections may decrease joint synovitis, thus allowing full extension at the elbow and preventing flexion contractures (Fig. 7.30). Olecranon bursae usually do not need to be injected, and injections in this frequently traumatized site may actually increase the risk of infection. While local steroid injections may diminish symptoms at antecubital cysts, complete cyst resection and joint synovectomy may be required (Ehrlich et al, 1973). Treatment of nerve compressions may involve surgical decompression and elbow synovectomy for complete restoration of extensor tendon function.

Conservative medical therapy is indicated for the majority of elbow problems. However, in those patients with severe disabling pain and marked limitation of motion, surgical in-

tervention should be considered. It has been suggested that combined synovectomy and radial head resection is the procedure of choice for relief of intractable elbow pain (Brumfield et al, 1985). Radial head resection may significantly reduce the pain of pronation and supination. Synovectomy may provide temporary pain relief (Inglis et al, 1971; Marmar et al, 1972; Brumfield et al, 1985). The combination of total capsulosynovectomy, muscle release, radial head resection, and partial resection of the olecranon and coronoid processes has been reported to improve pain and increase range of motion, even in advanced cases (Saito et al, 1986).

Earlier studies of constrained elbow prostheses have been found to have a high failure rate, with loosening occurring in approximately one third of cases (Dee et al, 1972). Recent attention has focused on nonconstrained elbow arthroplasty. These prostheses require an intact soft tissue envelope for stability at the elbow and may give

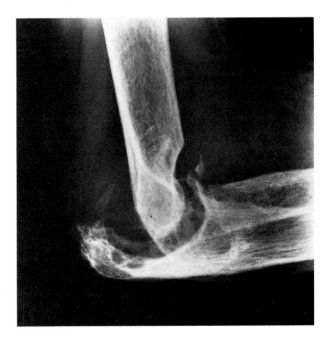

Figure 7.28 Severe destruction of the olecranon and distal humerus has led to the development of a pencil and cup elbow deformity. A large elbow effusion is evident.

pain relief and increased motion (Levy et al, 1985) (Fig. 7.31). However, there is a high complication rate, with infections, ulnar nerve palsies, dislocations, and prosthetic loosening occurring in all series (Morrey et al, 1981; Rosenberg et al, 1984; Lowe et al, 1984). The superficial location of the elbow joint with relatively little surrounding soft tissue has been suggested as a factor in the high infection rate.

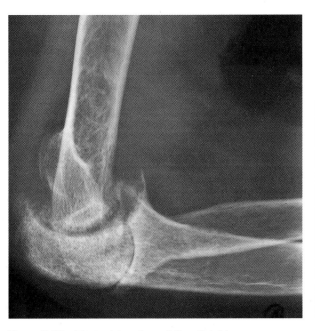

Figure 7.29 The subluxation of the distal humerus seen here has resulted from severe destructive erosive arthritis.

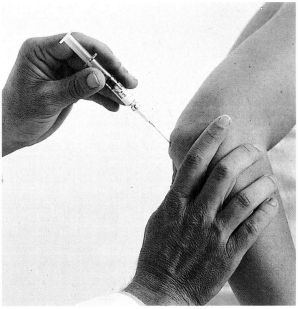

Figure 7.30 Intra-articular steroid injections may diminish synovitis and reduce early flexion contractures.

Figure 7.31 Lateral view of nonconstrained elbow prosthesis.

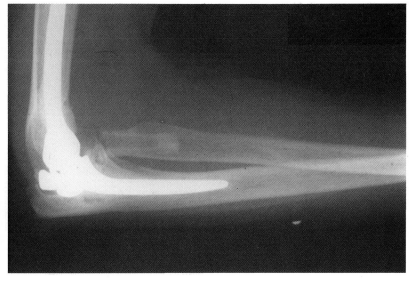

REFERENCES

Amis AA, Hughes SJ, Miller JH, et al: A functional study of the rheumatoid elbow. *Rheumatol Rehabil* 1982;21:151–157.

Balagtas-Balmaseda DM, Grabois M, Balmaseda PF, et al: Cubital tunnel syndrome in rheumatoid arthritis. *Arch Phys Med Rehabil* 1983;64:163–166.

Brumfield RH, Resnick CT: Synovectomy of the elbow in rheumatoid arthritis. *J Bone Joint Surg* 1985;67:16–20.

Chang LW, Gowans JD, Granger CV, et al: Entrapment neuropathy of the posterior interosseous nerve–a complication of rheumatoid arthritis. *Arthritis Rheum* 1972;15:350–352.

Dee R: Total replacement arthroplasty of the elbow for rheumatoid arthritis. *J Bone Joint Surg* 1972; 54:88–89.

Edwards JC, Edwards SE, Huskisson EC: The value of radiography in the management of rheumatoid arthritis. *Clin Radiol* 1983;34:413–416.

Ehrlich GE: Antecubital cysts in rheumatoid arthritis– a corollary to popliteal (Baker's) cysts. *J Bone Joint Surg* 1972;54:165–169.

Ehrlich GE, Guttmann GG: Valvular mechanisms in antecubital cysts of rheumatoid arthritis. *Arthritis Rheum* 1973;16:259–264.

Gerber NJ, Dixon A St J: Synovial cysts and juxta-articular bone cysts. *Semin Arthritis Rheum* 1974;3:323–348.

Goode JD: Synovial rupture of the elbow joint. *Ann Rheum Dis* 1968;27:604–609.

Hug G, Dixon A St J: Ankle joint synoviography in rheumatoid arthritis. *Ann Rheum Dis* 1977;36:532–539.

Inglis AE, Ranawat CS, Straub LR: Synovectomy and debridement of the elbow in rheumatoid arthritis. *J Bone Joint Surg* 1971;53:652–662.

Levy RN, Volz RG, Kaufer H, et al: Progress in arthritis surgery with special reference to the current status of total joint arthroplasty. *Clin Orthop* 1985; 200:299–321.

Lowe LW, Miller AJ, Allum RL, et al: The development of an unconstrained elbow arthroplasty–a clinical review. *J Bone Joint Surgery* 1984;66:243–247.

Marmar L: Surgery of the rheumatoid elbow: Follow-up study on synovectomy combined with radial head excision. *J Bone Joint Surg* 1972;55-A:573–578.

Millender LH, Nalebuff EA: Posterior interosseous nerve syndrome secondary to rheumatoid synovitis. *J Bone Joint Surg* 1973;55:375–377.

Morrey BF, Askew LJ, Chao EY: A biomechanical study of normal functional elbow motion. *J Bone Joint Surg* 1981;63:872–877.

Morrey BF, Bryan RS, Dobyns JH, et al: Total elbow arthroplasty. A five-year experience at the Mayo Clinic. *J Bone Joint Surg* 1981;63A:1050–1063.

Palmer DG: Synovial cysts in rheumatoid disease. *Ann Intern Med* 1969;70:61–68.

Pirani M. Lange-Mechlen I: Rupture of a posterior synovial cyst of the elbow. *J Rheumatol* 1982;9:94–96.

Rappoport AS, Sosman JL, Weissman BN: Spontaneous fractures of the olecranon process in rheumatoid arthritis. *Radiology* 1976;119(1):83–84.

Resnick D: Arthrography, tenography, and bursography, in Resnick D, Niwayama G (eds): *Diagnosis of Bone and Joint Disorders*. Philadelphia, WB Saunders, 1981, pp. 538–545.

Rosenberg GM, Turner RH: Nonconstrained total elbow arthroplasty. *Clin Orthop* 1984;187:154–162.

Saito T, Koshino T. Okamoto R, et al: Radical synovectomy with muscle release for the rheumatoid elbow. *Acta Orthop Scand* 1986;57:71–73.

Seeger MS: Splints, braces, and casts, in Riggs GK, Gall EP (eds): *Rheumatic Diseases–Rehabilitation and Management*. Boston, Butterworth Publishers, 1984, pp. 151–185.

Shaffer JW, Heiple KG: Surgery of the upper extremity, in Utsinger PD, Zvaifler NJ, Ehrlich GE (eds): *Rheumatoid Arthritis–Etiology, Diagnosis, Management*. Philadelphia, JB Lippincott Company, 1985, p 756.

Upton AR, McComas AJ: The double crush in nerve entrapment syndromes. *Lancet* 1973;2:359–362.

Vollertsen RS, Hunder GG: Approach to the patient and examination of the musculoskeletal system, in Utsinger PD, Zvaifler NJ, Ehrlich GE (eds): *Rheumatoid Arthritis-Etiology, Diagnosis, Management*. Philadelphia, JB Lippincott, 1985, p 273.

Weissman BN: Arthrography in arthritis. *Radiol Clin North Am* 1981;19:379–392.

Weissman BN, Sosman JL: The radiology of rheumatoid arthritis. *Orthop Clin North Am* 1975;6:653–667.

CHAPTER 8

THE SHOULDER

H. RALPH SCHUMACHER, Jr, MD

The shoulder is a key to the function of the entire upper limb. Although it has received little emphasis in the literature, the shoulder is involved in almost 50% of patients with rheumatoid arthritis (Laine, 1954). A recent study examining men with rheumatoid arthritis in a VA arthritis clinic showed that 84% had shoulder symptoms (Hozack et al, unpublished, 1986). Shoulders are more prominently involved in elderly patients than in younger individuals. The glenohumeral joint is the major site of rheumatoid arthritis involvement of the shoulder but is not the only affected area. The acromioclavicular and sternoclavicular joints and the scapulothoracic mechanism may also be involved. Primary or secondary changes in periarticular soft tissues are occasionally important. Because some limitation of joint motion is almost universal in chronic cases of rheumatoid arthritis, attention to range of motion exercises early in the course of the disease may minimize loss of motion and functional impairment. Clearly, further study of shoulder involvement in rheumatoid arthritis is justified by the frequency and documented effects of rheumatoid arthritis at this site.

JOINT INVOLVEMENT

Limitation of shoulder motion is extremely common in cases of rheumatoid arthritis. It is usually a result of glenohumeral synovitis (Fig. 8.1). When there is active glenohumeral rheumatoid inflammation, pain should be present with both active and passive motion. This, however, is not invariably true and evidence of subtle shoulder synovitis is often difficult to exclude or confirm on physical examination. Tenderness may be present anteriorly at the joint space, and often there is also tenderness in adjacent bursae. Crepitus may be palpated on glenohumeral motion;

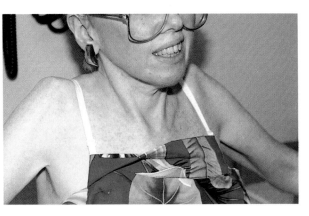

Figure 8.1 Severe limitation of shoulder abduction is shown in this young woman with advanced rheumatoid arthritis.

Hozack et al (unpublished, 1986) found that 80% of men with rheumatoid arthritis also have crepitus in the acromioclavicular area.

When detectable on physical examination, swelling of the glenohumeral joint is usually best appreciated anteriorly (Fig. 8.2). Occasionally there is massive swelling. Chronic rupture of a distended synovium can cause bulging in the anterior axillary fold (Fig. 8.3). Acute rupture has produced arm edema visible at the elbow and mimicking phlebitis or hemorrhage (DeJaeger, 1984) (Fig 8.4).

Rupture of the rotator cuff can occur. There was some suggestion of this upon physical examination of 40% of patients in a VA medical center (Hozack et al, unpublished, 1986). However, it may be very difficult to distinguish this from limitation caused by pain. It is easier to identify ruptures in cases with acute onset of inability to abduct the arm.

As noted above, Hozack et al have found shoulder involvement to be extremely common in a group of men with rheumatoid arthritis. Shoulder symptoms usually had not been the initial features but were causing important loss of function in 50% of the patients. Patients were having difficulty in reaching motions in their daily activities although they often had not complained of shoulder limitation. All had limitation of motion that seemed to have antedated their recognition of functional problems.

The great majority of patients with rheumatoid shoulder involvement have bilateral disease. Dominant arms have not been predictably more involved (Ennevaara, 1967). Night pain is common and is often a more prominent complaint than pain on activity. Patients seem to learn to avoid painful motions during much of their work; this avoidance may even foster the loss of motion that is so prominent. Night pain does not seem to correlate with loss of motion (Ennevaara, 1967) and may be more related to synovitis.

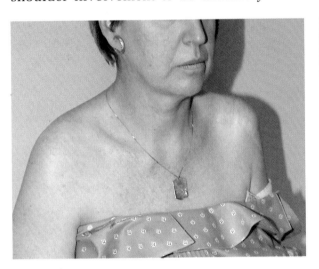

Figure 8.2 Moderate shoulder swelling is best seen as an anterior bulge as noted in the right shoulder of this woman.

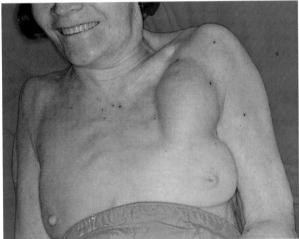

Figure 8.3 Massive bulging in the anterior axillary fold due to shoulder capsule rupture in a woman with psoriatic arthritis who had been bearing most of her weight on crutches. (Courtesy of Update Publications, Ltd).

Tenderness and swelling can also be seen at acromioclavicular and sternoclavicular joints (Fig. 8.5). Involvement of these joints also can contribute to avoidance of shoulder use and to nocturnal and other pain. Tenderness at the acromioclavicular joint is much more common than swelling (Ennevaara, 1967). Sternoclavicular swelling can be readily detected in many cases if sought, although studies of the shoulder have not provided good data on how often these joints are involved.

Synovial fluid occasionally can be aspirated from the glenohumeral joint to confirm the presence of synovitis. Manual pressure in the axilla may increase the yield of fluid when the joint is aspirated by the anterior approach.

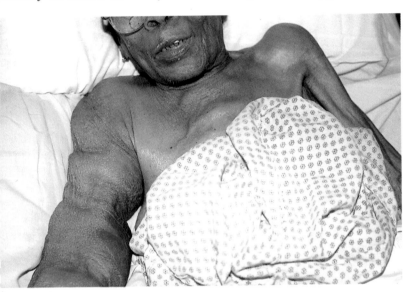

Figure 8.4 Edema and hemorrhage in right arm after synovial rupture. Note also swelling of left shoulder. This patient had renal failure and dialysis shoulder.

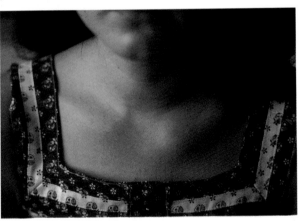

Figure 8.5 Left sternoclavicular joint swelling is prominent in this young patient from Spain. (Courtesy of Eliseo Pascual, MD).

PERIARTICULAR DISEASE

Muscular atrophy is the most common periarticular finding (Fig. 8.6). As motion decreases, atrophy can become extremely prominent. It is not yet known whether atrophy is due entirely to disuse, or whether the known type 2 muscle fiber atrophy and occasional cellular infiltration of muscle also contributes.

Pain on abduction is common and suggests the association of tendinitis and/or subacromial bursitis in many cases even without rotator cuff tear. There are still too few anatomic studies of these structures in rheumatoid arthritis. Arthrography as noted below can be helpful. Bicipital tenosynovitis has been seen but this has been difficult to separate from underlying joint disease using physical examination (Ennevaara, 1967). Rupture of the biceps tendon has been reported with resultant asymmetrical bulges in the biceps (Fig. 8.7).

Hand edema in rheumatoid arthritis patients has been reversed with aggressive local treatment of a very swollen shoulder. Lymphatic obstruction, disuse, and "shoulder-hand" syndrome can be considered factors contributing to such cases.

Rheumatoid nodules occasionally occur over the spine of the scapula and other bony prominences in bedridden patients. Lymphadenopathy in the axilla has rarely been symptomatic and it seems most often to be related to the severity of synovitis distally in the arm.

DIFFERENTIAL DIAGNOSIS

Other joint diseases may affect the glenohumeral joint (Fig. 8.8). There is little that is unique or characteristic of the shoulder involvement with most of these diseases. Gout, calcium pyrophosphate deposition disease, and seronegative spondyloarthropathies usually have additional features and manifestations in other joints that aid in differentiation. Gout usually involves the legs first but if allowed to progress without adequate therapy, can cause bone destruction due to massive tophaceous deposits at any site,

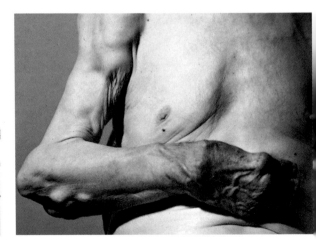

Figure 8.6 Severe muscle atrophy is seen around the shoulders in a young woman with rheumatoid arthritis.

Figure 8.7 Rupture of the biceps tendon with discrete bulges in the muscle mass is seen in a middle-aged man with severe rheumatoid arthritis.

DIFFERENTIAL DIAGNOSIS OF OTHER CAUSES OF SHOULDER PAIN

INTRINSIC CAUSES

EXTRINSIC CAUSES

JOINT DISEASE

Glenohumeral Arthritis:
infectious arthritis
osteoarthritis
gout
calcium pyrophosphate
disease
apatite crystal-induced arthritis
ochronosis
amyloidosis
seronegative
spondyloarthropathy
traumatic arthritis

Acromioclavicular arthritis:
osteoarthritis
hyperparathyroidism
multiple myeloma
amyloidosis
trauma

Sternoclavicular arthritis:
pustulosis palmaris et
plantaris
drug addiction (infection)
syphilis
polymyalgia rheumatica

PERIARTICULAR DISEASE

Bursitis, tendinitis
Adhesive capsulitis
Rotator cuff tear
Subacromial impingement

BONE DISEASE/DAMAGE

Avascular necrosis
Tumor, lymphoma
Fracture
Metabolic bone disease
Transient osteoporosis
Osteomyelitis

NEUROLOGIC DISEASE

Cervical Radiculopathy
Thoracic Outlet
Neuropathic Arthropathy
Syringomyelia

REFERRED PAIN

Diaphragmatic Area Lesions
Angina Pectoris

MUSCLE PAIN

Fibromyalgia
Polymyalgia Rheumatica

Figure 8.8 Differential diagnosis of causes of shoulder pain.

including the shoulder (Fig. 8.9). Calcium pyrophosphate disease may be associated with chondrocalcinosis of the humeral articular cartilage (Fig. 8.10). Both this and gout can occasionally cause chronic arthritis at the shoulder.

A destructive glenohumeral arthritis occurring especially in older women has been widely associated with apatite crystals (McCarty et al, 1981; Weiss et al, 1985). The original descriptions of "Milwaukee shoulder" emphasized an association with rotator cuff tears (Fig. 8.11). Similar destructive arthropathies can be seen with other crystals, including calcium pyrophosphate, in shoulders. Other joints in addition to shoulders can have a destructive arthritis associated with apatite. Glenohumeral swelling may be massive in apatite-related shoulder arthritis and joint effusions are often blood-tinged (Fig. 8.12). Pa-

tients with renal failure on chronic hemodialysis can also get large apatite-associated shoulder or other joint effusions (Fig. 8.13).

Osteoarthritis of the shoulder is often related to some repetitive trauma or, rarely, is a clue to an underlying metabolic disease, such as ochronosis. Idiopathic osteoarthritis also occurs more often than previously recognized (Sandler-Silver et al, 1984). Osteoarthritis commonly involves the acromioclavicular joint as well as the glenohumeral joint. Acromioclavicular changes can also be seen with hyperparathyroidism and multiple myeloma. Amyloid infiltration can produce massive shoulder swelling in primary amyloidosis, multiple myeloma and some hemodialysis patients.

Pustulosis palmaris et plantaris may be associated with a distinctive hyperostosis at the sternoclavicular joints (Sonozaki et al, 1981)

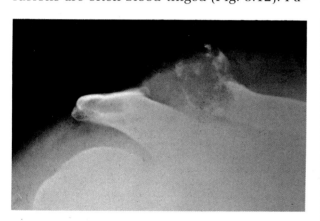

Figure 8.9 Lysis of a portion of the distal clavicle by a gouty tophus is seen in this patient with neglected tophaceous gout. (Courtesy of Murray Dalinka, MD).

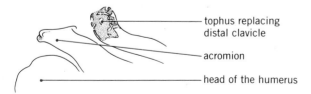

tophus replacing distal clavicle

acromion

head of the humerus

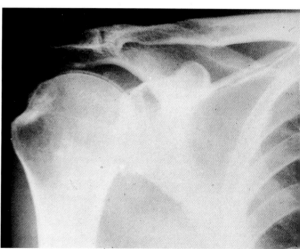

Figure 8.10 Chondrocalcinosis is seen in the articular cartilage of the humeral head. (Courtesy of Bernard Germain, MD and Duncan Owen, MD).

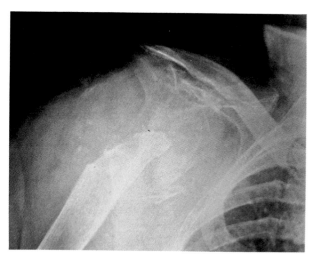

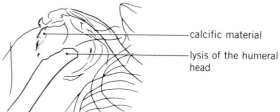

Figure 8.11 Destructive glenohumeral arthritis ("Milwaukee shoulder") in this patient was associated with apatite crystal deposition. Note the calcific material lining the synovial space.

calcific material

lysis of the humeral head

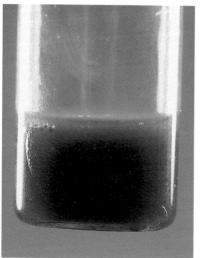

Figure 8.12 Blood-tinged shoulder effusion in a patient with apatite-associated destructive arthropathy.

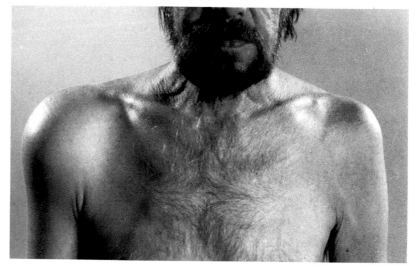

Figure 8.13 Huge right shoulder effusion in a man with "dialysis shoulder." (Courtesy of Armin Good, MD).

(Fig. 8.14). Infectious arthritis of the shoulder joints usually is monoarticular. Drug addicts have an increased incidence of sternoclavicular arthritis. The reason for this is unknown. There does not seem to be a clear relation to sites of intravenous injections. Infectious arthritis and periostosis at the sternoclavicular joint also occur in secondary syphilis (Reginato et al, 1979) and tuberculosis (Fig. 8.15). Sternoclavicular arthritis can be seen in polymyalgia rheumatica (Chou and Schumacher, 1984).

Pigmented villonodular synovitis usually involves only one joint but can produce erosions similar to those seen in rheumatoid arthritis (Fig. 8.16). Synovial fluid is often blood-tinged. Osteochondromas in the shoulder can produce locking. These can be distinguished from the calcifications seen in calcific tendinitis by the loose bodies located in the joint space and often by the identifiable bony trabeculae in the bodies (Fig. 8.17).

Pathologic conditions in the structures around the joint such as bursitis and tendinitis can be difficult to distinguish from rheumatoid arthritis. Such conditions are common and thus can also occur in some patients who already have rheumatoid arthritis. Limitation of active and passive motion (adhesive capsulitis or "frozen shoulder") or rupture of the rotator cuff with inability to actively hold the arm in abduction can result from many shoulder diseases as well as from rheumatoid arthritis (Schumacher and Hay, 1984). Periarthritis, with or without radiographically detectable calcification in the bicipital tendons or subacromial bursae, often causes severe, well-localized, unilateral pain with acute bouts. Pain is increased on active motion but passive motion is much less painful. Chronic periarthritis can lead to limited joint motion and adhesive capsulitis or rotator cuff disease (Fig. 8.18). Adhesive capsulitis usually develops slowly. Sudden onset and point

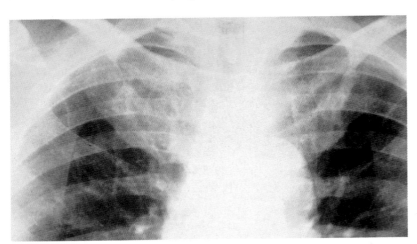

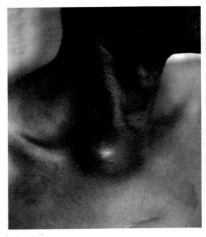

Figure 8.14 Extensive hyperostosis is seen in this radiograph of a patient with sternoclavicular hyperostosis. (Courtesy of Murray Dalinka, MD).

Figure 8.15 Very prominent right sternoclavicular swelling can be seen in tuberculous arthritis.

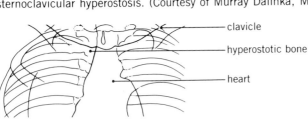

— clavicle

— hyperostotic bone

— heart

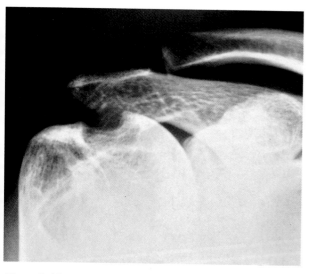

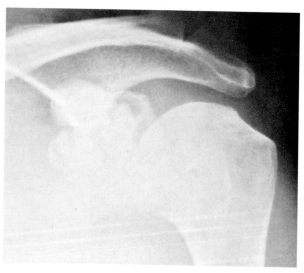

Figure 8.16 Pigmented villonodular synovitis typically causes erosive disease in single joints. The erosion of the humeral head seen here is similar to a rheumatoid erosion.

Figure 8.17 Osteochondromas appear as loose bodies with trabecular markings in this shoulder. (Courtesy of Murray Dalinka, MD).

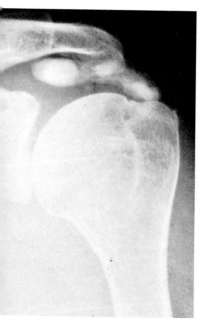

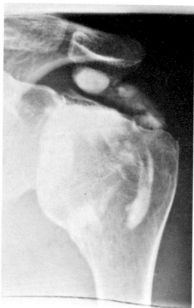

Figure 8.18 Unusually large calcific deposits are noted in this patient with calcific periarthritis *(left)*. The shoulder developed limited motion after a bout of painful calcific periarthritis. This arthrogram *(right)* shows a dramatically contracted joint space, typical of adhesive capsulitis. (Courtesy of Murray Dalinka, MD).

tenderness, if present, are helpful in diagnosis of rotator cuff tears although these tears can also occur gradually. Night pain is common with both adhesive capsulitis and rotator cuff tear. The cause or causes of much periarthritis are not known. Trauma may release calcium deposits into bursae but trauma is not likely to be the major factor in the initial deposition of the calcium. Similar attacks of periarthritis may also occur at other sites, so unknown systemic causes are likely.

Avascular necrosis of the shoulder must be considered in patients who have received high-dose systemic adrenocorticosteroids or who have other risk factors (Fig. 8.19). Other diseases primarily involving the bone can often only be distinguished by radiograph. At the shoulder these include metastatic tumors, transient osteoporosis, metabolic bone disease, fracture, lymphoma, and osteomyelitis.

Neurologic disorders are common extrinsic causes of shoulder pain. Pain in the thoracic outlet syndrome often involves the whole arm as well as the shoulder. Syringomyelia can cause neuropathic arthropathy (Charcot's joints) at the shoulders.

The shoulder is a common site for referred pain from the chest or diaphragmatic area or for radiating pain due to radiculopathy from the neck. Pancoast's tumors are notorious for producing neck and shoulder pain. Angina pectoris can be referred to the shoulder. Physical examination of the shoulder is normal early in this disease when pain is purely on a referred basis. Although neck motion is often limited in patients with rheumatoid arthritis Hozack et al (unpublished, 1986) could not confirm that this correlated with shoulder limitation.

Tender muscles seen in the poorly understood syndrome of fibromyalgia or the dramatic muscle pain of polymyalgia rheumatica can be distinguished by their localization to muscles rather than to the joint (Fig. 8.20). Joint effusions especially at sternoclavicular joints are seen in some patients with polymyalgia rheumatica. Some fibromyalgia-like muscle pain also occurs as a secondary problem in rheumatoid arthritis (Wolfe et al, 1984).

RADIOGRAPHIC FINDINGS

Radiographic changes at the shoulders have been noted in about two-thirds of rheumatoid patients who were studied. Ennevaara (1967) identified erosions in 46% (most often above the greater tuberosity or at either margin of the humeral head), osteopenia in 27%, superior subluxation of the humeral head in 24%, glenohumeral joint space narrowing in 19%, and bony sclerosis in 12%. DeSeze (1964) found similar findings although in slightly different distributions. Some erosions are seen primarily at the joint space (Fig. 8.21). Pressure erosions can occur along the humeral shaft after superior subluxation of the humerus (Fig. 8.22). Erosions can reach massive size and can totally destroy the joint

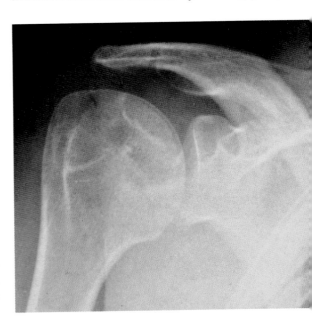

Figure 8.19 This radiograph shows early avascular necrosis with a crescent sign visible at the superior portion of the humeral head.

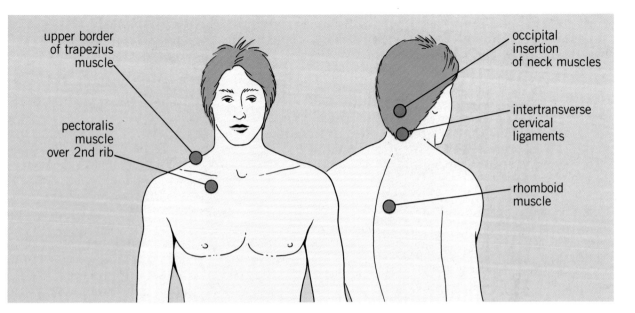

Figure 8.20 Trigger points characteristic of fibromyalgia syndrome.

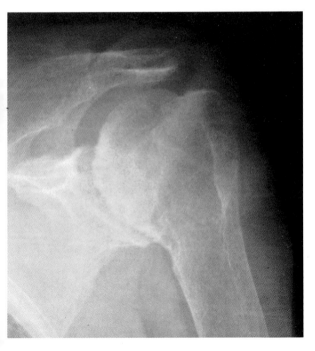

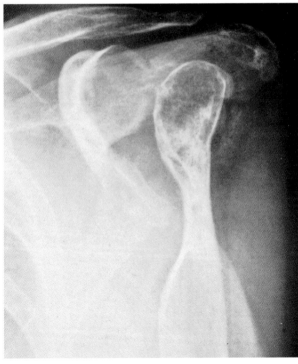

Figure 8.21 Erosions at the joint space, joint space narrowing and some secondary bony sclerosis are due to rheumatoid arthritis. There is an early pressure erosion at the medial shaft of the humerus. (Courtesy of Murray Dalinka, MD).

Figure 8.22 An extensive pressure erosion is seen along the humeral shaft in rheumatoid arthritis. (Courtesy of Murray Dalinka, MD).

(Fig. 8.23). Subtle joint space narrowing at the shoulder is difficult to document radiographically. Only fairly large cysts or erosions can be appreciated in the thick humeral head.

Arthrography shows thickened, irregular or corrugated synovium in rheumatoid arthritis or any other disease with synovial proliferation or inflammation (Resnick, 1981). Such findings were seen in up to 65% of cases with clinical shoulder involvement (Ennevaara, 1967). There may be nodular filling defects and loss of cartilage. Complete rupture of the rotator cuff by proliferated synovium can be shown by passage of the contrast medium from the joint into the subacromial bursa. Ennevaara found arthrographic evidence of rotator cuff tear in 26.5% of cases studied (Ennevaara, 1967). The arthrogram can also show cystic swellings arising from the shoulder but extending into the axillary area, the lateral aspect of the shoulder, or along the bicipital tendon. When adhesive capsulitis

has resulted from rheumatoid arthritis or other causes, the capacity for injection of contrast material is much decreased; only a few mL rather than the usual 10 to 15 mL can be injected (see also Fig. 8.18). Ennevaara (1967) found this in only about 15% of his cases. Rupture of the rotator cuff seems to prevent adhesive capsulitis.

Hozack et al (unpublished, 1986) found spurring and sclerosis to be common at acromioclavicular joints. Widening of the joint space and small erosions have also been reported (Ennevaara, 1967). The distal clavicle may be lysed, leading to a pencil-like lateral tip.

Interestingly, correlations between radiographic changes, function, and pain seem to be poor (Hozack et al, unpublished, 1986). Shoulder radiographs may be relatively unimportant in the day-to-day management of patients with rheumatoid arthritis so they often can be avoided except when concerns specifically about the shoulder are raised.

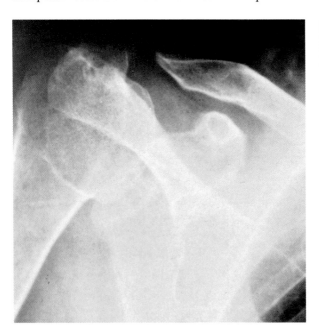

Figure 8.23 Advanced rheumatoid arthritis has resulted in superior subluxation of the humeral head and virtually total destruction of this shoulder joint. Note tapering of the distal clavicle.

IMPLICATIONS FOR THERAPY

Shoulder limitation seems to occur gradually. Because it is so common, more attention should be directed early in the disease at gentle movement of each shoulder through a full range of motion. Because osteopenia at the shoulder is common it seems best to avoid manipulation under anesthesia as it might cause fractures (Cruess, 1980). In addition to optimal systemic drug therapy, occasional intra-articular depot steroid injections may facilitate exercises. A recent study could not demonstrate any advantage of local steroid injection over anti-inflammatory medication and lidocaine infiltration in nonrheumatoid subacromial bursitis (White et al, 1986). Intra-articular steroids have not been studied as they apply to rheumatoid arthritis with its prominent joint involvement.

Various physical modalities such as heat, cold, massage, and ultrasound have been used to relieve pain as an antecedant to stretching exercises. Generally cold is considered less irritating and a better analgesic aid in acute pain although virtually no controlled studies have been done on any of these modalities. Passive range of motion seems better tolerated during painful exacerbations; active motion is emphasized later in the hope of improving muscle strength. Patients should be supervised to verify that they are moving the glenohumeral joint and not relying only on scapulothoracic motion.

Partial rotator cuff tears are common, seem to occur gradually, and have not been felt to be an indication for surgery. Most such rotator cuff tears in rheumatoid arthritis occur in patients with advanced shoulder joint disease, and have been handled adequately with nonsurgical therapy (Weiss, 1975).

Either intractable pain at the shoulder or severe loss of function should be considered as possible indications for surgical therapy, although there is much less experience with shoulder surgery than with operative procedures at most other peripheral joints in rheumatoid arthritis. Arthrodesis may still leave good function if scapulothoracic motion is good (Cruess, 1980). Prosthetic joint replacement has more recently been successful in some medical centers (Neer et al, 1982). Pain relief can be impressive. Neer (1983) did not consider either extent of rotator cuff or bone damage to be contraindications.

Recognition that some shoulder pain comes from the soft tissues and smaller shoulder joints can direct some local therapy to these sites. Night pain can be very difficult to relieve. More research might be directed at the problem of relief of night pain.

REFERENCES

Chou ET, Schumacher HR: Clinical and pathologic studies of synovitis in polymyalgia rheumatica. *Arthritis Rheum* 1984;27:1107–1117.

Cruess RL: Rheumatoid arthritis of the shoulder. *Orthop Clinics of North Am* 1980;11:333–342.

DeJaeger JP, Fleming A: Shoulder joint rupture and pseudothrombosis in rheumatoid arthritis. *Ann Rheum Dis* 1984;43:503–504.

DeSeze S, Debeyre N, Manuel R: The shoulder, in Carter E (ed): *Radiological Aspects of Rheumatoid Arthritis*. Excerpta Medica Foundation, 1964, pp 147–163.

Ennevaara K: Painful shoulder joint in rheumatoid arthritis. *Acta Rheum Scand* 1967; 11 (suppl):1–116.

Laine VAI, Vainio KJ, Pekanmaki K: Shoulder affections in rheumatoid arthritis. *Ann Rheum Dis* 1954;13:157–160.

McCarty DJ, Halverson PB, Carrera GF, et al: "Milwaukee shoulder"—association of microspheroids containing hydroxyapatite crystals, active collagenase and neutral protease with rotator cuff defects. I.Clinical aspects. *Arthritis Rheum* 1981;24:464–473.

Neer CS, Craig EV, Fukuda H: Cuff-tear arthropathy. *JBJS* 1983;65A:1232–1244.

Neer CS, Watson KC, Stanton J: Recent experience in total shoulder replacement. *JBJS* 1982;64A:319–337.

Reginato AJ, Schumacher HR, Jimenez S, et al: Synovitis in secondary syphilis. *Arthritis Rheum* 1979;22:170–176.

Resnick D: Shoulder arthrography. *Radiologic Clinics of North America* 1981;19:243–253.

Sandler-Silver F, Bridgeford PH, Espinoza LR, et al: Glenohumeral osteoarthritis associated with hydroxyapatite crystals. *Arthritis Rheum* (Abst) 1984;27:S52.

Schumacher HR, Hay EL: Toward more precise diagnosis and treatment of shoulder pain. *Fam Med Reports* 1984;2:49–56.

Sonozaki H, Mitsui H, Miyanaga Y, et al: Clinical features of 53 cases with pustulotic arthroosteolysis. *Ann Rheum Dis* 1981;40:547–553.

Weiss JJ, Thompson GR, Doust V, Burgener F: Rotator cuff tears in rheumatoid arthritis. *Arch Int Med* 1975;135:521–525.

Weiss, JJ, Good A, Schumacher HR: Four cases of "Milwaukee shoulder" with a description of clinical presentation and long-term treatment. *J Am Geriatrics Soc* 1985;33:202–205.

White RH, Paull DM, Fleming KW: Rotator cuff tendinitis: Comparison of subacromial injection of a long-acting corticosteroid versus oral indomethacin therapy. *J Rheum* 1986;13:608–613.

Wolfe F, Cathey MA, Kleinheksel SM: Fibrositis (fibromyalgia) in rheumatoid arthritis. *J Rheum* 1984;11:814–818.

CHAPTER 9

THE FOOT AND ANKLE

JOHN S. BOMALASKI, MD, AND H. RALPH SCHUMACHER, Jr, MD

The foot contains numerous small joints and bursae, and these structures are commonly affected early in the course of rheumatoid arthritis. Early involvement of the feet is almost as common as hand and wrist involvement (Vainio, 1956; Short et al, 1957; Fleming et al, 1976; Tillman, 1979; Spiegel and Spiegel, 1982). Patients with long-standing disease and those who are hospitalized have even more symptoms (Vidigal et al, 1975; Dixon, 1981b). A study of 50 hospitalized patients found that 28% recalled foot pain as the sole presenting symptom of their disease, 90% had intermittent foot complaints, and 86% had obvious clinical involvement (Minaker and Little, 1973). The foot is a major site of rheumatoid involvement and a major source of disability resulting from this disease.

JOINT INVOLVEMENT

The foot is a complex structure composed of 26 bones and many small joints (Fig. 9.1)

Figure 9.1 Bones of the foot (dorsal view).

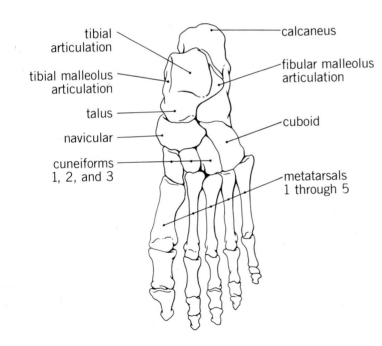

tibial articulation

calcaneus

tibial malleolus articulation

fibular malleolus articulation

talus

cuboid

navicular

cuneiforms 1, 2, and 3

metatarsals 1 through 5

(Sarrafian, 1983; Mann, 1986). The talus articulates at the ankle with the tibia and fibula. The small bones of the foot are held together by ligaments and are associated with a number of tendons (Fig. 9.2). The medial ankle or deltoid ligament is a strong, fan-shaped structure, while the lateral ligament has three small bands that run from the fibular malleolus to the calcaneus (inferior) and to the talus (posterior and anterior). Ligaments can

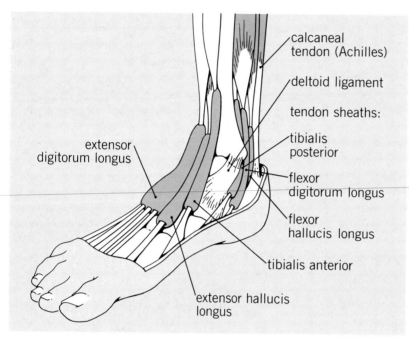

calcaneal tendon (Achilles)

deltoid ligament

tendon sheaths:

tibialis posterior

flexor digitorum longus

flexor hallucis longus

tibialis anterior

extensor hallucis longus

extensor digitorum longus

Figure 9.2 Bursae and tendon sheaths of the foot and ankle. Medial view (above) and lateral view (below).

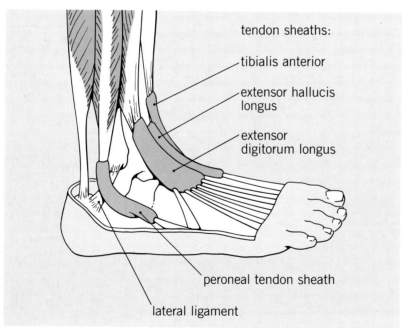

tendon sheaths:

tibialis anterior

extensor hallucis longus

extensor digitorum longus

peroneal tendon sheath

lateral ligament

become strained and sprained due to synovial disease with resultant instability. Numerous bursae are found in close approximation to the tendons. These structures may also be involved by the rheumatoid process. The posterior tibial nerve provides motor function to the foot and ankle, and divides to form the plantar digital nerves. Like the corresponding branches of the palmar ulnar and median nerves, the lateral and medial plantar nerves supply 1½ and 3½ digits, respectively, and are connected by a communicating branch.

Movements occur through two major axes in the foot, the vertical ankle axis and the horizontal subtalar axis. Major motions include inversion (supination), eversion (pronation), plantar flexion, and dorsiflexion.

The gait cycle has a stance phase and a swing phase (Gerber and Hunt, 1985). The swing phase normally consists of 40% of the cycle, while the stance phase comprises 60%. In patients with rheumatoid arthritis, a number of characteristic abnormalities in the gait are observed (Marshall et al, 1980). The earliest abnormality is usually a shortening of the entire gait cycle with greatest decrease in the stance phase leading to slower ambulation due to metatarsophalangeal (MTP) pain and swelling. Later midfoot and ankle pain tends to cause loss of ipsilateral knee flexion after heel strike.

Forefoot Involvement

The forefoot is the most common area of discomfort in patients with rheumatoid arthritis (Vainio, 1956; Calabro, 1962; Minaker et al, 1973; Luukkainem et al, 1983) (Fig. 9.3). In one study, forefoot pain was the initial

FOREFOOT PROBLEMS IN RHEUMATOID ARTHRITIS

Bursitis
Callosities and Corns
Cock-up toes and hammer toes
Cysts
Erosions
Fistulas
Infections
Fractures
Hallux valgus
Hallux rigidus
Hallux varus
Metatarsal spread
Metatarsalgia
Metatarsophalangeal subluxation
Rheumatoid nodules
Sesamoiditis
Synovitis
Trigger points
Quintus varus
Vasculitis and nailfold infarcts

Figure 9.3 Forefoot problems in rheumatoid arthritis.

symptom in 34% of rheumatoid patients and the only symptom in 16% of rheumatoid patients (Minaker et al, 1973). The most common clinical findings are soft tissue swelling, palpable first at the plantar surface of the MTP joints, and tenderness, elicited either by squeezing across all MTP joints or by palpating each separately. This synovitis can lead to spreading of the phalanges, hallux valgus and hammer toes (Fig. 9.4 and 9.5). Forefoot spread secondary to synovial proliferation and ligamentous laxity results in the sensation of progressive "shoe shortening," due to spreading and flattening of the phalanges medially and laterally. Patients commonly note each pair of new shoes is thus not wide enough. Tight shoes can also impair walking.

Progressive hallux valgus (with an angle of 20° to 40° deviated from the midline) is also a common, relatively early feature, and is usually associated with bunion development on the medial surface of the first metatarsal head. Quintus varus (fifth digit) also occurs, leaving the rheumatoid patient with painful bunions both medially and laterally (Dixon, 1981a, b). Cock-up toes and hammer toes also complicate rheumatoid arthritis (Calabro, 1962; Coughlin, 1987) (Fig. 9.6). Cock-up toe is a hyperextension of the toe at the MTP joint with subluxation of the phalange above the metatarsal head. The toe is thus elevated above the dorsum of the foot. Hammer toe deformity consists of the phalange at the distal or proximal interphalangeal joint pointing directly downward. The specific mechanisms for these deformities are not known, but appear to include ligament and tendon laxity and synovial bulging with resultant loss of both structural integrity and normal function.

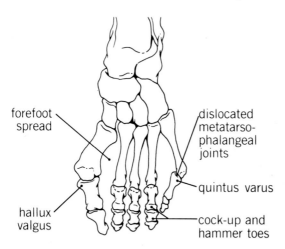

Figure 9.4 Common deformities of the forefoot in rheumatoid arthritis.

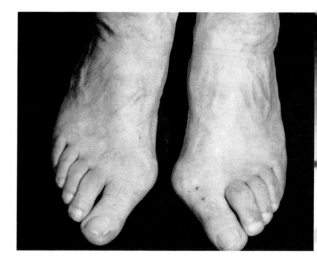

Figure 9.5 A rheumatoid foot with hallux valgus, early cock-up toes, and forefoot spreading.

Erosive synovitis of the first MTP joint causes discomfort due to both inflammation and later joint malalignment (Resnick, 1975). Acute exacerbations of joint pain reminiscent of gouty arthritis (pseudopodagra) may also occur (Bomalaski and Schumacher, 1984).

Midfoot Involvement

A flexible flat foot is the most common type of involvement in the midfoot and is found in approximately 50% of patients (Calabro, 1962; Minaker et al, 1973). It is caused by ligamentous laxity and shifting of inflamed joints, and complicated by intermittent postural changes dependent not only on the feet, but on the knees and hips. A rigid flat foot may also occur as a later feature.

Hindfoot/Ankle Involvement

The hindfoot joints are the least involved segment of the foot in rheumatoid arthritis. Ankle joint involvement occurs in approximately 20% of patients (Minaker et al, 1973; Vidigal et al, 1975), and almost always occurs with antecedant distal foot involvement (Vidigal et al, 1975). Rheumatoid inflammation in both the joints and bursae attenuates the ligaments supporting the ankle mortise. This results in instability, ankle sprains, and an abnormal gait. The ankles invert and, with midfoot flattening, result in weight being borne on the medial part of the midfoot (Fig. 9.7). Painful calcaneal plantar and posterior spurs and erosions may also develop (Monsees et al, 1985).

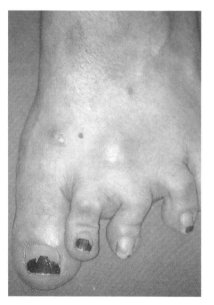

Figure 9.6 Cock-up and hammer toes with bulging dorsal synovium contributing to spreading of toes are seen in a rheumatoid foot.

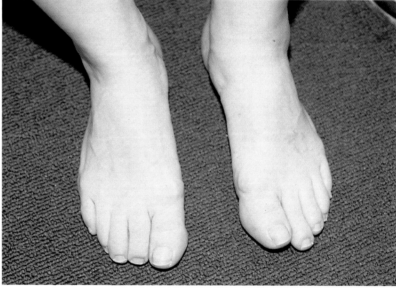

Figure 9.7 Forefoot swelling with midfoot flattening.

PERIARTICULAR FEATURES

Soft Tissue Changes

A variety of soft tissue components may be involved by the rheumatoid process (Fig. 9.8). There are numerous bursae and tendon sheaths in the foot, both intermetatarsal and at the plantar region. Inflammation of flexor tendons can produce swelling and tenderness in the digits or midfoot. Achilles tendon nodules and inflammation at the insertion and the pretendinous bursa can occur. As forefoot bone and joint involvement occurs early in rheumatoid arthritis, it is not surprising that adjacent bursae also become inflamed (Fig. 9.9). Such involvement may contribute to foot pain before erosions are visible on radiograph. Bursae also rarely may become infected, especially in patients with advanced deformities, bony protuberances, and chronic corticosteroid use.

As the bones and joints become progressively involved, increasing inflammation in tendon sheaths and biomechanical strain can lead to tendon rupture (Minaker et al, 1973; Helfet and Lee, 1980; Dixon, 1981b; Coughlin, 1984). The Achilles tendon is the most frequently ruptured but this is still rare (Rask, 1978).

Localized edema of the feet may also occur (Dixon, 1981a, b). This may be due in part to abnormal slow gait with less pumping action of the muscles and may also result from impaired venous return due to popliteal cysts. Ankle swelling and discoloration below the medial malleolus ("crescent sign") can result from popliteal cyst rupture with dissection of blood to the ankle area (Fig. 9.10).

Rheumatoid nodules may occur in the feet and tend to be most common at sites of irritation (Kaye et al, 1984). Nodules may be very painful, and excision may sometimes be necessary. Nodules are also very common in the Achilles tendon.

Callosities form on the plantar surface at

PERIARTICULAR INVOLVEMENT IN THE RHEUMATOID FOOT

Bursitis
Callosities
Edema
Fistulas
Plantar triggers
Rheumatoid nodules
Synovial cysts
Tendonitis/tendon rupture (especially
Achilles tendon)
Tarsal tunnel syndrome

Figure 9.8 Periarticular involvement in the rheumatoid foot.

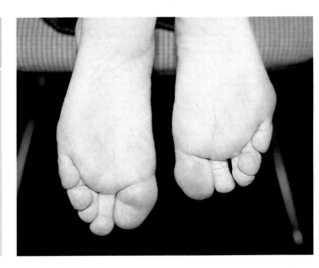

Figure 9.9 Unusually extensive soft tissue swelling of the plantar surface of the first toes caused mostly by tenosynovitis.

the MTP joints (Fig. 9.11), while corns may form at the intertarsal joints due to rubbing on shoe surfaces or malaligned adjacent digits (Calabro, 1962). Calluses are usually due to ill-fitting shoes early in the disease (Dixon, 1981a). With progressive disease, callosities develop at the medial and lateral aspects of the forefoot, the plantar surface of the MTP joints and on the dorsal surface where cock-up toes rub against the shoe.

Plantar or dorsal synovial cysts may also infrequently occur (Bienenstock, 1975). These outgrowths from the synovium may be painful and eventually require surgical removal. Corticosteroid injection may be a useful adjunctive therapy. Extensive debridement of corns and callosities surrounding the affected area should probably be avoided as the cyst may be scraped open, allowing fistulas to form with direct communication between the microbe-inhabited skin, shoe surfaces, and the synovial space. Aggressive rheumatoid synovium rarely may burrow spontaneously to the surface with resultant fistula devel-

opment (Shapiro et al, 1975). Such lesions can become infected, and may require surgical removal.

Plantar triggers are areas of tenderness on the weightbearing surface of the forefoot (Krout, 1982). It is unclear whether most of these areas are portions of inflamed synovium, tendon sheath, or bursae, or represent "triggers" reminiscient of fibromyalgia.

Infections of the foot are a dreaded complication of rheumatoid disease (Shapiro et al, 1975; Schnitzer, 1981). Deep abscesses most often occur in the central plantar spaces, while the more medial spaces are more often involved due to simple skin breakdown from shoe pressure. The dorsal foot space about the nails may also be involved. Although unusual, these abscesses are often difficult to manage, and may eventually necessitate surgical ankylosis or amputation. Ganglion cysts may develop. These painful protuberances may respond to corticosteroid injection, but sometimes require surgical relief.

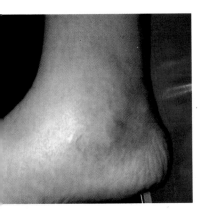

Figure 9.10 A ruptured popliteal cyst may lead to a "crescent sign" below the medial malleolus due to blood dissecting down the leg.

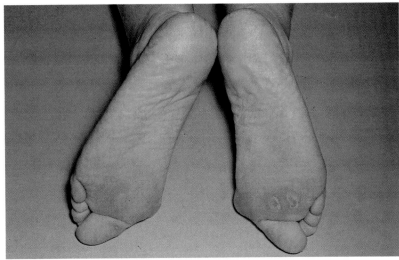

Figure 9.11 Callosities are present on the plantar surface of both feet, especially on the left foot.

Fractures

Patients with rheumatoid arthritis are at an increased risk for fractures of the small bones of the foot and ankle (Fig. 9.12). This is especially true for older female patients with long disease duration, osteopenia, and corticosteroid use (Hooyman et al, 1984). Metabolic bone disease is common in rheumatoid arthritis, and appears to include glucocorticoid-induced bone loss as well as a lesion not dependent on prior glucocorticoid therapy (Weisman et al, 1986).

Undisplaced stress fractures of the foot may be mistaken for rheumatoid synovitis (Fam et al, 1983; Fam, 1984). Clues to the diagnosis of rheumatoid stress fractures include acute onset of pain, tenderness, and swelling over bone rather than over a joint, and the presence of the risk factors mentioned above (Fam, 1984). Evaluation can include serial radiographs and bone scanning. CAT scan or MRI can help in diagnosis if the routine studies are negative yet significant suspicion persists.

Figure 9.12 Stress fracture at the fibula just above the ankle is present.

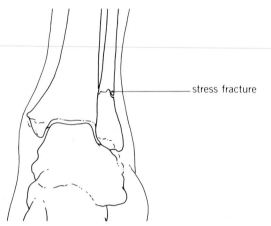

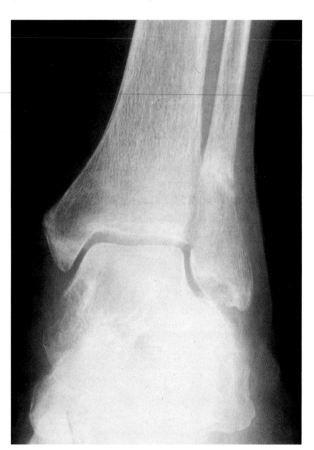

Skin and Vasculature

Rheumatoid vasculitis may produce large or small tender palpable ischemic lesions in the distal soft tissue or nail folds of the foot (Fig. 9.13) (White et al, 1986). These can progress to large ulcers (Fig. 9.14). Ankle area ulcers are especially common in Felty's syndrome.

Other skin manifestations include periungual erythema (Fig. 9.15), pyoderma gangrenosum (Fig. 9.16), and ulcerative lesions with evidence of both granulomatous vasculitis and rheumatoid nodule formation (Soderstrom, 1979; Hurd, 1979; Jorrizzo and Daniels, 1983; White et al, 1986).

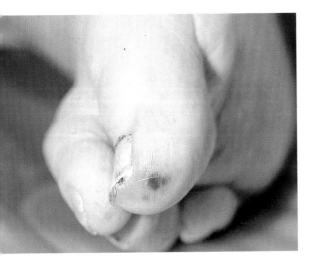

Figure 9.13 A tender red palpable infarction in the distal phalanx and a small nailfold infarct are seen in the great toe of a patient with rheumatoid vasculitis.

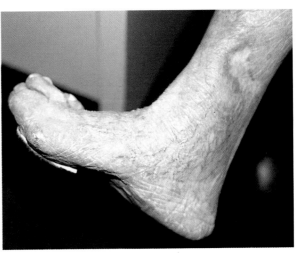

Figure 9.14 A large healed vasculitic ulcer is seen above the ankle. New ulcers are present on the plantar surface.

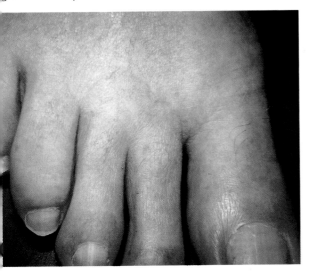

Figure 9.15 Periungual erythema of the forefoot and faint telangiectasias are present in this patient with rheumatoid arthritis.

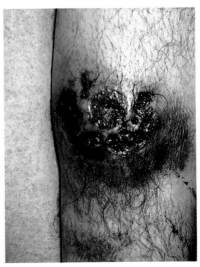

Figure 9.16 Pyoderma gangrenosum seen on the skin above the ankle in a patient with rheumatoid arthritis.

Neurologic Manifestations

Nerve involvement of the foot may complicate rheumatoid arthritis. The tarsal tunnel syndrome consists of entrapment of the plantar nerve by inflamed tendons, swollen joints or displaced bones (Goodgold et al, 1965; Nakano, 1975a) (Fig. 9.17). The symptoms depend on the duration and site of nerve compression. Both sensory and motor abnormalities may exist, so that the patient may complain of dysesthesias, paresthesias, and numbness, as well as weakness or paralysis. These symptoms may be intermittent, but are usually progressive. Like carpal tunnel syndrome, sometimes the symptoms are worse at night, and may be reproduced by tapping below the medial malleolus. Pain is also frequently exacerbated by standing, with relief on rest.

Other extra-articular neurologic manifestations may occur (Nakano, 1975; Edmonds et al, 1979). Diffuse stocking type peripheral neuropathy is characterized by a progressive loss of sensation in the feet and most often affects patients with long-standing disease. Vasculitis, with a mononeuritis multiplex pattern, can give patchy loss of motor or sensory function. Foot symptoms also rarely may be related to a space-occupying dural rheumatoid nodule (Nakano, 1975a, b).

DIFFERENTIAL DIAGNOSIS

The major disease processes to differentiate from rheumatoid arthritis foot involvement are osteoarthritis and the seronegative spondyloarthropathies but many other diseases can also involve the foot (Fig. 9.18). In osteoarthritis, first MTP joint involvement is common. Pain in osteoarthritis is mostly on use or weightbearing, in contrast to the more constant pain of rheumatoid disease. Joint motion is often severely limited (hallux ri-

gidis) and bony enlargement and crepitus are noted. Radiographs can show narrowing, sclerosis, cysts, and osteophyte formation (Fig. 9.19). Talonavicular osteoarthritis with a well-demarcated plantar calcaneal spur can also be seen (Roth, 1982). Occupational activities such as ballet dancing can predispose individuals to mechanical foot problems including MTP joint pain that must be distinguished from rheumatoid arthritis. Second as well as first metatarsal and phalange pain is very common in classical ballet dancers (Kravitz et al, 1985).

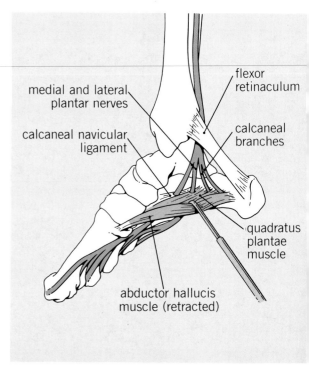

Figure 9.17 The relationship of the posterior tibial and plantar nerves. These nerves may be compressed by swollen bursae or tendons, or displaced bones, resulting in the tarsal tunnel syndrome. Both sensory and motor abnormalities may occur. Signs and symptoms may include numbness, paresthesias, burning pain or weakness of the small muscles of the foot. Sometimes a tender area is palpable at the margin of the medial malleolus. Tapping may trigger an attack of radiating pain. These symptoms may occur intermittently at first, but then occur constantly, especially at night. To obtain relief, patients may hang the foot over the edge of the bed.

DIFFERENTIAL DIAGNOSIS OF FOOT PAIN

Major Articular Etiologies	Other Articular Etiologies	Para-articular Etiologies
Rheumatoid arthritis	Crystal deposition disorders Gout Pseudogout (calcium pyrophosphate deposition) Apatite Oxalate	Thyroid acropachy
Osteoarthritis		Infection
Seronegative spondyloarthropathies ankylosing spondylitis psoriatic arthritis reactive arthritis Reiter's syndrome		Metatarsalgia (idiopathic)
		Sesamoiditis
	Fractures/dislocations	Skin disease
	Palindromic rheumatism	Tumors
	Paget's disease	Vasculitis
	Sarcoidosis	Scleroderma
	Infectious arthritis	Neurologic/neuropathic disorders
	Diabetes mellitus	Psychogenic rheumatism
	Hemochromatosis	
	Pancreatic disease	

Figure 9.18   Differential diagnosis of foot pain.

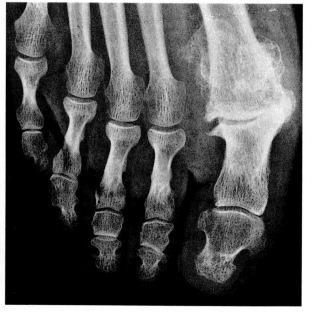

Figure 9.19   In osteoarthritis, the first MTP joint frequently shows joint space narrowing, bony sclerosis, and osteophyte formation. (Courtesy of PA Dieppe, MD).

The seronegative spondyloarthropathies have many features similar to those of rheumatoid foot involvement (Fig. 9.20). Prominent soft tissue swelling at the proximal interphalangeal (PIP) joints is much more often due to Reiter's syndrome of psoriatic arthritis than to gout. Oligoarthritis, or diffuse digital swelling ("sausage toes"), is much more common than in rheumatoid arthritis. Nail and skin abnormalities (Fig. 9.21) help in diagnosing psoriatic arthritis and Reiter's syndrome. Heel pain, especially at the Achilles tendon, is prominent in these disorders. The plantar calcaneal erosions and spurs seen in the seronegative disorders are more poorly marginated, fluffy, sclerotic, and larger than those seen in rheumatoid arthritis. While forefoot and ankle involvement, especially in the posterior calcaneal areas, occurs frequently in seronegative disorders and in rheumatoid arthritis, involvement of the subtalar region, midfoot, and metatarsal shaft are uncommon in the seronegative spondyloarthropathies (Steinback and Jensen, 1975 and 1976; Gerster et al, 1977 and 1978; Chand and Johnson, 1980; Capen and Schenk, 1981). Erosions can be large, crater shaped, and limited to fewer joints in the seronegative

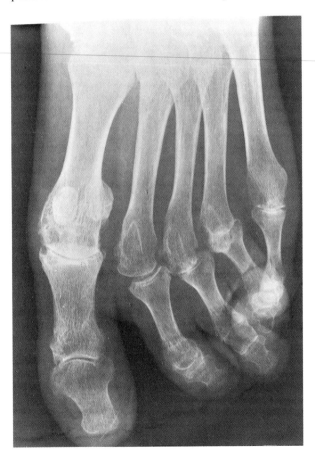

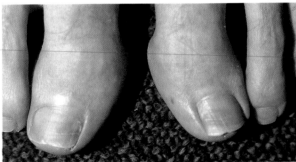

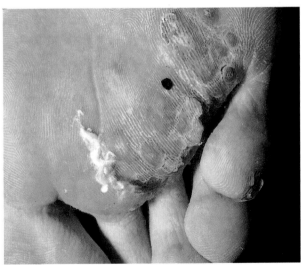

Figure 9.20 Ankylosing spondylitis seen in a patient who has foot arthritis with osteopenia, lateral deviation of several toes, erosions at several MTP joints and cystic lesions in the distal end of the metatarsal of the first digit.

Figure 9.21 Yellow necrotic material can be seen under the toenails in Reiter's syndrome (*top*). Keratodermia blenorrhagica on the soles (*bottom*) can be an important clue to Reiter's syndrome.

spondyloarthropathies but may be extremely destructive and associated with periostitis. Forefoot pencil and cup deformity and distal interphalangeal joint destruction are commonly seen in Reiter's syndrome and psoriatic arthritis (Fig. 9.22). However, note that all these changes are also seen in some patients with rheumatoid arthritis, so radio-graphic differences are suggestive but not diagnostic.

Other articular diseases to commonly affect the foot include the crystal deposition diseases. Gout is the classic cause of podagra (Bomalaski and Schumacher, 1984). The first MTP joint of the great toe is most commonly involved, although all other foot joints may

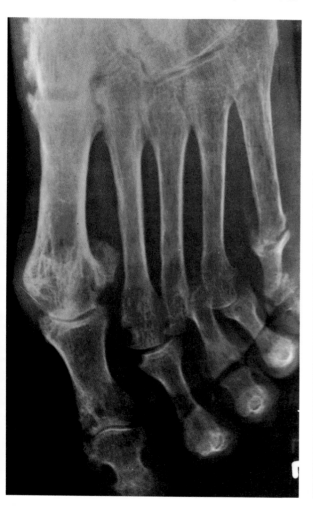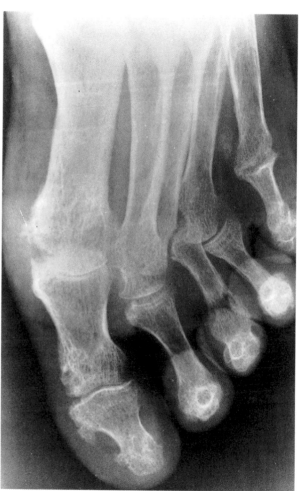

Figure 9.22 Patient (*left*) with severe pustular psoriasis has fluffy new bone formation about the cuboid-first metatarsal surfaces, fusion of that joint and periosteal new bone formation at the first MTP joint. Note marked subluxations, cysts, erosions, and a pencil and cup destructive lesion at the fifth MTP. Fluffy periosteal reaction as seen at the first MTP (*right*) are more common in the seronegative spondyloarthropathies than in rheumatoid disease.

be affected (Wallace et al, 1977). Classic acute arthritis caused by gout is dramatic with hot, red, cellulitis-like swelling that is rarely matched in rheumatoid arthritis (Fig. 9.23). Gouty tophi are common in the Achilles tendon (Fig. 9.24). They may be impossible to distinguish from rheumatoid nodules, xanthomas, and other lesions without biopsy. Chronic arthritis can evolve after the early self-limited dramatic attacks. In contrast to the erosions seen in rheumatoid arthritis, the gouty radiographic lesion may have a characteristic "overhanging edge" (Martel, 1970) (Fig. 9.25). Patients with rheumatoid disease may rarely have a secondary acute arthritis due to complicating apatite, calcium pyrophosphate deposition disease (CPPD), or cholesterol crystals that mimic acute gout (Fig. 9.26). Primary CPPD or "pseudogout" may also affect the foot, and even can involve the first MTP joint, although it occurs more commonly at the knees and wrists (Dieppe et al, 1982). Apatite crystal disease can cause acute or chronic tendinitis or arthritis of the feet that can mimic gout or rheumatoid arthritis (Fig. 9.27). There are usually periarticular calcifications but cases have been reported with apatite synovitis with no radiographically visible calcifications (Schumacher et al, 1977). Tarsal involvement may be especially common (Dieppe et al, 1984); and changes may be very destructive. Oxalosis may also result in foot involvement (Reginato et al, 1986). Calcium oxalate crystal deposition can cause podagra, midtarsal pain, and Achilles tendinitis. Radiographs may demonstrate periarticular, Achilles tendon, and plantar fascial calcifications. In most patients with articular oxalosis the deposition is due to chronic renal failure treated with

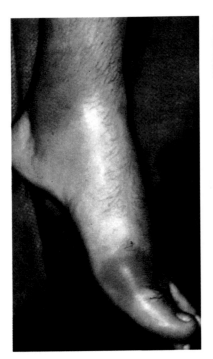

Figure 9.23 Acute gout involving both the first MTP joint and ankle with a dramatic cellulitis-like inflammation.

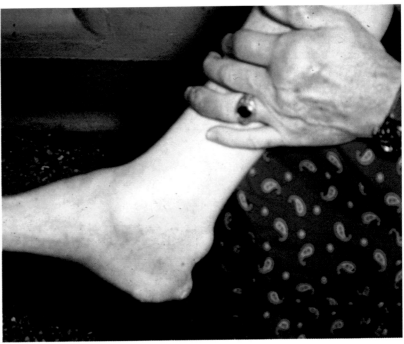

Figure 9.24 Gouty tophi in the Achilles tendon and hand.

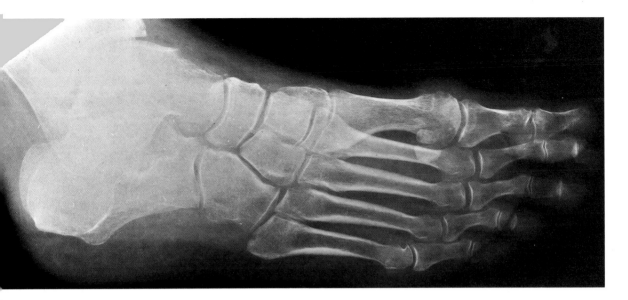

Figure 9.25 Small bony tophus showing cystic changes with a small distal overhanging edge at first MTP typical of gout (oblique view).

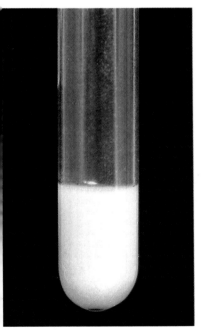

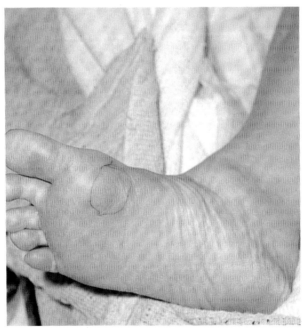

Figure 9.26 Cholesterol crystals in synovial fluid from a rheumatoid patient with a swollen red bursa and first MTP joint.

Figure 9.27 Acute nodular plantar tenosynovitis due to apatite crystal disease.

hemodialysis (Hoffman et al, 1982).

Paget's disease, a disorder of bone modeling and remodeling that results in increased bone turnover, may also affect the foot. Swelling may cause confusion with rheumatoid arthritis but radiographic findings of new bone are diagnostic (Franck et al, 1974;

Altman and Collins, 1980) (Fig. 9.28). Sarcoidosis may also affect the foot, especially the digits, with punched out areas, cysts, dactylitis, and destructive lesions resulting in fracture (James et al, 1976; Lovy and Hughes, 1981). Fleeting migratory polyarthralgias, chronic granulomatous synovitis, tenosynovi-

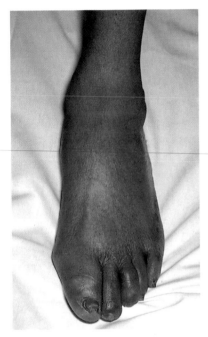
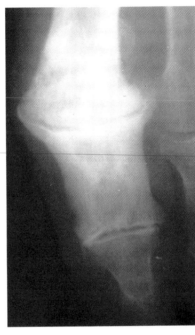

Figure 9.28 A grossly enlarged great toe seen in a patient with Paget's disease (*left*). Radiograph (*right*) reveals the typical coarsened trabeculae and bone expansion of Paget's disease.

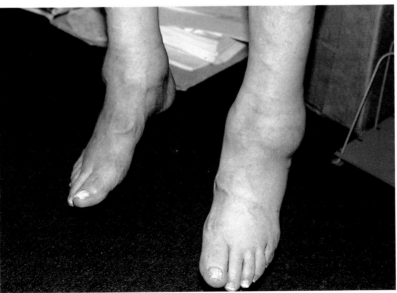

Figure 9.29 Though painless, the extreme ankle and tarsal destruction seen here resulted from the neuropathic arthropathy of diabetes.

tis, asymmetric fusiform swelling of the toes with onycholysis and gout-like podagra may also occur. Adult onset Still's disease can cause acute arthritis of the foot, most frequently involving the intertarsal and MTP joints. Tarsal ankylosis can occur (Larson, 1984).

Various metabolic disorders may also affect the foot. Diabetes mellitus can cause osteolysis, dactylitis, monoarthritis and tarsometatarsal neuropathic joint destruction (Holt, 1981) (Fig. 9.29). Hemochromatosis may also affect the foot. Frequently first it manifests as

mild hand arthritis, but may progress to a widespread degenerative arthritis also involving the MTP and tarsal joints (M'Seffer et al, 1977, Baker et al, 1984). CPPD and apatite deposition disease commonly complicates hemochromatosis (Schumacher, 1982a) (Fig. 9.30). Pancreatic disease, especially when associated with skin nodules and fat necrosis may also affect the foot. There may be lipid-laden effusions particularly at the ankle, and osteolytic lesions in the small bones of the feet (Gibson et al, 1975). Joint pain may precede overt abdominal and skin

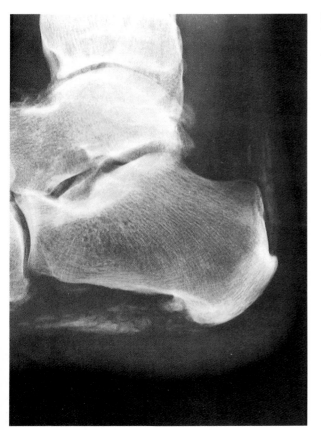

Figure 9.30 Hemochromatosis with plantar and Achilles tendon calcification due to apatite and CPPD deposition is here causing chondrocalcinosis in the ankle and subtalar joints.

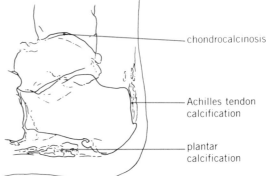

manifestations, or occur concurrently. Thyroid acropachy causes a distinctive painless swelling of the toes (Fig. 9.31) and periosteal new bone formation in the diaphyses of the metatarsals (Kinsella and Beck, 1968).

A subset of elderly patients with rapid onset of seronegative polyarthritis appear particularly prone to edema fluid accumulation in the feet (McCarty et al, 1985). Infection may occur in the absence of rheumatoid ar-

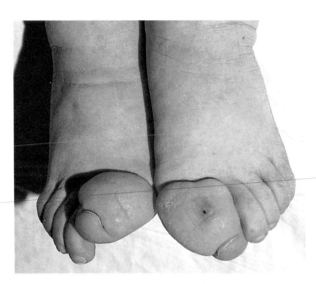

Figure 9.31 Diffuse soft tissue swelling of the first toes due to thyroid acropachy.

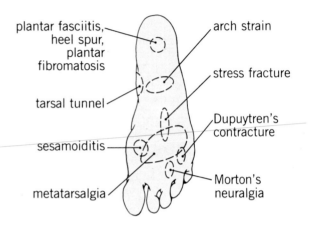

Figure 9.32 Plantar pain. The differential diagnosis can often be narrowed by physical examination and radiographic evaluation.

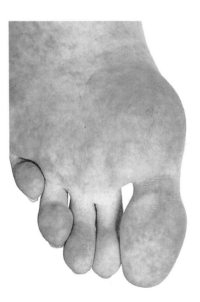

Figure 9.33 Livedo reticularis of the foot is seen in vasculitis.

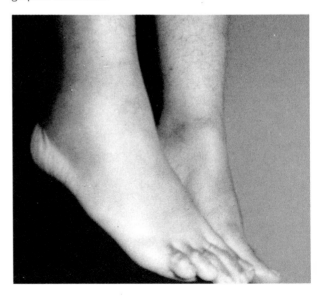

Figure 9.34 Ankle swelling caused by an acute allergic arthritis with urticaria.

hritis, but may also occur in the foot of the rheumatoid patient, thus posing a sometimes difficult dilemma in distinguishing a rheumatoid flare from microbiological invasion (Mastaglia et al, 1980). Persistent synovitis despite increased antiinflammatory therapy suggests that synovial fluid should be cultured for possible infecting organisms.

Metatarsalgia and sesamoiditis may be associated with rheumatoid arthritis, but these disorders frequently present idiopathically with localized pain and palpable bony protuberances (Fig. 9.32). Vasculitis of various causes may produce a variety of skin changes in the foot including palpable purpura and livedo reticularis (Fig. 9.33). Acute allergic arthritis with urticaria can cause ankle swelling (Fig. 9.34). Scleroderma can affect the feet although such involvement occurs less often than in the hands (Fig. 9.35).

Linear scleroderma with melorrheostosis is a rare, nonfamilial lesion resulting in hyperostosis that resembles wax dripping down a candle (Fig. 9.36). Patients may have pain, limitation of motion, or deformity. Other secondary causes of metatarsalgia include stress fractures, dislocations, nerve entrapment (tarsal tunnel syndrome), Morton's neuralgia, vascular disease, verrucae, shortened ipsilateral limb, and sesamoiditis (DuVries, 1956; Berlin et al, 1975; Scranton, 1980; Mann, 1986; Alexander et al, 1987). Sesamoid bones may develop erosions, ankylosis, painful dislocation and juxtaposition secondary to ligamentous laxity and infection (Vidigal et al, 1975; Resnick et al, 1977; Cartlidge and Gillespie, 1979; Gray, 1981). Other foot problems not directly related to rheumatoid arthritis involving bony structures include plantar fasciitis, Dupuytren's con-

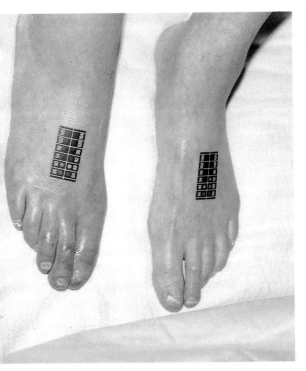

Figure 9.35 Raynaud's phenomenon in a patient with the CREST variant of scleroderma. Temperatures of the feet are being measured in a patient before treatment.

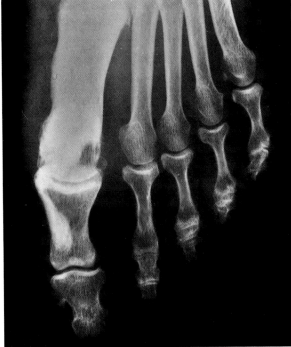

Figure 9.36 Melorrheostosis of the first toe is seen complicating linear scleroderma.

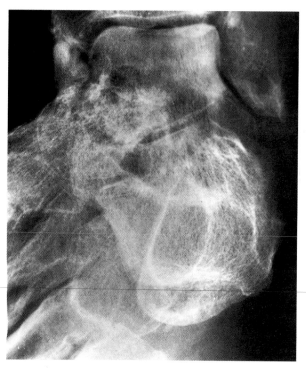

tracture, and plantar fibromatosis. This latter condition may be a cause of plantar triggers. Avascular necrosis may also occur (Fig. 9.37).

Deformities mimicking those seen in rheumatoid arthritis should be differentiated from the pseudorheumatoid deformity with lateral deviation seen in parkinsonism (Bissonnette 1986). Other neurologic diseases can cause hammer toes (Fig. 9.38). Systemic lupus erythematosus with Jaccoud's type arthritis can also produce toe and ankle deformities without erosions. Changes appear to be due to fibrous capsule weakness (Fig. 9.39).

Psychogenic rheumatism includes a heterogeneous group of disorders in which "functional" complaints occur without any apparent organic illness. The foot has been the focus of such complaints in some patients (Rotes-Querol, 1979). Palindromic rheumatism is a condition in which acute arthritis of various sites including the feet waxes and wanes, usually over years, and which eventually may more fully express itself as rheumatoid arthritis (Schumacher, 1982b). A variety of tumors may also affect the foot, both as primary or metastatic lesions (Zindrick et al, 1982). Fortunately, most primary bone tumors of the foot are benign.

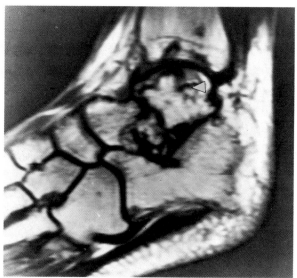

Figure 9.37 This patient complained of persistent midfoot pain. Radiograph (*top*) showed mild joint space narrowing, sclerosis and osteopenia. Pain was not relieved by drug therapy and shoe insert. MRI (*bottom*) revealed avascular necrosis of the talus. (Courtesy of Murray Dalinka, MD).

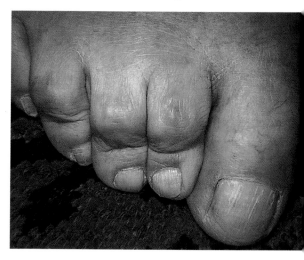

Figure 9.38 Hammer toes in a patient with chronic brain syndrome.

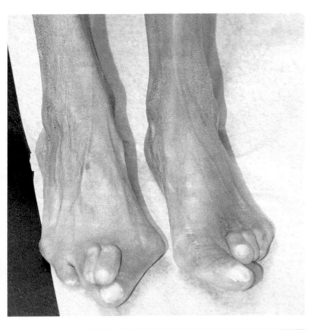

RADIOGRAPHIC FINDINGS

Abnormalities of the foot in rheumatoid arthritis are extremely common and are frequently the earliest radiologic changes noted. The forefoot is usually affected first and most severely. Osteopenia and soft tissue swelling are followed by erosions. Initial erosions are generally at the MTP joints, and are most common on the medial aspect (Fig. 9.40). Lateral erosions also may occur at the fifth digit. The interphalangeal joint of the first toe is also frequently involved, especially with an irregular and elongated medial erosion (Martel, 1970).

Another relatively early radiologic change may be joint space narrowing. Subchondral radiolucent cystic areas are common, especially on the medial aspects of the metatarsal

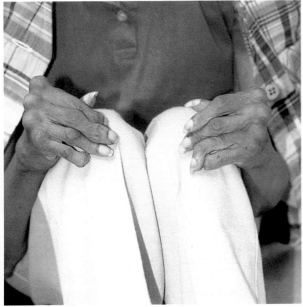

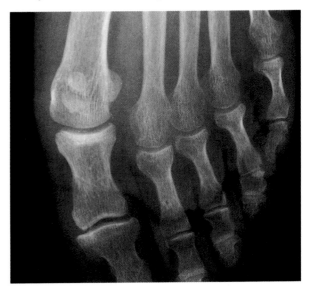

Figure 9.39 Jaccoud's type deformities are seen in the feet (*top*) and hands (*bottom*) of a patient with systemic lupus erythematosus. The left foot had soft tissue surgery but deformities are seen returning. Radiographs show no erosions.

Figure 9.40 In early rheumatoid arthritis there is periarticular demineralization. The first erosion in this foot is at the medial aspect of the fifth MTP joint.

heads. Erosions increase with time and can cause joint instability (Fig. 9.41). Later, less common findings can include progressive bony sclerosis, osteolysis, and periostitis. The latter is clearly less common than in the seronegative spondyloarthropathies. Gross deformities can be seen in some patients. These include hammer toes, cock-up toes, hallux valgus, and forefoot spread. Sesamoid displacement and sesamoid erosions may develop.

The most common abnormalities seen in the midfoot are soft tissue swelling and pes valgoplanus with talocalcaneonavicular joint space narrowing and sclerosis (Fig. 9.42).

Midfoot erosions are unusual, although joint space obliteration and marked sclerosis do develop in some patients.

The hindfoot is not as frequently involved as the forefoot. Synovial effusions are common, but large erosions are uncommon. Calcaneal cysts (Fig. 9.43) can occasionally be massive enough to even raise the question of multiple myeloma or other malignancy. Plantar or posterior calcaneal spurs can occur (Gerster et al, 1977 and 1978).

Radiographic changes in the ankle (tibiotalar joint) appear less frequently than in the foot. Loss of joint space, erosions and sclerosis may develop (Fig. 9.44).

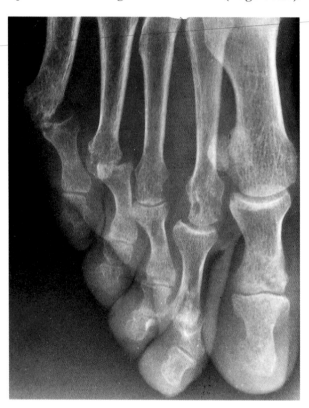

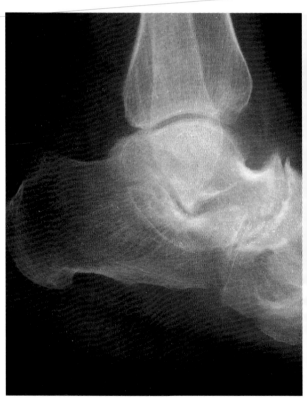

Figure 9.41 Cysts and erosions have developed at the second, third, and fourth MTP joints. The fourth and fifth joints are unstable and subluxed. These disease manifestations develop over time. This is the same patient as Figure 9.40 seen 16 years later.

Figure 9.42 A lateral view of the midfoot and hindfoot demonstrates osteopenia, loss of the metatarsal, cuneiform, and cuboid margins, marked sclerosis, and erosions of the talonavicular joint margins with superior new bone formation, some navicular compression, and talocalcaneonavicular joint narrowing.

IMPLICATIONS FOR THERAPY

Along with pharmacologic therapy for rheumatoid arthritis, education of the patient, especially concerning the often ignored importance of foot protection, will have long lasting benefits. Podiatrists, orthopedists, and occupational and physical therapists may be helpful in reaffirming the importance of good foot care, and may also instruct the patient in foot protection. These maneuvers will help the patient continue the activities of daily living that require steady foot movement (Bardwick and Swezey, 1982; Cracchiolo, 1982; Dimonte and Light, 1982). In some cases, a cane or walker will be useful.

Early on, the patient should consider molded shoe inserts (Barrett, 1976; Dixon, 1981a,b; D'Ambrosia, 1987). If the disease progresses, a set of orthotic shoes should be considered. These shoes should be of high quality material, and fitted to the shape of each foot. Imprints for molding inserts may be performed in the office or clinic and then sent to a company specializing in such shoes. If a shop with experience exists in the patient's metropolitan area, the patient may be referred directly there. Early models of or-

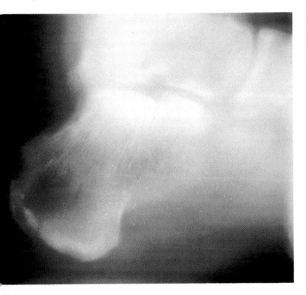

Figure 9.43 A massive calcaneal cyst is present in this tomogram of a patient with severe, rheumatoid arthritis. Note also small talocalcaneal erosions.

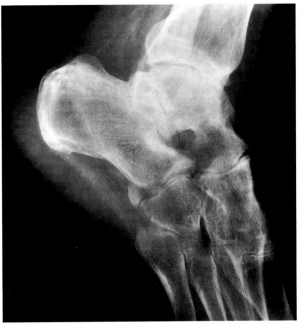

Figure 9.44 Rheumatoid arthritis involving the hindfoot and ankle manifested by osteopenia, subchondral sclerosis and erosions in the calcaneus, and narrowing and sclerosis of joint margins. Note the early spurs on both the inferior and superior lateral aspects of the calcaneus.

thopedic shoes were drab, and many patients refused to wear them. Newer more fashionable models are now available (Fig 9.45). Athletic shoes may also be helpful.

A podiatrist with a special interest in arthritic feet may provide padding and gently trim callosities. A podiatrist may also insert an internal metatarsal bar or a wedge to help provide MTP joint protection. Considerations for bunionectomy and corrective surgery should also be entertained with an orthopedic surgeon with an interest in arthritic feet. Several surgical approaches have been suggested to treat rheumatoid forefoot involvement. However, it is important to also treat the patient with non-operative measures as discussed above (Craxford et al, 1982; Gould, 1982).

Surgical treatment of the great toe has usually consisted of excising all or part of the MTP joint (Barton, 1973; Bordelon, 1987; Mann, 1987). Recent investigations have confirmed the utility of this treatment using the Fowler or Kates procedures (Vahvanen et al, 1980; Goldie et al, 1983). Excision of other metatarsals and MTP joints may be combined with this procedure. With a mean follow-up of approximately five years in 132 patients representing 238 feet from two studies, 66% to 93% of patients were satisfied or considered the results good or fair (Vahvanen et al, 1980; Goldie et al, 1983). Complications included joint swelling for longer than two months, hypoesthesia, infection, delayed healing, scarring and a sensation of cold (Goldie et al, 1983). Surgical treatment of the great toe should be considered early before significant hallux valgus (20° deviation) and painful bunion, corns, and erosions develop.

Arthrodesis and flexible silicone implant arthroplasty are useful treatments, but primarily are of value for only the great toe

(Mann and Thompson, 1984; Cracchiolo et al, 1981). Nonetheless, early treatment with one of these procedures may allow a rheumatoid patient to wear normal shoes for a longer period of time and markedly slow the development of progressive deformities.

A variety of surgical treatments may be useful to treat hindfoot involvement, including ankle arthrodesis and replacement, subtalar fusion with grafting, tibiotalar fusion (Fig. 9.46), supramalleolar osteotomy, and synovectomy (Tillman, 1979; Heywood, 1983; Ruff and Turner, 1984). The precise indications for these procedures remain unclear, but include progressive articular destruction, severe pain on weightbearing and gait instability. Total ankle replacement has been proposed as an alternative to osteotomy and arthrodesis to preserve functional range of motion at the ankle and compensatory gait movement at the distal hindfoot and forefoot (Lachiewicz et al, 1984). Experience with this procedure is still very limited.

Undisplaced stress fractures of the foot may be mistaken for rheumatoid synovitis (Fam et al, 1983; Fam, 1984). Treatment consists primarily of casting, with size and duration of cast dependent on fracture location and its severity, although ambulation with crutches and elastic bandage wraps may be tried first.

Ligamentous laxity is generally treated with orthopedic shoes, and sometimes by ankle fusion. Corticosteroid injection has been used, but rupture, especially of the Achilles tendon, may occur (Bedi and Ellis, 1970; Rask, 1978). Corticosteroid injection may be a useful adjunct to physical therapy in the early treatment of tarsal tunnel syndrome; in some patients, surgical division of the roof of the tarsal tunnel is required (Goodgold et al, 1965).

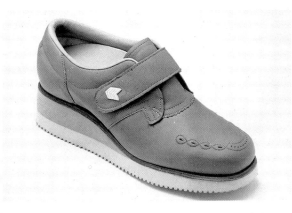

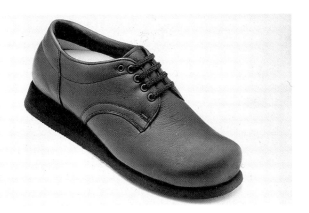

Figure 9.45 Shoes now available for treatment of the arthritic foot not only provide more support but are more normal looking than older models. (Courtesy of Sabel Shoe Co., Jenkintown, PA).

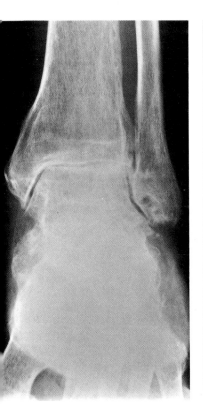

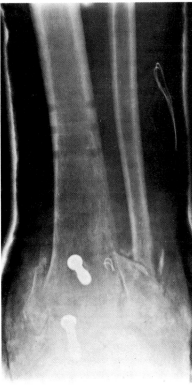

Figure 9.46 Preoperative view (*left*) of severe rheumatoid arthritis with ankle joint space narrowing and fibular cysts and erosions. Ankle fusion (*right*) has been performed because of persistent pain and poor mobility. Intraoperative fracture of the talus and fibula was used to aid the fusion and increase stability.

REFERENCES

Alexander IJ, Johnson KA, Parr JW: Morton's neuroma: A review of recent concepts. *Orthopedics* 1987;10:103–105.

Altman RD, Collins B: Musculoskeletal manifestations of Paget's disease of bone. *Arthritis Rheum* 1980;23:1121–1127.

Baker ND, Jahss MH, Leventhal GH: Unusual involvement of the feet in hemochromatosis. *Foot Ankle* 1984;4:212–215.

Bardwick PA, Swezey RL: Physical modalaties for treating the foot affected by corrective tissue diseases. *Foot Ankle* 1982;3:41–44.

Barrett JP: Plantar pressure measurements: Rational shoe-wear in patients with rheumatoid arthritis. *JAMA* 1976;235:1138–1139.

Barton NJ: Arthroplasty of the forefoot in rheumatoid arthritis. *J Bone Joint Surg* 1973;55B:126.

Bedi SS, Ellis W: Spontaneous rupture of the calcaneal tendon in rheumatoid arthritis after local steroid injection. *Ann Rheum Dis* 1970;29:494–495.

Berlin SJ, Donick II, Block LD, et al: Nerve tumors of the foot: Diagnosis and treatment. *J Am Podiatry Assoc* 1975;65:157–166.

Bienenstock H: Rheumatoid plantar synovial cysts. *Ann Rheum Dis* 1975;34:98–99.

Bissonnette B: Pseudorheumatoid deformity of the feet associated with parkinsonism. *J Rheumatol* 1986;13:825–826.

Bomalaski JS, Schumacher HR: Podagra is more than gout. *Bull Rheum Dis* 1984;34(6):1–8.

Bordelon RL: Evaluation and operative procedures for hallux valgus deformity. *Orthopedics* 1987;10:38–44.

Calabro JJ: A critical evaluation of the diagnostic features of the feet in rheumatoid arthritis. *Arthritis Rheum* 1962;5:19–29.

Capen D, Scheck M: Seronegative inflammations of the ankle and foot: Diagnostic challenges. *Orthop Clin* 1981;155:147–155.

Cartlidge IJ, Gillespie WJ: Hematogenous osteomyelitis of the metatarsal sesamoid. *Br J Surg* 1979;66:214–216.

Chand Y, Johnson KA: Foot and ankle manifestations of Reiter's syndrome. *Foot Ankle* 1980;1:167–172.

Coughlin MJ: The rheumatoid foot: Pathophysiology and treatment of arthritic manifestations. *Postgraduate Medicine* 1984;75(5):207–216.

Coughlin MJ: Lesser toe deformities. *Orthopedics* 1987;10:63–75.

Cracchiolo A III: Management of the arthritic forefoot. *Foot Ankle* 1982;3:17–23.

Cracchiolo A III, Swanson A, Swanson GD: The arthritic great toe metatarsophalangeal joint: A review of flexible silicone implant arthroplasty from two medical centers. *Clin Orthop* 1981;157:64–69.

Craxford AD, Stevens J, Park C: Management of the rheumatoid forefoot: A comparison of conservative and surgical methods. *Clin Orthop* 1982;166:121–126.

D'Ambrosia RD: Conservative management of metatarsal and heel pain in the adult foot. *Orthopedics* 1987;10:137–142.

Dieppe PA, Alexander GJM, Jones HE, et al: Pyrophosphate arthropathy: A clinical and radiological study of 105 cases. *Ann Rheum Dis* 1982;41:371–376.

Dieppe PA, Doherty M, MacFarlane DS, et al: Apatite associated destructive arthritis. *Br J Rheumatol* 1984;23:84–91.

Dimonte P, Light H: Pathomechanics, gait deviations, and treatment of the rheumatoid foot: A clinical perspective. *Phys Ther* 1982;62:1148–1156.

Dixon A St J: Footwear for arthritic feet. *Clin Rheum Dis* 1981a;7:377–394.

Dixon A St J: The physician's foot. *J Royal Soc Med* 1981b;74:101–110.

DuVries HL: Dislocation of the toe. *JAMA* 1956;160:728.

Edmonds ME, Jones TC, Saunders WA, et al: Autonomic neuropathy in rheumatoid arthritis. *Br Med J* 1979;2:173–175.

Fam AG: Another look at stress fractures in rheumatoid arthritis. *J Rheumatol* 1984;11:867–868.

Fam AG, Shuckett R, McGillivray DC, et al: Stress fractures in rheumatoid arthritis. *J Rheumatol* 1983;10:722–726.

Fleming A, Crown JM, Corbett M: Early rheumatoid disease: I. Onset. *Ann Rheum Dis* 1976;35:357–360.

Franck WA, Buss NM, Singer FR, et al: Rheumatic manifestations of Paget's disease of bone. *Am J Med* 1974;56:592–603.

Gerber LH, Hunt GC: Evaluation and management of the rheumatoid foot. *Bull NY Acad Med* 1985;61:359–368.

Gerster JC, Vischer TL, Bennai A, et al: The painful heel: Comparative study in rheumatoid arthritis ankylosing spondylitis, Reiter's syndrome, and generalized osteoarthritis. *Ann Rheum Dis* 1977;36:343–348.

erster JC, Saudan Y, Fallet GH: Talalgia: A review of 30 severe cases. *J Rheumatol* 1978;5:210–216.

ibson TJ, Schumacher HR, Pascual E, et al: Arthropathy, skin disease and bone lesions in pancreatic disease. *J Rheumatol* 1975;2:7–13.

oldie I, Bremell T, Althoff B, et al: Metatarsal head resection in the treatment of the rheumatoid forefoot. *Scand J Rheumatology* 1983;12:106–112.

oodgold J, Kopell HP, Spielholz NI: The tarsal tunnel syndrome. *N Engl J Med* 1965;273:742–745.

ould JS: Conservative management of the hypersensitive foot in rheumatoid arthritis. *Foot Ankle* 1982;2:224–229.

ray PF: Osteomyelitis of the metatarsal sesamoid. *Am Fam Physician* 1981;24:131–133.

elfet AJ, Lee OMG: *Disorders of the Foot.* Philadelphia, JB Lippincott Co., 1980.

eywood AWB: Supramalleolar osteotomy in the management of the rheumatoid hindfoot. *Clin Orthop* 1983;177:76–81.

offman GS, Schumacher HR, Paul H, et al: Calcium oxalate microcrystalline-associated arthritis in end stage renal disease. *Ann Intern Med* 1982;97:36–42.

olt PJL: Rheumatological manifestations of diabetes mellitus. *Clin Rheum Dis* 1981;7:423–476.

ooyman JR, Melton LJ III, Nelson AM, et al: Fractures after rheumatoid arthritis: A population based study. *Arthritis Rheum* 1984;27:1353–1361.

urd ER: Extraarticular manifestations of rheumatoid arthritis. *Semin Arthritis Rheum* 1979;8:152–176.

ames DG, Neville E, Carstairs LS: Bone and joint sarcoidosis. *Semin Arthritis Rheum* 1976;6:53–81.

orizzo JL, Daniels JC: Dermatologic conditions reported in patients with rheumatoid arthritis. *J Am Acad Dermatol* 1983;8:439–457.

aye BR, Kaye RL, Bobgrove A: Rheumatoid nodules: Review of the spectrum of associated conditions and proposal of a new classification, with a report of four seronegative cases. *Am J Med* 1984;76:279–292.

insella RA, Beck DF: Thyroid acropachy. *Med Clin North Am* 1968;52:395–403.

ravitz SR, Fink KL, Huber S, et al: Osseous changes in the second ray of classical ballet dancers. *J Am Podiatr Assoc* 1985;75:346–348.

Krout RR: Arthritis–an attempt to gain insight on the great crippler. *Current Podiatry* 1982;3010:9–17.

Lachiewicz PF, Inglis AE, Ranawat CS: Total ankle replacement in rheumatoid arthritis. *J Bone Joint Surg* 1984;66A;340–343.

Larson EB: Evolution of a clinical syndrome and diagnosis, treatment and follow-up of 17 patients. *Medicine* 1984;63:82–91.

Lovy MR, Hughes GRV: Sarcoidosis presenting as subacute polydactylitis. *J Rheumatol* 1981;8:350–352.

Luukkainem R, Kaarela K, Isomaki H, et al: The prediction of radiological destruction during the early stage of rheumatoid arthritis. *Clin Exp Rheumatol* 1983;1:295–298.

Mann RA: *Surgery of the Foot,* ed 5. St. Louis, CV Mosby Co, 1986.

Mann RA: Treatment of the bunion deformity. *Orthopedics.* 1987;10:49–55.

Mann RA, Thompson FM: Arthrodesis of the first metatarsophalangeal joint for hallux valgus in rheumatoid arthritis. *J Bone Joint Surg* 1984;66A:687–692.

Marshall RN, Myers PB, Palmer DG: Disturbance of gait due to rheumatoid disease. *J Rheumatol* 1980;7:617–623.

Martel W: Acute and chronic arthritis of the foot. *Semin Roentgenol* 1970;5:391–406.

Mastaglia GL, Edelman J, Owen ET: Beware of acute podagra rheumatoid arthritis. *Med J Aust* 1980;2:44–45.

McCarty DS, O'Duffy JD, Pearson L, Hunter JB: Remitting symmetrical synovitis with pitting edema: RS_3PE syndrome. *JAMA* 1985;254:2763–2767.

Minaker K, Little H: Painful feet in rheumatoid arthritis. *Can Med Assoc J* 1973;109:724–730.

Monsees B, Destouet JM, Murphy WA, et al: Pressure erosions of bone in rheumatoid arthritis: A subject review. *Radiology* 1985;155:53–59.

M'Seffer A, Fornasier VL, Fox IH: Arthropathy as the major clinical indicator of occult iron storage disease. *JAMA* 1977;238:1825–1828.

Nakano KN: The entrapment neuropathies of rheumatoid arthritis. *Orthop Clin* 1975a;6:837–860.

Nakano KN: Neurologic complications of rheumatoid arthritis. *Orthop Clin* 1975b;6:861–880.

Rask MR: Achilles tendon rupture owing to rheumatoid disease: Case report with a nine-year follow-up. *JAMA* 1978;239:435–436.

Reginato AJ, Seoane JLF, Alvarez CB, et al: Arthropathy and cutaneous calcinosis in hemodialysis oxalosis. *Arthritis Rheum* 1986;29: 1387–1396.

Resnick D: The interphalangeal joint of the great toe in rheumatoid arthritis. *J Can Assoc Radiol* 1975;26:255–262.

Resnick D, Niwayama G, Feingold ML: The sesamoid bones of the hands and feet: Participators in arthritis. *Radiology* 1977;123:57–62.

Rotes-Querol J: The syndromes of psychogenic rheumatism. *Clin Rheum Dis* 1979;5:797–805.

Roth RD: Talonavicular osteoarthritis. *J Am Podiatry Assoc* 1982;72:237–243.

Ruff ME, Turner RH: Selective hindfoot arthrodesis in rheumatoid arthritis. *Orthopedics* 1984;7:49–54.

Sarrafian SK: *Anatomy of the Foot and Ankle*. Philadelphia, JB Lippincott Co, 1983.

Schnitzer J: Soft tissue infections of the foot (possible source of spread and treatment). *Current Podiatry* 1981;30(11):25–27.

Schumacher HR: Articular cartilage in the degenerative arthropathy of hemochromatosis. *Arthritis Rheum* 1982a;12:1460–1468.

Schumacher HR: Palindromic onset of rheumatoid arthritis: Clinical, synovial fluid, and biopsy studies. *Arthritis Rheum* 1982b;25:361–369.

Schumacher HR, Somlyo AP, Tse RL, et al: Arthritis associated with apatite crystals. *Ann Intern Med* 1977;87:411–416.

Scranton PE: Metatarsalgia: Diagnosis and treatment. *J Bone Joint Surg* 1980;62A:723–732.

Shapiro RF, Resnick D, Castles JJ, et al: Fistulization of rheumatoid joints: Spectrum of identifiable syndromes. *Ann Rheum Dis* 1975;34:489–498.

Short CL, Bauer W, Reynolds WE: *Rheumatoid Arthritis*. Cambridge, Harvard University Press, 1957.

Soderstrom CW: Cutaneous manifestations of rheumatoid arthritis. *Cutis* 1979;24:533–562.

Spiegel TM, Spiegel JS: Rheumatoid arthritis in the foot and ankle–diagnosis, pathology, and treatment. The relationship between foot and ankle deformity and disease duration in 50 patients. *Foot Ankle* 1982;2:318–324.

Steinbach HL, Jensen PS: Roentgenographic changes in the arthritides (Part I). (Rheumatoid arthritis, Still's disease, ankylosing spondylitis, Felty's syndrome, psoriatic arthritis, Sjögren's syndrome). *Semin Arthritis Rheum* 1975;5:167–202.

Steinbach HL, Jensen PS: Roentgenographic changes in the arthritides (Part II) (Reiter's syndrome, gout, osteoarthrosis, chondrocalcinosis, sarcoidosis, hemochromatosis, systemic lupus erythematosus, progressive systemic sclerosis). *Semin Arthritis Rheum* 1976;5:203–246.

Tillman K: *The Rheumatoid Foot. Diagnosis, Pathomechanics, and Treatment*. Littleton, Mass, Wright-PSF, 1979.

Vahvanen V, Piirainen H, Kettunen P: Resection arthroplasty of the metatarsophalangeal joints in rheumatoid arthritis: A follow-up study of 100 patients. *Scand J Rheumatol* 1980;9:257–265.

Vainio K: The rheumatoid foot: A clinical study with pathological and roentgenological comments. *Annales Chirurgiae et Gynaecologiae Fenniae* 1956;(Suppl 1)45:1–107.

Vidigal E, Jacoby RJ, Dixon A St J, et al: The foot in chronic rheumatoid arthritis. *Ann Rheum Dis* 1975;34:292–297.

Wallace SL, Robinson H, Masi AT, et al: Preliminary criteria for the classification of the acute arthritis of primary gout. *Arthritis Rheum* 1977;20:895–900.

Weisman MH, Orth RW, Catherwood BD, et al: Measures of bone loss in rheumatoid arthritis. *Arch Intern Med* 1986;146:701–704.

White R, Wegman A, Bulpitt P, et al: Facial rash with scarring due to granulomatous vasculitis in rheumatoid arthritis. *Ann Rheum Dis* 1986;45:75–77.

Zindrick MR, Young MP, Daley RJ, et al: Metastatic tumors of the foot: Case report and literature review. *Clin Orthop* 1982;170:219–225.

CHAPTER 10

THE KNEE

MARGARET M. MILLER, MD

The knee joints are commonly affected in rheumatoid arthritis. Although the knee joint is not usually the initial joint affected, 30% of patients will have knee involvement early in their disease course (Fleming et al, 1976). Most patients with severe rheumatoid arthritis (class III or class IV disease) will have knee involvement that restricts ambulation and that is a major factor in their functional disability and impaired quality of life.

JOINT INVOLVEMENT

The knee joint can be thought of as comprising three compartments: the medial, the lateral, and the patellofemoral compartments of the femorotibial joint (Fig. 10.1). The synovial lining of the joint has several recesses and bursae extending from it. These bursae may or may not communicate with the joint space. The recesses and bursae include the supra-

Figure 10.1 The knee joint is comprised of three compartments.

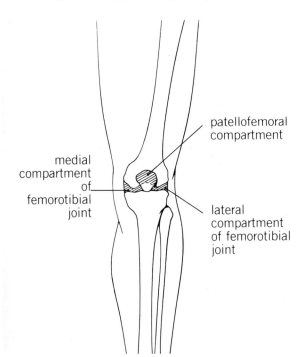

patellofemoral compartment

medial compartment of femorotibial joint

lateral compartment of femorotibial joint

patellar pouch lying beneath the quadriceps femoris muscle, the subpopliteal recess, the semimembranous bursa, the gastrocnemius bursa, and the popliteal bursa (Fig. 10.2). Bursae surrounding the gastrocnemius head may fuse to form a composite bursa, which when distended is referred to as a popliteal cyst or Baker's cyst. Other bursae include the prepatellar, the superficial infrapatellar, the deep infrapatellar, and the anserine. The stability of the knee is maintained by the anterior and posterior cruciate ligaments and by the medial and lateral collateral and patellar ligaments.

The synovial lining of all three joint compartments can be affected by rheumatoid arthritis. This is in contrast to the unilateral damage that typically occurs in osteoarthritis. Synovial hypertrophy, proliferation, and inflammation results in joint effusion, capsular and bursal distention, bony erosion and subchondral cyst formation, cartilage destruction, and eventual loss of joint space (Fig. 10.3). The ligaments, which are crucial for normal joint mechanics and stability, become lax, resulting in an unstable knee. The knee may assume either a varus or valgus position (Fig. 10.4).

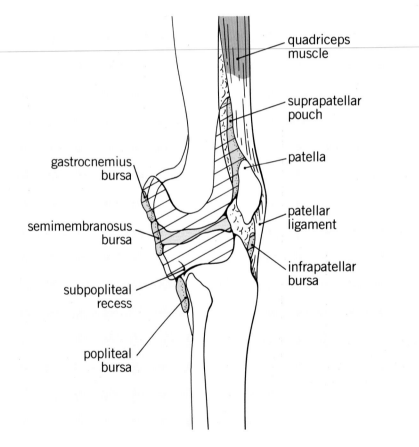

quadriceps muscle

suprapatellar pouch

patella

patellar ligament

infrapatellar bursa

gastrocnemius bursa

semimembranosus bursa

subpopliteal recess

popliteal bursa

Figure 10.2 The synovial membrane of the knee extends to form the suprapatellar pouch and the subpopliteal recess. Several bursae surround the knee joint.

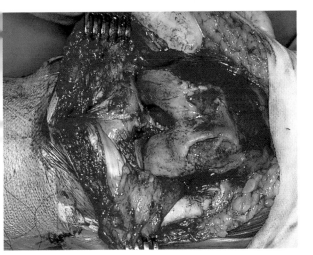

Figure 10.3 The rheumatoid knee may show extensive erosions and synovial hypertrophy.

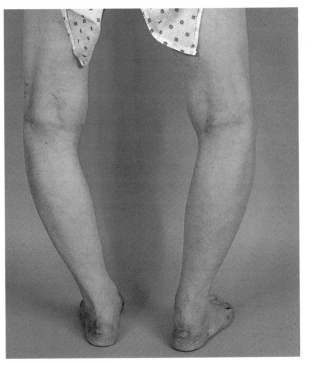

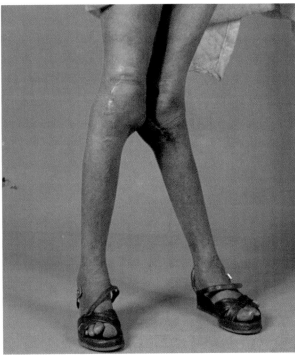

Figure 10.4 Varus deformity (*left*) of the knees in a rheumatoid arthritis patient contributes to knee instability and difficulty with ambulation. Valgus deformity (*right*) can also result from rheumatoid knee involvement. Marked ligamentous laxity is present. Note the marked quadricep atrophy.

Inflammation of the knee invariably results in effusion. Small amounts of synovial fluid can be detected by the "bulge sign" (Fig. 10.5). Fluid from the medial side of the joint is manually expressed to the lateral side. The lateral side is then stroked quickly and movement of fluid can be detected as the medial side bulges. With larger amounts of fluid the patella becomes ballotable and can be tapped against the femoral condyles. This can be most easily done while compressing the fluid downward from the suprapatellar pouch. The patella can also be balloted when there is synovial thickening without effusion or when there is a large fat pad, and therefore ballottement is not specific for intra-articular fluid. Very large amounts of fluid can accumulate in the knee. It is not unusual to aspirate greater than 100 mL of fluid. As the fluid accumulates it fills the subpopliteal recess and distends the suprapatellar pouch. Fluid under pressure furthermore may reach communicating popliteal bursae through a valve mechanism, resulting in formation of popliteal or Baker's cyst (Raushing, 1980).

These cysts are susceptible to both dissection and rupture. The fluid in these cysts is inflammatory synovial fluid that is thick and concentrated, presumably because its water content has diffused out through the semipermeable membrane, resulting in gelatinous material analogous to that in a ganglion cyst of the wrist. The clinical presentation of popliteal cysts is varied; cysts may be asymptomatic. Some patients feel a tightness or pressure sensation behind the knee. Often a soft tissue mass can be palpated in the popliteal space (Fig. 10.6); occasionally this can be transilluminated.

SOFT TISSUE CHANGES AND PERIARTICULAR INVOLVEMENT

The quadriceps muscle, particularly the vastus medialis, undergoes atrophy quickly when articular inflammation occurs. Muscle mass may be measured by using the edges of the tibial plate as a bony reference and measuring the circumference of the knee 7.5 cm above the knee. This may be compared with the contralateral side to discover differences and can be followed over time to determine the efficacy of treatment and of muscle-strengthening exercises. Quadriceps atrophy further compromises ligamentous stability, and with continued weightbearing and inflammation can lead to worsening deformity. Keeping the knee in flexion is the most comfortable position when the joint is swollen and painful. Thus, patients will walk with knees kept in slight flexion and often sleep with a pillow tucked under the painful knees. Fixed flexion contracture and further quadriceps atrophy often results (Fig. 10.7). Unless aggressive treatment is begun, these patients will continue to deteriorate to the point that they are wheelchair bound and have difficulty with weightbearing transfers. Modalities to decrease pain, such as heat, cold, and transcutaneous nerve stimulation in addition to stretching exercises and serial splinting can often be successful in restoring full extension to the knee.

Knee discomfort in some cases may be referred pain from hip disease. This should be suspected when knee pain is out of propor-

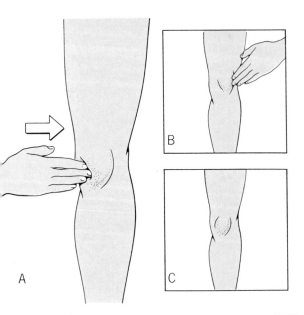

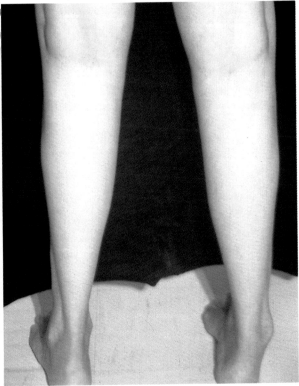

Figure 10.5 The bulge sign may be used to detect the presence of fluid in the knee. **A.** Fluid from the medial side of the knee is expressed to the lateral side. **B.** Promptly the lateral side is stroked. **C.** Movement of fluid can be detected as a bulge appears on the medial side.

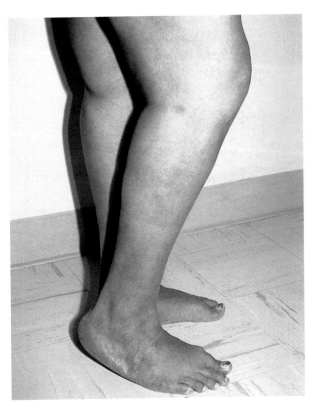

Figure 10.6 A popliteal cyst of the right leg presents as a soft tissue mass in the popliteal space.

Figure 10.7 Persistent synovitis of the knee and quadriceps atrophy can result in fixed flexion deformity.

tion to physical findings and radiographic changes. Underlying flexion contracture of the hip may secondarily cause knee contractures, and must be corrected.

Popliteal cysts may dissect or rupture causing marked soft tissue and periarticular abnormalities (Fig. 10.8). With dissection, there may be soft tissue swelling of the calf, or masses in the thigh, lateral lower leg, or anterior tibial surface (O'Dell, 1984) (Fig. 10.9). With dissection into the calf, patients often experience a tightness in the calf that worsens with walking and improves with rest. Ischemic claudication may mistakenly be diagnosed in such patients (Wigley, 1982). However, there has been one case reported in which there was true claudication caused by popliteal artery obstruction from a popliteal cyst (Katz, 1977). Rarely, a cystic degeneration of the popliteal artery occurs, which is thought to result from synovial extensions from popliteal cysts into the popliteal artery (Shute, 1973). Although arterial obstruction is rare, venous obstruction resulting in pitting edema in the lower extremity is common. Nerve palsies have also been described involving the lateral popliteal, superficial peroneal, tibial, and sural nerves.

When popliteal cyst rupture occurs, the clinical presentation is often dramatic. When rupture occurs, the inflammatory fluid causes an intense reaction in the soft tissues of the leg. Ruptured popliteal cysts in an osteoarthritic knee, in contrast, cause much less soft tissue reaction, suggesting that the enzymes in the rheumatoid knee account for the inflammatory response (Bacon, 1974). Patients may give a history of a pressure sensation behind the knee for some time and then explosive calf pain following sudden knee extension and weightbearing on the leg. The fluid usually ruptures downward into the calf, but rupture into the thigh is also possible. The clinical presentation is of acute deep venous thrombosis with heat, erythema, and calf swelling (Fig. 10.10). Homans' sign is often present. Although inactive patients with rheumatoid arthritis and venous disease may also develop deep venous thrombosis, their nonsteroidal anti-inflammatory medication probably provides some protection because of platelet-aggregation inhibition. The crescent sign, a curved discoloration from a hematoma beneath one of the malleoli, may be present if cyst rupture occurs (Kraag et al, 1976) (Fig. 10.11). Ruptured Bakers' cysts should be the prime consideration in rheumatoid arthritis patients with swollen and painful calves. Mistaken diagnosis of deep venous thrombosis is common. Anticoagulatory treatment of patients with ruptured popliteal cysts often causes bleeding into the cyst and hematoma formation and should be avoided if possible.

Diagnosis of popliteal cysts can be made by either arthrography or ultrasound scanning. Arthrography of the knee will clearly delineate the anatomy of the joint and its com-

MANIFESTATIONS AND COMPLICATIONS OF POPLITEAL CYSTS

Soft tissue masses or swelling

Neuropathy

Pseudothrombophlebitis syndrome

Venous obstruction

Popliteal artery obstruction

Cystic degeneration of popliteal artery

Figure 10.8 Manifestations and complications of popliteal cysts.

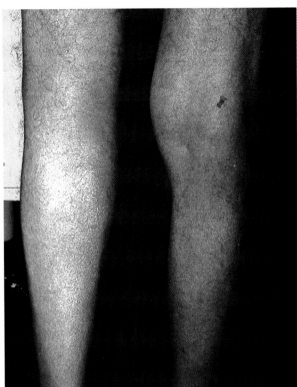

Figure 10.10 Swelling and inflammation of the left calf from a ruptured popliteal cyst is mimicking acute thrombophlebitis.

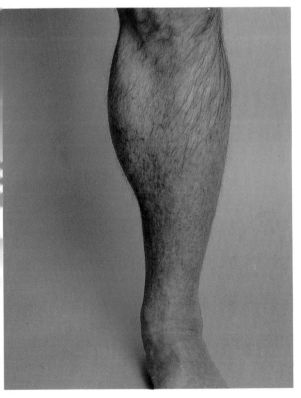

Figure 10.9 This medial soft tissue mass is a dissected popliteal cyst.

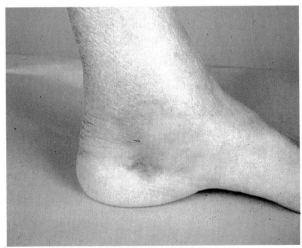

Figure 10.11 The crescent sign may be present in the event of ruptured hemorrhagic popliteal cyst.

munications with most cysts and will demonstrate rupture if present (Fujikawa, 1981) (Fig. 10.12). Exercising the leg is usually necessary to facilitate diffusion of the dye into cysts. However, movement for patients with severe arthritis may be quite limited, thus compromising the accuracy of the examination. In some instances in which there is little or no joint communication with the cysts the examination may be falsely nega-

tive. An alternative technique, ultrasound scanning, avoids this problem in addition to having the advantage of being painless and noninvasive (Fig. 10.13). Ultrasound is accurate and reliable in detecting popliteal cysts that have an intraluminal anteroposterior diameter of more than 0.5 cm (Gompels and Darlington, 1982). There is good correlation with arthrography results. Venography results will be negative for deep venous

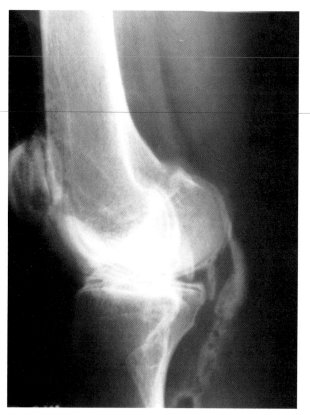 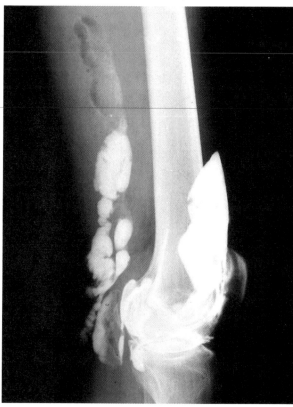

Figure 10.12 A typical popliteal cyst (*left*) is outlined by arthrogram. Another arthrogram (*right*) shows dissection of a popliteal cyst superiorly into the posterior thigh.

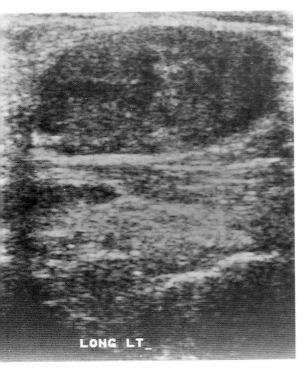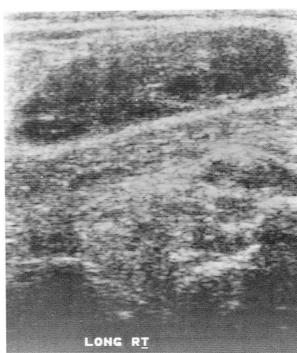

Figure 10.13 Longitudinal ultrasound scans showing
bilateral popliteal cysts.

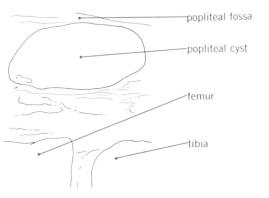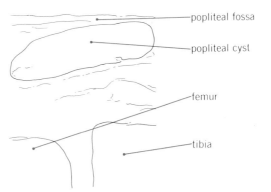

poplibeal fossa

popliteal cyst

femur

tibia

popliteal fossa

popliteal cyst

femur

tibia

thrombosis and may also clearly demonstrate displacement of blood vessels by the popliteal cyst (Fig. 10.14).

Infectious cellulitis must also be considered in the differential diagnosis, particularly if results of venography and ultrasound studies are negative. To complicate things further, there are reports of infected popliteal cysts causing soft tissue infection (Rubin et al, 1982).

DEFORMITIES

The most common deformity of the knee is fixed flexion contracture with either varus or valgus deformity. Valgus deformity is more common. Invariably there is marked atrophy of the quadriceps muscle and ligamentous instability. Subluxation of the tibia and femur or tibia and fibula can occur, although this is

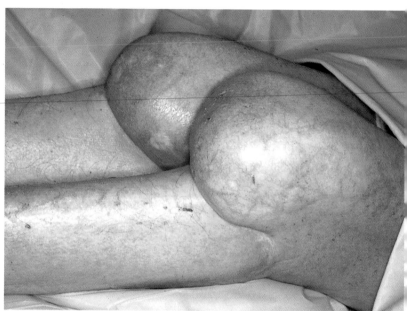

Figure 10.15   This patient has severe subluxation of both femurs and tibias.

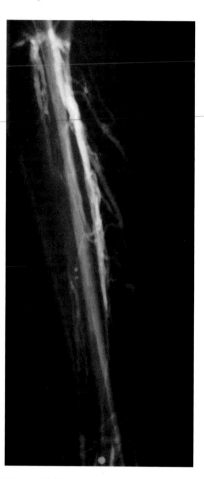

Figure 10.14   Venogram ruled out thrombophlebitis, and showed displacement of vessels by a popliteal cyst.

unusual (Fig. 10.15). Rupture of the infra-patellar tendon has been reported. Rheuma-toid nodules may occur on the knee surface, particularly over the patella (Fig. 10.16).

DIFFERENTIAL DIAGNOSIS

Rheumatoid involvement of the knee joint generally causes synovial thickening and/or fluid that is inflammatory. Synovial fluid aspiration of the knee is technically easy and can be an important diagnostic aid. The knee is often the easiest joint to aspirate, particularly for a primary care physician. Synovial fluid white blood cell counts higher than $2000/mL^3$ indicate an inflammatory effusion and exclude uncomplicated noninflammatory disorders such as osteoarthritis, meniscal tears, traumatic arthritis, and amyloidosis. Effusions in systemic lupus erythematosus usually have synovial fluid white blood cell counts lower than $3000/mL^3$, although they can be higher. Rheumatoid synovial fluid has white blood cell counts in the range of $10,000/mL^3$ to $30,000/mL^3$. Much higher counts can be seen but those higher than $50,000/mL^3$ suggest consideration of an infectious etiology, and in such a case, fluid should be cultured.

Synovial fluid always should be examined for crystals, particularly calcium pyrophosphate and sodium urate. Pseudogout frequently presents as an inflammatory knee effusion and can be mistaken for rheumatoid arthritis, particularly if there is bilateral knee and wrist involvement.

Mechanical and local syndromes which can cause knee pain, such as bursitis and tendi-

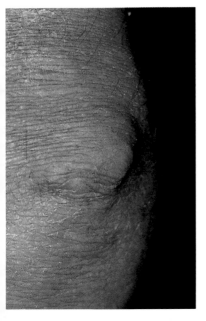

Figure 10.16 Rheumatoid nodules may appear on the anterior patellar surface.

MECHANICAL AND LOCAL SYNDROMES CAUSING KNEE PAIN

Bursitis	**Septic arthritis**
Anserine	**Referred pain from hip or other joint**
Prepatellar	
	Osteochondromatosis
Tendinitis	
	Arthritis
Internal derangements	
	Inflammatory
Meniscal tear	Noninflammatory
Ligament tear	
	Neoplasm
Avascular necrosis	
	Hemarthrosis
Osteochondritis	
Osgood-Schlatter disease	Trauma
	Bleeding disorders
Cellulitis	

Figure 10.17 Mechanical and local syndromes causing knee pain.

nitis, also must be considered in the differential diagnosis of knee pain (Fig. 10.17).

Once noninflammatory disorders and crystalline arthritis have been ruled out, the differential diagnosis includes not only rheumatoid arthritis but Reiter's syndrome, anklyosing spondylitis, psoriasis, inflammatory bowel disease, pigmented villonodular synovitis, and hemophilic arthropathy. The pattern of other joint involvement, radiographic evaluation, extra-articular manifestations, and laboratory data can usually point to the correct diagnosis.

Arthroscopic examination of the knee may be helpful if the diagnosis is unclear and/or other anatomic pathology, such as meniscal tear or synovial plicae, is suspected. Histologic examination and culture of synovium can be done to rule out other disorders including indolent infections such as coccidioidomycosis, or pigmented villonodular synovitis.

RADIOGRAPHIC FINDINGS

The earliest radiographic abnormality is often the presence of a synovial complex on the lateral projection of the knee radiograph. This may be either fluid or hypertrophied synovium and appears as a radiographically dense area between two radiolucent fat collections (Fig. 10.18). Increased radiodensity can also be seen in the posterior aspect of the knee

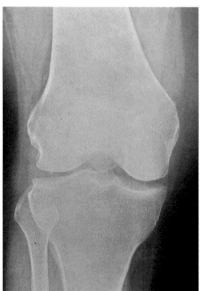

Figure 10.19   A bony erosion is present at the articular margin of the lateral tibia and femur.

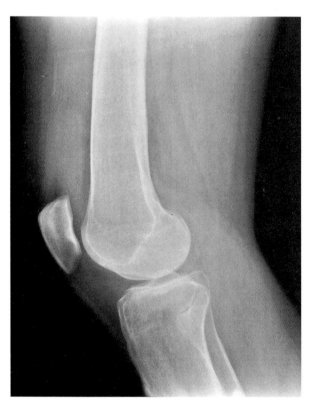

Figure 10.18   The radiodense area in the suprapatellar area indicates fluid or synovial thickening.

joint. Initial erosion of bony cortex occurs at articular margins at the medial and lateral aspects of the tibia, femur, or fibula (Fig. 10.19). Pressure erosions can also occur as focal erosions of the anterior distal femoral shaft underlying a sharp edge of an adjacent patella (Monsees et al, 1985) (Fig. 10.20).

With more severe involvement the interosseous distance between the femur and tibia narrows, reflecting articular cartilage destruction. Similarly, the distance between patella and femur may narrow. Typically both medial and lateral joint spaces are symmetrically narrowed (Fig. 10.21). This feature

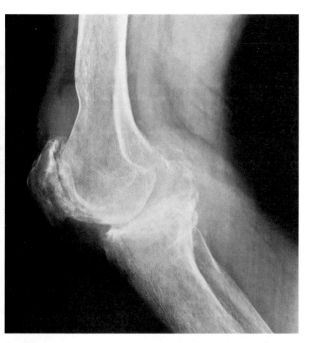

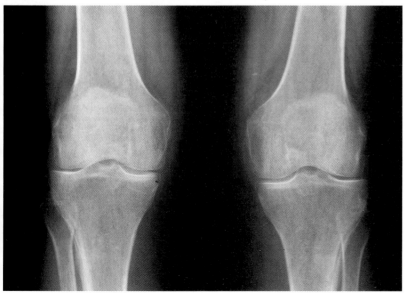

Figure 10.20   A large pressure erosion of the femoral shaft is present in addition to marked joint space loss at the patellofemoral joint.

Figure 10.21   Radiographs show typical bicompartmental narrowing caused by rheumatoid arthritis.

is a radiographic aid in distinguishing rheumatoid arthritis from the asymmetric involvement of osteoarthritis. Weightbearing views of the knees sometimes demonstrate the joint space narrowing when routine views do not, and should be part of the radiographic examination.

Varus and valgus deformities of the knee can be easily recognized on radiographs, and can sometimes give the false impression of asymmetric narrowing (Fig. 10.22).

Other radiographic findings include subchondral erosions and cysts that may be quite large (Magyar et al, 1974) (Fig. 10.23), and subchondral bone collapse that may mimic aseptic necrosis. Loose bodies are unusual but some can be seen on radiographs (Moldofsky and Dalinka, 1979). Subluxation of femur and

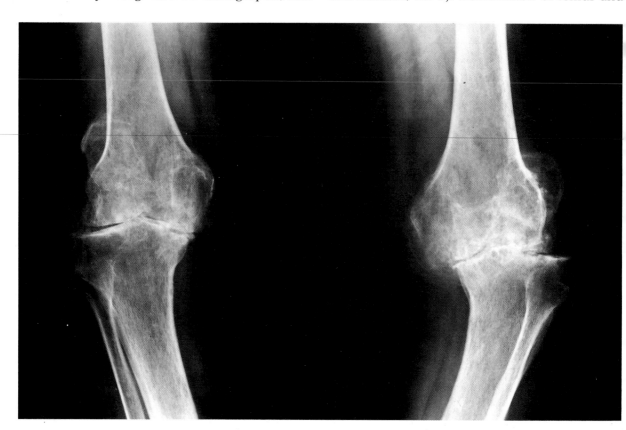

Figure 10.22 Varus deformities are seen at both knees. Subchrondal cysts are evident.

ibia, and tibia and fibula can occur rarely. Bony ankylosis of the knee is extremely unusual in rheumatoid arthritis.

Although most of these radiographic changes in the knee can be seen in any type of inflammatory arthritis, the presence of certain additional features may point to a different diagnosis. Cartilaginous calcification is seen with calcium pyrophosphate deposition disease, and patellofemoral disease is often more severe than femorotibial disease. Subchondral eburnation and osteophytes are more often features of osteoarthritis. Rapid and extensive cortical loss is seen in infectious arthritis. Hemophilic arthritis causes widening of the intracondylar notch and irregular narrowing of the joint space and sclerosis of the bone (Fig. 10.24). Pigmented villonodular

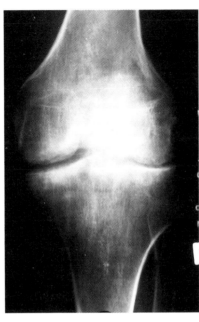

Figure 10.24 Sclerosis and irregular joint space narrowing in the knee of a patient with hemophilia and repeated hemarthroses.

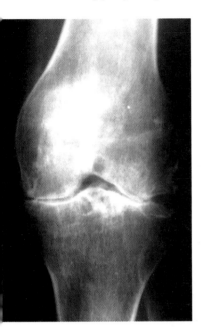

Figure 10.23 Subchondral cysts are present in the tibia and the femur.

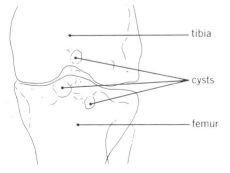

tibia

cysts

femur

synovitis may appear radiographically as a synovial mass or as a destructive bone lesion (Fig. 10.25).

IMPLICATIONS FOR THERAPY

Knee synovitis should be treated aggressively. Physical therapy is vital and should begin at the onset of knee involvement. Quadriceps mass and strength should be maintained and flexion contractures avoided. Quadriceps exercises should be a part of the patient's daily routine. Nonweightbearing exercises such as swimming and bicycling may also be useful. Bracing of the knee may be helpful if liga-

mentous instability exists. Drainage of knee effusions and occasional intra-articular injection of steroids not only relieves pain but may help prevent the cycle of quadriceps atrophy and flexion deformity.

Popliteal cysts and cyst rupture can usually be treated effectively with intra-articular injection of steroids. Surgical excision can also be done but the recurrence rate is high unless complete anterior and posterior synovectomy is done.

Because persistent synovitis in the knee is such a significant problem, synovectomy has been proposed as a valuable adjunctive treatment (Ranawat et al, 1972). The procedure can be performed with relative ease on the knee joint and large amounts of proliferative synovium may be removed. Results of syno-

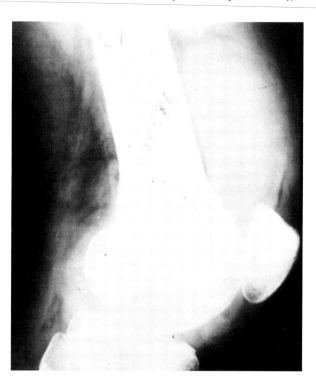

Figure 10.25 The large suprapatellar mass turned out to be due to pigmented villonodular synovitis.

ectomy are variable and the procedure itself may have significant morbidity (Marmor, 1979). Arthroscopic synovectomy has been described and may reduce the morbidity of surgical synovectomy (Aritomi, 1984). However, synovectomy is palliative at best because the pathologic synovium will recur unless the systemic disease activity is controlled. Investigations using intra-articular radioactive gold (^{198}Au) and radioactive yttrium (^{90}Y) have had favorable outcomes in some patients (Bridgman, 1984). However, larger studies and long-term follow-up are needed to assess overall effectiveness of such medical synovectomies."

Knee replacement surgery has been a major advance for the rheumatoid knee. Patients with end-stage knee disease can walk again without pain and have an improved quality of life. Because rheumatoid arthritis almost always involves both medial and lateral joint compartments, bicompartmental arthroplasty is usually necessary. Rarely, osteotomy or unicompartmental arthroplasty is sufficient. Recent advances in prosthetic materials and cementing technique have resulted in a high success rate and low morbidity (Volz, 1982) (Fig. 10.26). Complications, including prosthetic loosening and infection, are low at approximately 1%. A cementless prosthesis may further decrease the incidence of loosening (Bobyn, 1984; Hungerford and Kenna, 1983). When both knees are severely damaged, bilateral total knee replacements can be done, which minimizes rehabilitation and surgical morbidity.

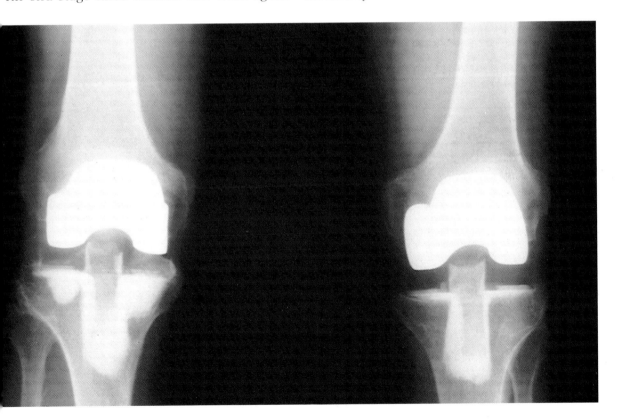

Figure 10.26   Postoperative radiograph following total knee replacement.

REFERENCES

Aritomi H: Arthroscopic synovectomy of the knee joint with the electric resectoscope. *Scand J Haematol* 1984;33:249–262.

Bacon PA, Gerber NJ: Popliteal cysts and synovial rupture in osteoarthritis. *Rheumatol Rehabil* 1974;13:98–100.

Bobyn JD: Human histology of the bone-porous metal implant surface. *Orthopedics* 1984;7 (September):1410–1421.

Bridgman JF, Bruckner FE, Bleehen NM: Radioactive yttrium (^{90}Y) in the treatment of rheumatoid knee effusions. *Ann Rheum Dis* 1971;30:180–182.

Fleming A, Benn RT, Cobett M, Wood PHN: Early rheumatoid disease. II. Patterns of joint involvement. *Ann Rheum Dis* 1976;35(4):361–364.

Fujikawa K: Arthrographic study of the rheumatoid knee. I. Synovial proliferation. *Ann Rheum Dis* 1981;40:332–343.

Gompels BM, Darlington LG: Evaluation of popliteal cysts and painful calves with ultrasonography: comparison with arthrography. *Ann Rheum Dis* 1982;41:355–359.

Haid SP, Conn J, Bergan JJ: Cystic adventitial disease of the popliteal artery. *Arch Surg* 1970;101:652–670.

Hungerford D, Kenna RV: Preliminary experience with a total knee prosthesis with porous coating used without cement. *Clin Orthop* 1983;176:95–107.

Katz RS, Zizic TM, Arnold WP, et al: The pseudothrombophlebitis syndrome. *Medicine* 1977;56:151–164.

Kraag G, Thevathasan EM, Gordon DA, Walker IH: The hemorrhage crescent sign of acute synovial rupture. *Ann Intern Med* 1976;85:477–478.

Magyar E, Telerman A, Feher M, Wouters HW: Giant bone cysts in rheumatoid arthritis. *J Bone Joint Surg Br* 1974;56:121–129.

Marmor L: Synovectomy of the knee joint. *Ortho Clin North Am* 1979;1:10:211–222.

Moldofsky PJ, Dalinka MK: Multiple loose bodies in rheumatoid arthritis. *Skeletal Radiol* 1979;4:219–22?.

Monsees B, Destouet JM, Murphy WA, Resnick D: Pressure erosions of bone in rheumatoid arthritis: a subject review. *Radiology* 1985;155:53–59.

O'Dell JR, Anderson PA, Hollister JR, West SG: Anterior tibial mass: an unusual complication of popliteal cysts. *Arthritis Rheum* 1984;1:75:113–115.

Ranawat CS, Ecker M, Straub LR: Synovectomy and debridement of the knee in rheumatoid arthritis. A study of 60 knees. *Arthritis Rheum* 1972;6:15:571–580.

Rausching W: Anatomy and function of the communication between knee joint and popliteal bursae. *Ann Rheum Dis* 1980;39:354–358.

Rubin BR, Gupton VP, Levy RS, Marmar E, Ehrlich G: Anaerobic abscess of a popliteal cyst in a patient with rheumatoid arthritis. *J Rheumatol* 1982;9:733–734.

Shute K, Rothnie NG: The aetiology of cystic arterial disease. *Br J Surg* 1973;60:397–400.

Volz R: Recent strides in total joint replacement. *Drug Ther Hosp* December 1984, pp 35–46.

Wigley RD: Popliteal cysts: Variations on a theme of Baker. *Sem Arthritis Rheum* 1982;1:82:1–10.

CHAPTER 11

THE HIP

JOHN S. BOMALASKI, MD

linical involvement of the hip joint in pa-ents with rheumatoid arthritis is difficult to iagnose early, and may follow a varied pat-rn of progression or remission in untreated atients and in response to drug therapy.

Radiographic surveys have noted that ap-roximately half of the patients with estab-shed disease will have radiographic evi-ence of inflammatory hip disease (Duthie nd Harris, 1969; Glick et al, 1963; Isdale, 962). Progressive changes in hip radiographs nay also occur in up to 20% of patients who ave had the disease for only 18 months Duthie and Harris, 1969). Involvement of the eriarticular tissues is occasionally impor-ant. Because some limitation of motion is lmost always present in patients with long-tanding disease, the use of range of motion xercises early on may minimize muscle vasting, loss of motion, and functional im-airment.

JOINT INVOLVEMENT

Pain, tenderness, discomfort on walking or olling over in bed, limb shortening, gait ab-normalities (especially "waddling"), and imitation of range of motion (especially ab-duction, internal rotation, and extension) are common symptomatic clinical manifesta-ions. Physical examination may occasionally eveal signs of soft tissue swelling anteriorly t the joint space or laterally, due to bursitis. Classically detectable signs of inflammation

such as warmth and redness, however, are frequently absent at this deeply placed joint. As the disease progresses, contractures and muscle wasting can occur. A mass in the medial portion of the groin due to synovial cyst formation rarely may develop. These alterations result in difficulty in ambulation, as well as other activities requiring hip motion, such as using a commode or engaging in sexual intercourse (Yoshino and Uichida, 1981).

PERIARTICULAR INVOLVEMENT

In addition to joint involvement, other significant causes of hip area pain in the rheumatoid patient include trochanteric bursitis (Raman and Haslock, 1982), "lipid nodules" (Mittal et al, 1968), dissecting synovial cysts (Peters et al, 1980; Pellman et al, 1986), and flexion contractures. Lipid nodules and synovial cysts are probably due to synovial distension in rheumatoid arthritis. In some chronic cysts, degenerating cells produce lipid collections. Synovial cysts at the hip frequently occur as an enlarging mass in the femoral–inguinal area. They may cause compression of adjacent structures, including the iliac vein, which may produce leg swelling and pseudothrombophlebitis. The cause of such cysts in so few patients is controversial, but may be due to synovial fluid herniation at a weak spot, or natural commu-

DIFFERENTIAL DIAGNOSIS OF CAUSES OF HIP PAIN

Arthropathies

Rheumatoid arthritis

Osteoarthritis

Seronegative arthropathies
Ankylosing spondylitis
Reiter's syndrome
Psoriatic arthropathy
Reactive arthropathies:
Acne
Enteropathic:
ulcerative colitis; Crohn's disease;
Whipple's disease; Behçet's disease;
postdysentery

Crystal-induced diseases
Gout
Pseudogout
(Calcium pyrophosphate dihydrate
crystal deposition)
Apatite crystal deposition
Oxalate crystal deposition

Amyloidosis

Lyme disease

Still's disease

Endocrine and metabolic disorders

Ochronosis

Hemochromatosis

Acromegaly

Paget's disease

Gaucher's disease

Familial Mediterranean fever

Local periarticular disease and neurologic disorders

Trauma
Bursitis

Fascia lata syndrome

Abductor and adductor
muscle strain

"Snapping hip syndrome"

Piriform muscle spasm

Fibromyalgia

Coccygodynia

Radiculopathy

Spinal stenosis

Entrapment neuropathies
Meralgia paresthetica
(lateral femoral
cutaneous nerve)
Obturator nerve
Abdominal cutaneous nerve
Sciatic nerve

Distant Referred Pain

Pelvic inflammatory disease

Testicular disease

Abdominal aortic aneurysm

Nephrolithiasis

Bone disease/damage

Fractures

Avascular necrosis

Hematologic disorders

Malignancy

Metabolic bone disease

Transient osteoporosis

Infection

Local Referred Pain

Sacral cysts

Episacroiliac lipomas

Osteitis condensans ilii

Osteitis pubis

Sacroiliac joint disease

Figure 11.1 Differential diagnosis of causes of hip pain.

nication of the joint with the iliopsoas bursa, with resultant bursal enlargement. Surgical excision is often necessary.

Fractures occur frequently in the hips of rheumatoid patients, especially those patients with giant cystic erosions, but fractures may occur even in the absence of cysts (Hadden et al, 1982; Williams et al, 1986). Transcervical and extracapsular lesions occur in rheumatoid patients in approximately the same ratio as in control populations of patients with hip fractures who do not have rheumatoid arthritis. In contrast to control patients, rheumatoid patients tend to have fractures at an earlier age and have them more spontaneously, but tend to survive the 2-month postfracture period at a rate greater than that of the general population. The reasons for this increased survival are unknown, but may be related to the lower frequency of multisystem trauma as the precipitating factor for the fracture and a lower incidence of other serious medical illnesses in the rheumatoid group.

Other patients may have low-back disease producing hip area pain (Terry and DeYoung, 1979; Heywood and Meyers, 1986). These patients may also complain of radiculopathy. Radiographs rarely may show lumbar rheumatoid disk disease. Coincidental degenerative disk disease is much more common. Patients with hip pain due only to back disease will have normal hip range of motion.

DIFFERENTIAL DIAGNOSIS

Arthropathies other than rheumatoid arthritis may affect the hip joint (Fig. 11.1). Most offer some general or local clues to their etiology.

Osteoarthritis of the hip is caused by various anatomic defects (either acquired, developmental, or congenital), trauma, or metabolic disorders (Peyron, 1986). Osteoarthritic pain is often clearly exacerbated by motion, whereas the rheumatoid patient also has morning stiffness. Osteoarthritis is loosely defined by radiologic abnormalities, including joint space narrowing, subchondral cysts, subchondral sclerosis, and osteophyte development (Fig. 11.2). Osteoarthritis of the hip is common and may affect 5% to 10% of the

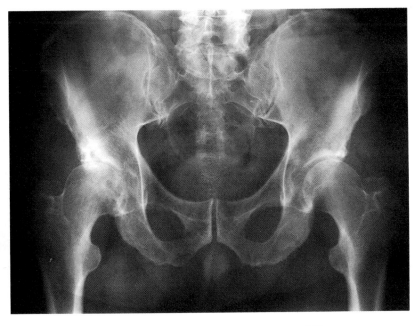

Figure 11.2 This patient with osteoarthritis has subchondral cysts, osteophyte formation, subchondral sclerosis, and joint space narrowing of the hip joint, especially on the right.

population. A particularly severe form of osteoarthritis-like hip disease may develop in patients with familial Mediterranean fever (Kaushansky et al, 1981).

The so-called "seronegative spondyloarthropathies" are a group of interrelated disorders that includes ankylosing spondylitis, Reiter's syndrome, psoriatic arthropathy, and reactive arthropathies associated with acne and inflammatory bowel diseases (Moll, 1974; Neumann and Wright, 1983; Calin, 1984). Many patients with these disorders have the HLA-B27 antigen on peripheral blood lymphocytes. They typically do not have serum rheumatoid factor or subcutaneous nodules, and may show familial aggregation. In contrast to rheumatoid arthritis, these disorders are often "enthesiopathic," with inflammation at the entheses or ligamentous insertions into bone, especially the sacroiliac joints, and are especially likely to have sacroiliac involvement.

Radiographic features that are useful in distinguishing ankylosing spondylitis hip involvement from rheumatoid arthritis include a greater frequency of asymmetric involvement, less periarticular demineralization, smaller erosive changes, and a propensity for bony ankylosis and marginal periostitis (Resnick et al, 1976) (Fig. 11.3).

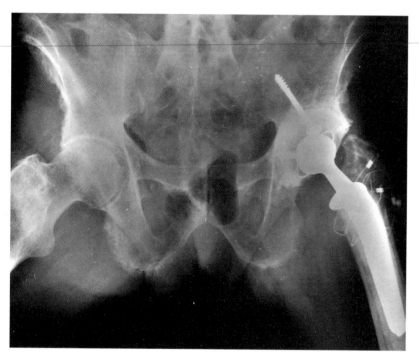

Figure 11.3 Anklosing spondylitis has resulted in joint space narrowing, subchondral sclerosis, and mild periarticular osteopenia of the right hip. However, the left hip was severely involved and joint replacement was required. Note the marginal periostitis about the hip joints and symphysis pubis, and the fused sacroiliac joints.

A variety of crystal induced diseases may affect the hip. Hip involvement in gout is unusual, and accounts for less than 5% of all sites of involvement (Barthelemy et al, 1984). Gouty attacks may even occur in the area of a prosthetic hip joint (Healy et al, 1984). Rare radiographic findings are marginal bone erosions with an overhanging edge at the periphery of the lesion.

Calcium pyrophosphate crystal deposition (CPPD) involves the hip more frequently. Approximately one third of cases with severe, destructive osteoarthritis are complicated by deposition of CPPD crystals (Fam et al, 1981). Rapid hip destruction in primary CPPD dep-

osition disease may also occur (Menkes et al, 1985). The hip joint is involved in approximately one third of patients during the course of the illness, especially in women, and is the most troublesome joint in approximately 8% of patients. Radiographs may show joint space narrowing, cysts, bony sclerosis, and chondrocalcinosis (Fig. 11.4).

The apatite crystal deposition syndrome commonly occurs as a periarthritis, or arthritis. Large joint areas such as the hip are commonly affected (Fam et al, 1979; Schumacher et al, 1981). In hip arthritis a rapidly destructive arthritis may follow and can lead to protrusio acetabuli, atrophic changes, and

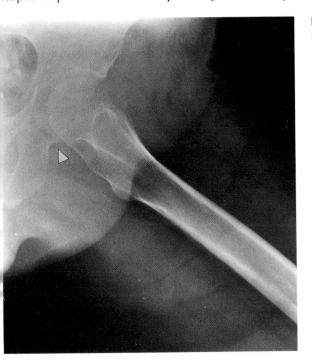

Figure 11.4 Pseudogout involvement of this hip joint is manifested by subchondral sclerosis, joint space narrowing, cysts, and chondrocalcinosis (arrow).

severe joint destruction that may necessitate total hip replacement (Dieppe et al, 1984) (Fig. 11.5).

Hip involvement may also be observed with oxalate crystal deposition (Reginato et al, 1986). This may be impossible to distinguish radiographically from apatite disease and requires study of joint fluid or tissue for diagnosis.

Amyloid deposition and infection may be other causes of severe destructive hip arthritis, especially in patients on dialysis.

In Lyme disease chronic synovitis may occur rapidly during the months after the onset of illness, with resultant joint destruction and erosion of cartilage and bone (Lawson and Steere, 1985). Radiographs often reveal loss of cartilage space, diffuse calcification, periarticular ossification at entheses, osteophytes, osteopenia, and large cysts (Fig. 11.6).

Still's disease (acute febrile juvenile rheumatoid arthritis in adults) affects the hip in approximately 10% of cases (Neumann and Wright, 1983). Bony sclerosis, erosions, and ankylosis may develop (Fig. 11.7).

Paget's disease of bone may also secondarily affect the hip joint (Hadjipavlou et al, 1986). Radiographs show bony expansion

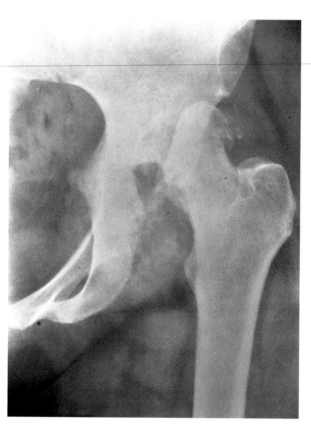 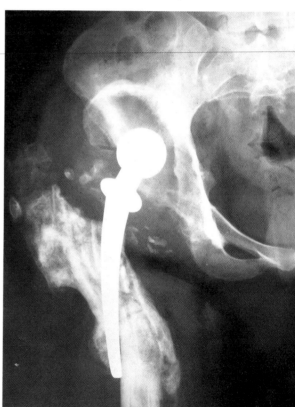

Figure 11.5 Apatite crystal deposition has resulted in severe joint destruction. The left hip (*left*) shows extensive bone resorption and obliteration of joint space, as well as osteophytes. The right hip had become so severely destroyed that a total hip replacement was performed (*right*) to relieve pain and increase hip range of motion.

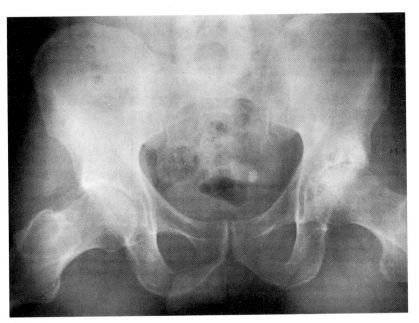

Figure 11.6 Chronic Lyme disease involving the hips can produce marked diffuse joint space narrowing and subchondral sclerosis. (Courtesy of Murray Dalinka, MD)

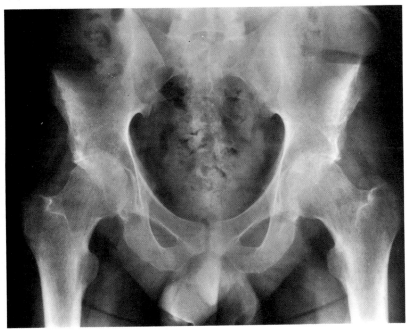

Figure 11.7 Still's disease affecting the hips has resulted in erosions and bony sclerosis, especially of the right hip.

and a remodeling phase with coarse trabeculae. The adjacent joint can become narrowed (Fig. 11.8). Protrusio acetabuli can occur, partially due to the softened bone.

Several endocrine and metabolic disorders with an arthropathic component affect the hip. Ochronosis (alkaptonuria) is a rare, hereditary disorder resulting from the deficiency of the enzyme homogentistic acid oxidase. A progressive degenerative arthropathy first involving the hip and lumbar spine may develop, with symptoms beginning in the fourth decade of life. Osteophyte formation is sparse. Gaucher's disease primarily involves the bone and may cause a severe secondary form of osteoarthritis with avascular necrosis. Hemochromatosis is characterized by excessive deposition of iron in parenchymal tissues. Chondrocalcinosis and osteoarthritis-like hip joint involvement are common. Acromegaly results from excessive growth hormone. The hip is the most frequently involved joint, with disease manifested by initial extensive hypertrophy of bone and cartilage followed by cartilage degeneration and the development of large osteophytes (Fig. 11.9).

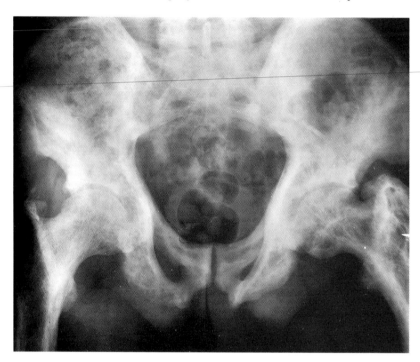

Figure 11.8 Diffuse Paget's disease of bone has resulted in early joint space narrowing bilaterally and disordered trabeculi in the bone.

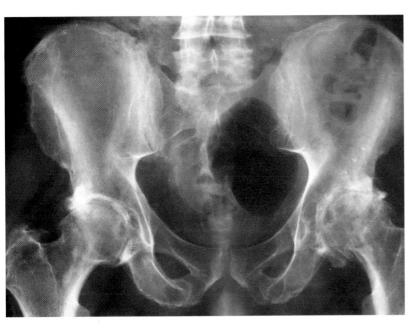

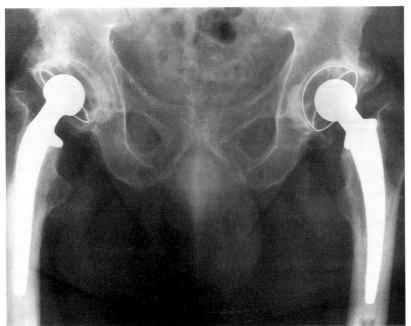

Figure 11.9 Progressive acromegaly involving the hips resulted in extensive hypertrophy of bone and cartilage with degenerative changes, including large osteophyte formation (*top*) associated with significant pain. Following bilateral total hip replacement (*bottom*), the patient experienced pain relief and increased hip motion.

Avascular necrosis of the femoral head produces femoral changes before any joint-space narrowing occurs (Fig. 11.10), and should be considered in all patients who have received high-dose corticosteroids or who have other risk factors such as alcoholism and vascular disease. Other diseases that may primarily involve the bone include hemophilia (Fig. 11.11), hemoglobinopathies, malignancies, metabolic bone disease, and transient osteoporosis and osteomyelitis.

Numerous bursae have been described in the hip (Fig. 11.12). Pathologic involvement of these structures is common. Most bursitis

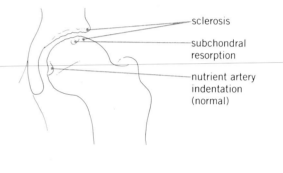

Figure 11.10 Avascular necrosis of the femoral head produces femoral abnormalities before joint space narrowing occurs. A tomographic view shows mild sclerosis and early subchondral resorption (*top*). A magnetic resonance image (*bottom*) depicts the medial superior subchondral resorption in even better detail.

sclerosis

subchondral resorption

nutrient artery indentation (normal)

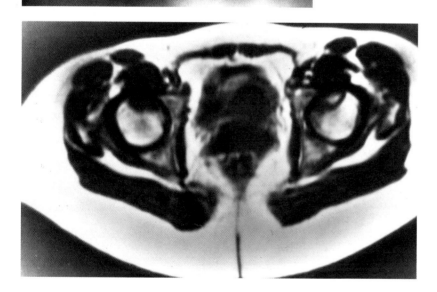

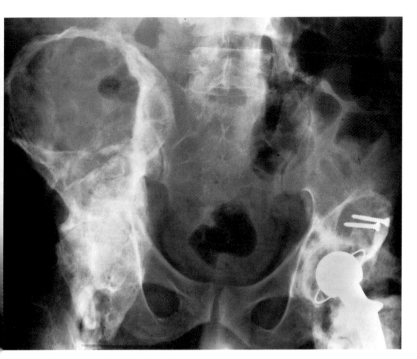

Figure 11.11 Hemophilia has resulted in joint space narrowing and sclerosis of the right hip and destruction of the left hip, necessitating total hip replacement. Note the pseudotumor in the right iliac and acetabular region. (Courtesy of Murray Dalinka, MD)

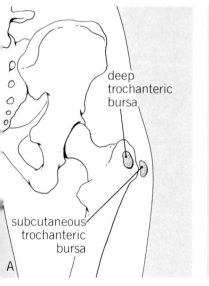
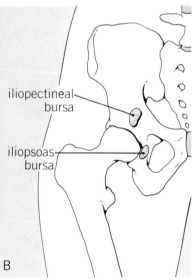

Figure 11.12 A. The superficial (subcutaneous or adventitial) and deep trochanteric bursae may be inflamed. **B.** The iliopectinal and iliopsoas bursae may also be inflamed and swollen, due to synovial fluid accumulation.

is idiopathic but disease of these bursae also can occur in patients with rheumatoid disease. The trochanteric bursa lies over the posterolateral prominence of the greater trochanter; a more superficial (adventitial) bursa is also often found in this region. Night pain and point tenderness, usually 2.5 cm posterior and superior to the greater trochanter, are found. The iliopectineal bursa lies between the iliopsoas muscle and the iliopectineal eminence. The iliopectineal and iliopsoas bursa may communicate with the hip joint, so that intrinsic hip disease may result in bursal pain. Palpation on the anterior thigh in Scarpa's triangle will reproduce iliopsoas bursal pain. The ischial (ischiogluteal) bursa lies more posteriorly along the ischial prominence near the sciatic nerve. The patient often experiences pain with bursitis at this site when sitting or lying down, and exquisite point tenderness is often found on palpation.

Meralgia paresthetica is an entrapment neuropathy of the lateral femoral cutaneous nerve (Fig. 11.13). Intermittent paresthesias occur over the anterior thigh. Other entrapment neuropathies include involvement of

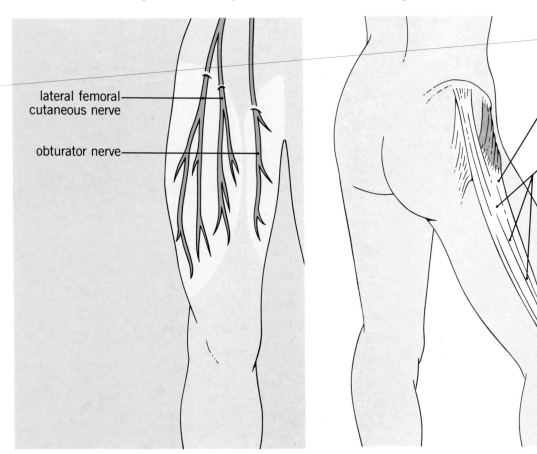

Figure 11.13 Meralgia paresthetica is entrapment of the lateral femoral cutaneous nerve that results in dysesthesias along the superior anterolateral area of the thigh.

Figure 11.14 Inflammation of the fascia lata results in tenderness along any point of the lateral portion of the thigh.

the obturator nerve with pain down the inner aspect of the groin and thigh, and of the abdominal cutaneous nerve with pain across the lower pelvis bridging the superior hip joint. Entrapment of the sciatic nerve at the hip is unusual.

Fascia lata fasciitis results in a dull ache over the lateral portion of the hip and lower back area that extends to the knee, which increases with walking or other mild exercise (Fig. 11.14). When the affected leg is held tightly across the other leg, dimpling or tenderness to palpation may result. Abductor and adductor muscle strain usually occur af-

ter strenuous exercise or following the commencement of a new form of exercise by a previously sedentary individual. The "snapping hip syndrome" describes a painless, nonpathologic clicking noise that results from a taut iliotibial band crossing the greater trochanter. Piriform muscle spasm can occur in the poorly understood syndrome of fibromyalgia (Sinaki et al, 1977). Other trigger points may be present in the hip and the lower back area, including involvement of the gluteus medius, multifidus, and iliocostal muscles (Fig. 11.15). Coccygodynia can be due to numerous disorders, but all result in

Figure 11.15 Multiple myofascial trigger points exist in the lower back area. These areas of tenderness may be present following mechanical back injury, or as part of the fibromyalgia/fibrositis syndrome.

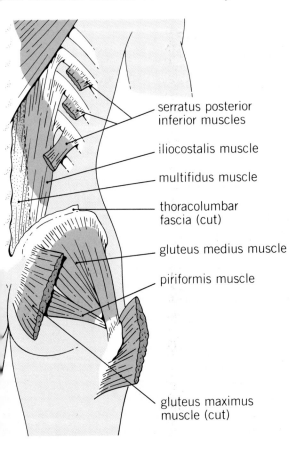

serratus posterior inferior muscles

iliocostalis muscle

multifidus muscle

thoracolumbar fascia (cut)

gluteus medius muscle

piriformis muscle

gluteus maximus muscle (cut)

pain in the coccyx region. Aching discomfort in this region following defecation or sexual intercourse is often diagnostic.

Radiculopathy frequently produces pain in the posterior hip, buttock, and thigh. The pain can be either more lateral if primarily L-5 is involved, or medial if the S-1 root is affected. Spinal stenosis, a disorder resulting from narrowing of the neural canal, frequently results in posterior hip pain and pseudoclau-dication. Patients will frequently complain of pain while standing or walking, and often find relief of pain with sitting, leaning forward, or lying down with flexed legs.

Pain in the hip may also be due to locally referred pain. Most such pain is from the sacroiliac joint and due to the seronegative spondyloarthropathies described above. Sacral cysts and episacroiliac lipomas should also be considered. Episacroiliac lipomas are

Figure 11.16 An anatomical approach to hip pain.

AN ANATOMICAL APPROACH TO HIP PAIN	
LOCATION OF PAIN	CAUSES OF PAIN
Anterior and medial thigh	Hip joint Arthropathies Bone disease/damage Local periarticular disease Iliopectineal bursitis Meralgia paresthetica Obturator neuropathy Abdominal cutaneous neuropathy Adductor/quadriceps muscle strain Distant referred pain
Lateral hip and thigh	Local periarticular disease Trochanteric bursitis Meralgia paresthetica Fascia lata syndrome Abductor muscle strain "Snapping hip syndrome"
Posterior hip, thigh, and buttock	Local periarticular disease Radiculopathy: L-5 (lateral) or S-1 (medial) Piriform muscle spasm Fibromyalgia Coccygodynia Spinal stenosis Local referred pain

fleshy, soft nodules occurring near the sacro-iliac joint at the insertion of the spinal erector muscles. Although these nodules frequently occur in the normal population, some patients have localized pain and tenderness (Singewald, 1966).

Pain syndromes of the pelvis may also result in pain referred to the hip. Osteitis condensans ilii is a sclerosing disorder on the iliac side of the pubis at the sacroiliac joint. Some patients with this radiographic finding complain of sciatica or fibromyalgia symptoms. Symptoms are usually self-limited. Osteitis pubis is inflammation of the periosteal bone of the symphysis pubis that is detected clinically by the location of the pain and radiographic findings of sclerosis, erosions, and symphysis widening. Although osteitis pubis may also occur following direct spread of prostate or bladder disease, it is more frequently seen in patients with seronegative spondyloarthropathy or chondrocalcinosis (Scott et al, 1979). In some cases, patients have no predisposing condition for the development of this disorder.

Pelvic inflammatory disease in women and testicular diseases, including torsion and malignancy, are disorders of reproductive organs that may result in pain radiating to the buttocks, thighs, and hip region. Retroperitoneal disease, including psoas abscess and fibrosis, nephrolithiasis, and abdominal aortic aneurysm, may result in referred pain. An anatomical approach to the differential diagnosis of hip pain is also presented (Fig. 11.16).

RADIOGRAPHIC FINDINGS

Radiographic abnormalities of the rheumatoid hip usually are bilaterally symmetric, although unilateral asymmetric lesions may occur (Isdale, 1962; Glick et al, 1963; Duthie and Harris, 1969; Resnick, 1975). The most typical finding is loss of joint space (Duthie and Harris, 1969; Resnick 1975); narrowing is usually concentric, reflecting a diffuse loss of cartilage (Fig. 11.17). This results in axial

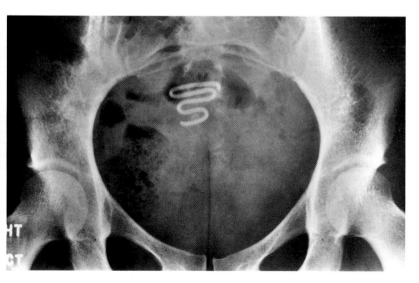

Figure 11.17 This patient with early rheumatoid arthritis has mild, concentric loss of hip joint space bilaterally.

migration toward the midline of the femoral head. However, loss of joint space in rare cases may occur only superiorly, and the femoral head may shift only upward, a pattern commonly seen in osteoarthritis. The pattern of wear in rheumatoid patients is also more posterior compared with osteoarthritic patients (Barrie, 1986).

As the disease progresses, the loss of joint space also usually progresses until the femoral head and acetabulum abut (Fig. 11.18). Loss of acetabular bone results in protrusio acetabuli and disruption of Shenton's line, with eventual collapse of the acetabular roof (Fig. 11.19). Medial migration of the acetabulum of 3 mm or more in men and 6 mm or more in women can be considered protrusio acetabuli. Protrusio acetabuli is particularly common in rheumatoid arthritis. In one study of 694 unselected consecutive rheumatoid-factor–positive patients, 5% had some degree of protrusio. Bilateral protrusio was present in approximately half of the patients. Interestingly, there was a significant association with prior treatment with corticosteroids (Hastings and Parker, 1975).

Protrusio in rheumatoid disease may be distinguished from primary or idiopathic protrusio (Otto's pelvis) by the older age of onset in the rheumatoid patient and by the lack of gross changes in the femoral head in most patients with the primary variety (Edelstein and Murphy, 1983). Other disorders that may cause protrusio include osteoarthritis, the seronegative spondyloarthropathies, radiation therapy, Paget's disease, and neoplasm.

Cysts and erosions have also been well described in rheumatoid disease of the hip (Duthie and Harris, 1969; Resnick, 1975). The earliest erosions occur near the femoral neck, and usually are seen later than erosions of the small bones of the hand and foot. This may be due to the thicker bone in the hip. Giant granulomatous cysts may predispose to hip fracture (Colton and Darby, 1970).

Progressive bony sclerosis, bone resorption and collapse, and/or eventual osteophyte formation may also occur as the joint attempts to repair itself. These changes suggest primary osteoarthritis, but the presence of symmetric joint space loss, significant osseous resorption, and the "brushed away" appearance of osteopenia surrounding the inflamed joint are more typical of rheumatoid disease.

Untreated hip disease may eventually lead to complete obliteration of the joint space with fibrous, but not bony, ankylosis. Interestingly, recovery of joint space has occurred when the contralateral hip joint has been replaced (Pascual et al, 1975). The mechanism of this repair is unknown.

Avascular necrosis of the femoral head is not uncommon in patients treated with high-dose corticosteroids (Bossingham et al, 1978). Radiographic detection of avascular necrosis in the rheumatoid patient is difficult when the patient also has signs of rheumatoid disease; however, significant osseous collapse, cyst formation, and sclerosis are also characteristic of avascular necrosis.

In addition to imaging of the hip with radiographs and bone scans, computerized axial tomography (CAT) scans and magnetic resonance imaging (MRI) may be valuable modalities to image this deep joint.

IMPLICATIONS FOR THERAPY

Nonoperative, nonpharmacologic modes of therapy for rheumatoid hip disease include range of motion exercises and physical therapy to maintain motion and strength, weight reduction where appropriate, and the use of crutches or other supportive devices. The primary indications for operative therapy are significant pain and disability that remains after aggressive nonoperative approaches. Disability in general should be so great that the patient is willing to take perhaps a 5%

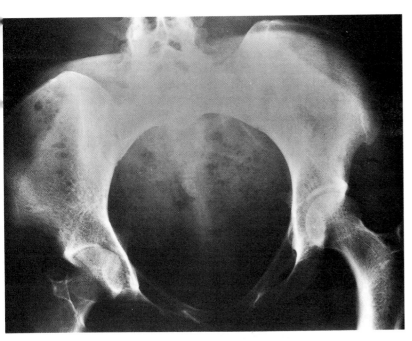

Figure 11.18 Progressive rheumatoid arthritis has resulted in further axial migration (to the midline) of the hips, further joint space narrowing, and the development of erosions.

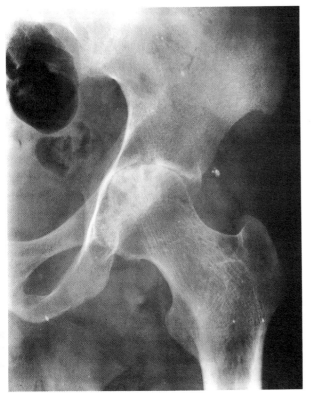

Figure 11.19 Protrusio acetabuli in this patient with rheumatoid arthritis is evident in the left hip. Also note the erosions, cysts, sclerosis, and loss of joint space.

chance of being worse after surgery. Other causes of hip pain, including lumbar spine disease and soft tissue involvement, should be ruled out.

Hip replacement has begun to be used more frequently in rheumatoid arthritis, and it is now not uncommon to have patients with replacement of both hips and both knees (McElwain and Sheehan, 1985; Yoshino, 1985) (Fig. 11.20).

The most common operative procedures used to treat the patient with rheumatoid arthritis are noted in Figure 11.21. The choice of the specific procedure is based on the functional status and age of the patient, and the experience of the surgeon. More than 90% of rheumatoid patients experience symptomatic improvement following surgery (Liang and Cullen, 1984; Poss et al, 1984).

Complications of hip replacement in rheumatoid arthritis are the same as those encountered in patients with other diseases. However, rheumatoid patients tend to have more intraoperative fractures, difficulties with anesthesia, and malposition of prosthetic components (Poss et al, 1984).

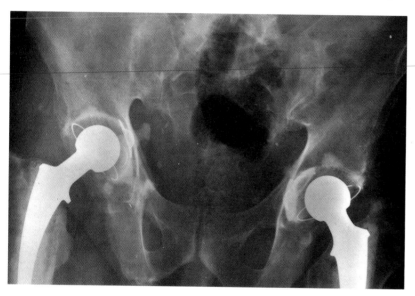

Figure 11.20 This patient with rheumatoid arthritis affecting the hips underwent bilateral hip replacements with excellent results.

MOST COMMON OPERATIVE PROCEDURES USED TO TREAT RHEUMATOID ARTHRITIS OF THE HIP

Arthroplasties	Girdlestone pseudoarthrosis
Cup	Osteotomy
Femoral endoprosthesis Bipolar Unipolar	Soft tissue release
	Surgical revision
Surface replacement	Synovectomy
Total hip replacement	Fusion

Figure 11.21 Most common operative procedures used to treat rheumatoid arthritis of the hip.

REFERENCES

Barrie HJ: Unexpected sites of wear in the femoral head. *J Rheumatol* 1986;13:1099–1104.

Barthelemy CR, Nakayama DA, Carrera GF, et al: Gouty arthritis: a prospective radiographic evaluation of sixty patients. *Skeletal Radiol* 1984;11:1–8.

Bossingham DH, Schorn D, Morgan G: Patterns of hip involvement in rheumatoid arthritis *Ann Rheum Dis* 1978; 37:293 (abstract).

Calin A (ed): *Spondyloarthropathies.* Orlando, FL, Grune & Stratton, 1984.

Colton CL, Darby AJ: Giant granulomatous lesions of the femoral head and neck in rheumatoid arthritis. *Ann Rheum Dis* 1970;29:626–633.

Dieppe PA, Doherty M, MacFarlane DG, et al: Apatite associated destructive arthritis. *Br J Rheumatol* 1984;23:84–91.

Duthie R, Harris C: A radiographic and clinical survey of the hip joints in sero-positive rheumatoid arthritis. *Acta Orthop Scand* 1969;40:346–364.

Edelstein G, Murphy WA: Protrusio acetabuli: Radiographic appearance in arthritis and other conditions. *Arthritis Rheum* 1983;1511–1516.

Fam AG, Pritzker KPH, Stein JL, et al: Apatite-associated arthropathy: A clinical study of 14 cases and of 2 patients with calcific bursitis. *J Rheumatol* 1979;6:461–471.

Fam AG, Topp JR, Stein HB, et al: Clinical and roentgenographic aspects of pseudogout: A study of 50 cases and a review. *Can Med Assoc J* 1981;124:545–551.

Glick EN, Mason RM, Wenley WG: Rheumatoid arthritis affecting the hip joint. *Ann Rheum Dis* 1963;22:416–423.

Hadden WA, Abernethy PJ, Haw C: Hip fractures in rheumatoid arthritis. *Clin Orthop* 1982; 170:252–259.

Hadjipavlou A, Lander P, Srolovitz H: Pagetic arthritis: Pathophysiology and management. *Clin Orthop* 1986;208:15–19.

Hastings DE, Parker SM: Protrusio acetabuli in rheumatoid arthritis. *Clin Orthop* 1975;108:76–83.

Healey JH, Dines D, Hershon S: Painful synovitis secondary to gout in the area of a prosthetic hip joint. *J Bone Joint Surg Am* 1984;66:610–611.

Heywood AWB, Meyers OL: Rheumatoid arthritis of the thoracic and lumbar spine. *J Bone Joint Surg Br* 1986;68:362–368.

Isdale IC: Femoral neck destruction in rheumatoid arthritis and osteoarthritis: A clinical review of 27 cases. *Ann Rheum Dis* 1962;21:23–30.

Kaushansky K, Finerman GAM, Schwabe AD: Chronic destructive arthritis in familial Mediterranean fever: The predominance of hip involvement and its management. *Clin Orthop* 1981;155:156–161.

Lawson JP, Steere AC: Lyme disease: Radiographic findings. *Radiology* 1985;154:37–43.

Liang MH, Cullen KE: Evaluation of outcomes in total joint arthroplasty for rheumatoid arthritis. *Clin Orthop* 1984;182:41–45.

McElwain JP, Sheehan JM: Bilateral hip and knee replacement for rheumatoid arthritis. *J Bone Joint Surg Br* 1985;67:261–265.

Menkes CJ, Decraemere W, Postel M, Forest M: Chondrocalcinosis and rapid hip destruction. *J Rheumatol* 1985;12:130–133.

Mittal A, Block MA, Wylie JH Jr: Lipoid nodules of chronic rheumatoid arthritis presenting in the groin. *Am Surgeon* 1968;34:309–310.

Moll JMH, Haslock I, Macrae I, et al: Associations between ankylosing spondylitis, psoratic arthritis, Reiter's disease, the intestinal arthropathies, and Beçhet's syndrome. *Medicine* 1974;53:343–364.

Neumann V, Wright V: Arthritis associated with bowel disease. *Clin Gastroenterol* 1983;12:767–795.

Pascual E, Steinberg ME, Schumacher HR: Restoration of the hip joint space in long-standing rheumatoid arthritis following contralateral cup arthroplasty. *Clin Orthop* 1975;111:121–123.

Pellman E, Kumari S, Greenwald R: Rheumatoid iliopsoas bursitis presenting as unilateral leg edema. *J Rheumatol* 1986;13:197–200.

Peters JC, Coleman BG, Turner ML, et al: CT evaluation of enlarged iliopsoas bursa. *AJR* 1980; 135:392–394.

Peyron JG: Osteoarthritis: The epidemiologic viewpoint. *Clin Orthop* 1986;213:13–19.

Poss R, Maloney JP, Ewald FC, et al: Six- to 11-year results of total hip arthroplasty in rheumatoid arthritis. *Clin Orthop* 1984;182:109–116.

Raman D, Haslock I: Trochanteric bursitis-a frequent cause of "hip" pain in rheumatoid arthritis. *Ann Rheum Dis* 1982;41:602–603.

Reginato AJ, Seoane JLF, Alvarez CB, et al: Arthropathy and cutaneous calcinosis in hemodialysis oxalosis. *Arthritis Rheum* 1986;29:387–396.

Resnick D: Patterns of migration of the femoral head in osteoarthritis of the hip: Roentgenographic-pathologic correlation and comparison with rheumatoid arthritis. *AJR* 1975;124:62.

Resnick D, Dwosh IL, Georgen TG, et al: Clinical and radiographic abnormalities in ankylosing spondylitis: A comparison of men and women. *Radiology* 1976;119:293–297.

Schumacher HR, Miller JL, Ludivico C, et al: Erosive arthritis associated with apatite crystal deposition. *Arthritis Rheum* 1981;24:31–37.

Scott DL, Eastmond CJ, Wright V: A comparative study of the pubic symphysis in rheumatic disorders. *Ann Rheum Dis* 1979;38:529–534.

Sinaki M, Merritt JL, Stillwell GK: Tension myalgia of the pelvic floor. *Mayo Clin Proc* 1977;52:717–722.

Singewald ML: Sacroiliac lipomata: An often unrecognized cause of low back pain. *Johns Hopkins Med J* 1966;118:492–498.

Terry AF, DeYoung R: Hip disease mimicking low back disorders. *Orthop Rev* 1979;8:95–104.

Williams PL, Amin NK, Young A: Unsuspected fractures of the femoral neck in patients with chronic hip pain due to rheumatoid arthritis. *Br Med J* 1986;292:1125–1126.

Yoshino S: Multiple replacements of major joints in rheumatoid arthritis. *Orthopedics* 1985;8:57–59.

Yoshino S, Uichida S: Sexual problems of women with rheumatoid arthritis. *Arch Phys Med Rehabil* 1981;62:122–123.

CHAPTER 12

THE SPINE

MICHAEL J. MARICIC, MD

In the presence of rheumatoid synovitis, increased motion of a joint may be responsible for increased susceptibility to damage. The cervical spine, especially the synovial atlantoaxial joint, has a higher frequency of significant clinical and radiographic involvement in rheumatoid arthritis than the dorsal, lumbar, or sacroiliac joints, probably due to its greater use and motion.

JOINT INVOLVEMENT

In 1890, Garrod was the first to describe clinical involvement of the cervical spine in rheumatoid arthritis, noting its presence in 28% of his patients. Current estimates of clinical involvement vary from 40% to 70% (Conlon and Markely, 1966; Bland, 1974), while estimates of the prevalence of radiographic changes secondary to rheumatoid

arthritis vary from 50% to 86%, depending on the technique for detection and attentiveness to such changes (Bland, 1974). A lack of correlation between radiographic and clinical abnormalities may be present, and some patients with significant radiographic evidence of disease may be entirely asymptomatic, necessitating a thorough neurological examination and strict correlation of symptoms and signs with radiographic changes.

In order to describe the specific clinical abnormalities of the cervical spine in rheumatoid arthritis, it will be useful to divide the cervical spine into the occipitoatlantoaxial articulation and the subaxial articulations, and to review their respective anatomy.

The occiput rests on the superior articulating surfaces of the lateral masses of the atlas, permitting anteroposterior motion of the head (Fig. 12.1). The inferior articulating surfaces of the atlas articulate with the axis

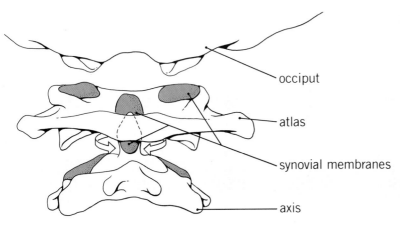

occiput

atlas

synovial membranes

axis

Figure 12.1 The relationship between the occiput, atlas, and axis in the anteroposterior view is shown. (The separation of the bones is exaggerated for better visualization.)

and permit rotatory movement. The odontoid process of the axis acts as the pivot upon which the atlas, carrying the head, rotates. Immediately posterior to the odontoid is the transverse ligament, which serves to hold the odontoid in firm proximity to the anterior arch of the atlas (Fig. 12.2). The odontoid is also held in position by the cruciform ligament, which is derived from the transverse ligament and connects the odontoid to the base of the occiput and the body of the axis, and the alar ligaments, which extend from the odontoid process to the occipital condyles. The anterior and posterior articulating surfaces of the odontoid, the articulating surfaces connecting the lateral masses of the occiput and atlas, and the atlas and axis, are lined by synovial membranes. Rheumatoid inflammation of these synovial structures may lead to erosions of the lateral masses or the odontoid, and may weaken and cause destruction of the transverse, cruciform, or alar ligaments, and leading subsequently to varying types of subluxation.

SUBLUXATION

There are four main types of subluxations which may occur: anterior, posterior, vertical (basilar invagination or cranial settling), and lateral (rotary). Anterior atlantoaxial sublux-

ation (AAS) is the most common type and is thought to be secondary to laxity or rupture of the transverse ligament due to synovial inflammation and hyperemia of the adjacent articulations. During flexion, the atlas separates anteriorly from the axis, and the spinal canal is compressed by the posterior arch of the atlas. The patient may be entirely asymptomatic or may exhibit any of a number of symptoms (Fig. 12.3). Synovitis may cause local pain and muscle spasm. Irritation or compression of the first and second cranial nerves may cause referred pain or headache, usually prominent in the occiput, but may also be referred to the temporal or retro-orbital regions. If spinal cord compression results, long tract signs may occur, such as paresthesia of the hands and feet, quadriparesis of varying degrees of severity, or dysfunction of the bowel or bladder. These will usually be accompanied by hyperreflexia and a Babinski sign, although these neurological abnormalities may be difficult to detect in the rheumatoid patient with advanced joint deformities. Because the vertebral arteries pass through the foraminae transversariae of C-1, anterior AAS may cause kinking and/or occlusion of the arteries, leading to a variety of vertebrobasilar symptoms, such as nausea, vomiting, dysarthria, dysphagia, blurred or double vision, or transient loss of consciousness (Fig. 12.4).

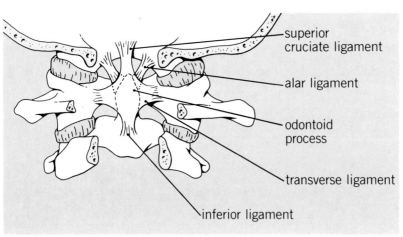

superior cruciate ligament

alar ligament

odontoid process

transverse ligament

inferior ligament

Figure 12.2 The relationship of the transverse ligament to the posterior surface of the odontoid process is seen in this posterior view.

CLINICAL MANIFESTATIONS OF ANTERIOR ATLANTOAXIAL SUBLUXATION

Secondary to synovial inflammation

Neck pain

Cervical muscle spasm

"Clicking"

Secondary to nerve root compression

Neck pain

Radicular pain (occipital,
temporal, retro-orbital)

Secondary to cord compression

Paresthesia

Paresis

Bowel or bladder dysfunction

Hyperreflexia, extensor plantar reflexes

Secondary to vertebral artery compression

Nausea, vomiting

"Drop attacks"

Opthalmoplegia

Cerebellar signs
(dysarthria, dysphagia, ataxia)

Figure 12.3   Clinical manifestations of anterior atlantoaxial subluxation.

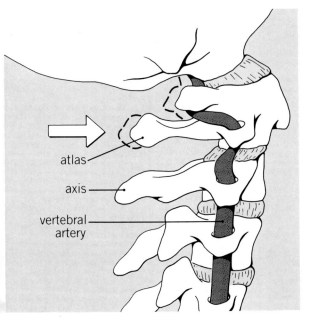

Figure 12.4   The vertebral arteries pass through the foraminae transversariae and are predisposed to "kinking" in the event of anterior subluxation.

atlas

axis

vertebral
artery

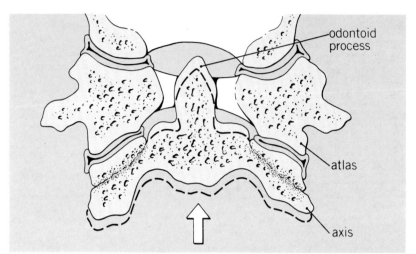

Figure 12.5 The odontoid process tends to migrate upward in the event of destruction of the supporting structures between the occiput and the atlas, or between the atlas and the axis.

odontoid process

atlas

axis

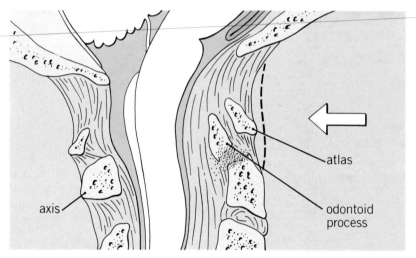

Figure 12.6 Erosion of the odontoid process can lead to posterior subluxation of the atlas over the axis. The anterior portion of the spinal cord can then be compressed by the anterior arch of the atlas.

atlas

odontoid process

axis

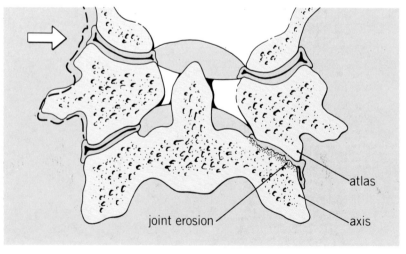

Figure 12.7 Lateral subluxation of the atlas to the right occurs as a result of erosion and collapse of the right C1-2 facet joint as seen in posterior view.

joint erosion

atlas

axis

Vertical subluxations (cranial settling and/or basilar invagination) may occur as a result of erosion and collapse of the bony and articular supporting structures between either the occiput and the atlas or between the atlas and the axis (Fig. 12.5). The vertically subluxed odontoid may compress the brain stem and cause sudden death. Fortunately erosion and lysis of the odontoid process by synovitis frequently coexists with vertical subluxation and this may protect the brain stem from this compression. Upper cervical and occipital pain are frequently present. Since vertical and anterior subluxation often coexist, the symptoms or signs of anterior AAS may also be present.

Posterior subluxation (Fig. 12.6) arises as a result of complete erosion of, or fracture through, the odontoid process. These changes allow posterior movement of C-1 upon C-2, especially in extension. As with anterior AAS, local pain, long tract signs or vertebrobasilar symptoms may be present.

Lateral or rotary subluxation (Fig. 12.7) occurs as a result of erosion and collapse of the lateral C1-2 facet joints with subsequent disruption of the articular capsules and lateral shift of the atlas upon the axis (Halla and Fallahis, 1982.) Lateral subluxation accompanies approximately 20% of all anterior AAS. Because it further reduces the spinal canal, it is more frequently seen in neurologically abnormal patients (Weissman et al, 1982). If the degree of subluxation is severe enough, lateral subluxation may actually cause a noticeable tilting of the head to the left or right (Fig. 12.8).

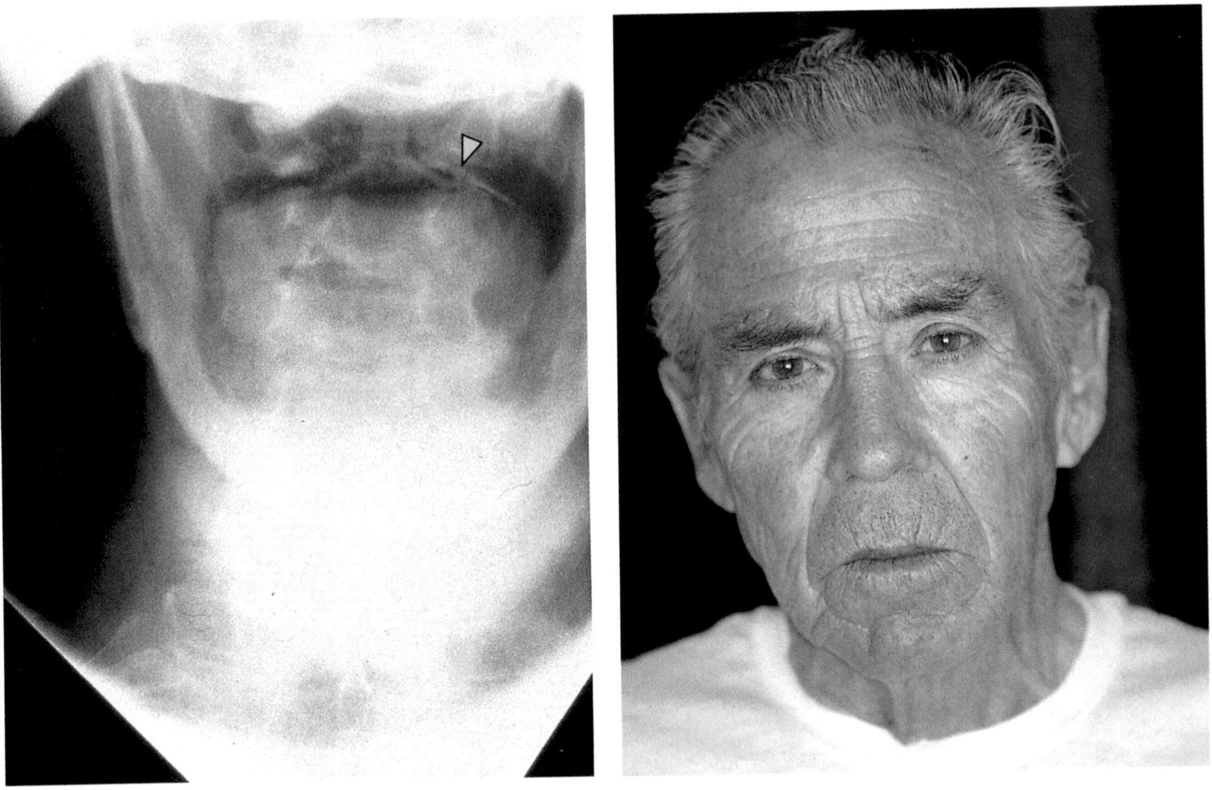

Figure 12.8 A patient with lateral subluxation of C-1 upon C-2 (arrow). C-1 has shifted to the right as a result of erosion and collapse of the C1-2 facet joints (*left*). The head is held tilted to the right (*right*).

Discovertebral joint abnormalities (joint space narrowing and end plate erosions) are a much more prominent feature of the cervical spine than of the dorsal and lumbar spines in rheumatoid arthritis. These lesions originate in the neurocentral joints of Luschka, which are found only in the cervical spine (Fig. 12.9). These joints are clefts lined by synovium located at the posterolateral margin of the disc. Whether the discs are damaged by pannus extending from the joints of Luschka (Ball, 1971) or by intravertebral herniation of discal material as a result of apophyseal joint instability (Martel, 1977) is still a subject of debate. In either case, the resultant damage to the disc predisposes it to subluxation. Particularly characteristic of rheumatoid arthritis are subluxations at the C3-4 and C4-5 levels, which are typically serial and produce a "staircase" appearance. Subaxial disease may also be characterized by spinous process erosions and apophyseal joint narrowing and erosions.

Signs and symptoms of subaxial disease may be due to local inflammation, nerve root compression, or spinal cord compression. Pain may be felt over the spinous processes and the cervical musculature, or it may radiate into the chest, the interscapular area, or down the arms. Subaxial subluxation may cause cord compression and result in long tract signs and symptoms.

PERIARTICULAR DISEASE

As opposed to appendicular joints where obvious swelling and erythema of adjacent soft tissues may be visible, there is usually a paucity of soft tissue change observable in cervical spine disease due to the position of the joints deep within the cervical musculature. Tilting or "guarding" of the neck toward the site of pain may be seen and palpation of the musculature will often reveal tenderness and spasm. Fasiculations may suggest local nerve root irritation and atrophy of the muscles may be evident secondary to long-standing inflammation and disuse.

Rheumatoid nodules may occasionally be found along the posterior aspect of the cervical spine. They are usually found there only in patients with extensive nodulosis.

DIFFERENTIAL DIAGNOSIS

A number of other arthritic disorders may mimic rheumatoid involvement of the spine (Fig. 12.10). In the cervical spine, other chronic inflammatory diseases, such as juvenile onset arthritis, ankylosing spondylitis,

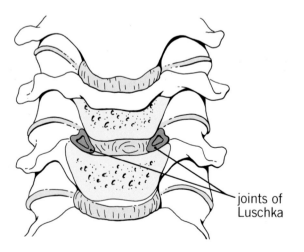

Figure 12.9 The joints of Luschka are located posterolaterally in the cervical spine. They are lined with synovium and are thought to play a significant role in the genesis of discovertebral disease.

joints of Luschka

psoriatic arthritis, and Reiter's syndrome, may cause erosions, discovertebral disease, and subluxation.

Juvenile onset rheumatoid arthritis, especially the polyarticular seropositive form, may cause atlantoaxial subluxation (Ansell, 1977), although it can also be observed in Still's disease and juvenile ankylosing spondylitis (Fig. 12.11). Other characteristic features of rheumatoid arthritis of juvenile onset which help differentiate it from the adult onset form include apophyseal joint space narrowing and bony ankylosis, most commonly seen at the C2-3 and C3-4 levels.

Atlantoaxial subluxation may be found in up to 2% of adult ankylosing spondylitis patients (Sharp, 1961). Erosions and subaxial subluxations may also be present. Extensive

DIFFERENTIAL DIAGNOSIS OF ATLANTOAXIAL SUBLUXATION

Rheumatoid Arthritis

Atlantoaxial subluxation with subaxial subluxation

Diffuse osteopenia

Erosions of the subchondral plates

Juvenile Rheumatoid Arthritis

Atlantoaxial subluxation (polyarticular, seropositive type)

Apophyseal joint narrowing and fusion (especially at C2-3 and C3-4)

Idiopathic Ankylosing Spondylitis

Extensive apophyseal joint ankylosis

Ossification of the anterior longitudinal ligament

"Squaring" of the vertebral bodies

Psoriatic Arthritis

Scattered syndesmophyte formation producing "skip" lesions

Lack of osteopenia (differentiation from ankylosing spondylitis/rheumatoid arthritis)

Reiter's Disease

Lesions similar to psoriatic arthritis

Figure 12.10   Differential diagnosis of atlantoaxial subluxation

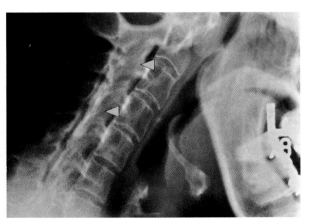

Figure 12.11   Anterior AAS in juvenile onset rheumatoid arthritis is associated with extensive apophyseal joint fusion (arrows).

ankylosis of apophyseal joints and ossification of interspinous and supraspinous ligaments in the cervical spine (Fig. 12.12), thoracic spine, and lumbar spine, along with bilateral fusion of the sacroiliac joints, should help to differentiate this disease from rheumatoid arthritis.

Atlantoaxial subluxation also may be seen rarely in psoriatic arthritis (Killibrew et al, 1973) (Fig. 12.13) and even less commonly in Reiter's syndrome (Latchaw and Mayer, 1978). Syndesmophyte formation, apophyseal joint fusion, and sacroiliac abnormalities are all seen more commonly in these diseases than in rheumatoid arthritis and may give a clue to the proper diagnosis.

All of the diseases discussed above may cause discovertebral joint abnormalities. However, septic discitis in particular may cause a great deal of difficulty for those attempting to differentiate its discovertebral changes from those of rheumatoid arthritis, and it may coincide with rheumatoid arthritis. Disc space narrowing, end plate erosions (which may be wide-based), and lack of reactive sclerosis are characteristics of both

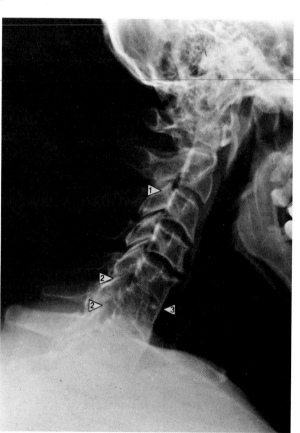

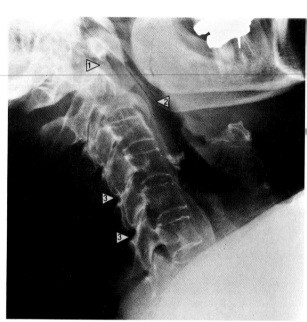

Figure 12.13 Anterior AAS in psoriatic arthritis. The odontoid and dens axis are separated by a distance of 4 mm (arrow 1). Note the large syndesmophyte (arrow 2) at the base of C-2 and extensive apophyseal joint erosion and fusion (arrows 3).

Figure 12.12 Cervical spine in ankylosing spondylitis. Note the apophyseal joint erosion at C2-3 (arrow 1) and fusion at C5-6 and C6-7 (arrows 2) Ossification of the anterior longitudinal ligament bridges the lower cervical vertebrae (arrow 3).

diseases. Tomographic and radionuclide studies may be helpful in differentiating the two. A high index of suspicion, correlation of films with the clinical picture, and comparison of old films (to estimate the progression of disease) are the most important tools for proper diagnosis.

Osteoarthritis may cause discovertebral abnormalities. These abnormalities are usually accompanied by end plate sclerosis and osteophyte formation, and usually affect the lower cervical spine, especially C5-6 and C6-7 (Fig. 12.14). Osteoarthritis rarely should be a cause for confusion with rheumatoid arthritis, although the two diseases may coexist and thereby alter the radiographic picture.

While diffuse idiopathic skeletal hyperostosis (DISH) most commonly affects the thoracic and lumbar spines, cervical spine involvement may be seen in up to 80% of cases. Hyperostosis of the anterior cortex of the vertebrae and flowing ossification of the anterior longitudinal ligament with preservation of the joint spaces are hallmarks of this disease (Fig. 12.15), and rarely may cause confusion with rheumatoid arthritis. The two diseases may

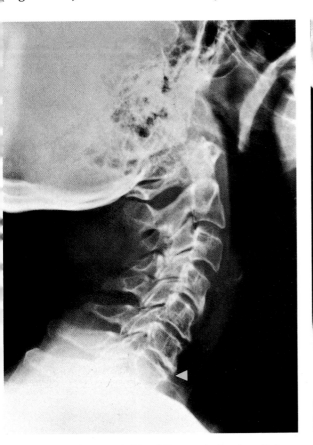

Figure 12.14 Osteoarthritis of the cervical spine. Note that the discovertebral narrowing involves predominantly the lower cervical spine and is accompanied by end plate sclerosis and osteophytes (arrow).

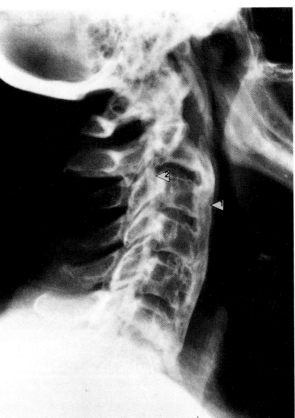

Figure 12.15 Diffuse idiopathic skeletal hyperostosis. There is flowing ossification of both the anterior (arrow 1) and posterior (arrow 2) longitudinal ligaments. Note that the joint spaces are preserved.

coexist, however. In these instances, the vertebral sclerosis, proliferative osseous change around erosions, and the degree of bony ankylosis are greater than that seen in rheumatoid arthritis alone (Resnick, 1978).

Calcium pyrophosphate dihydrate deposition disease (CPPD) may occasionally involve the cervical spine, producing disc space narrowing, end plate sclerosis, and subluxations, including atlantoaxial subluxation (Resnick, 1977). Calcification of the intervertebral discs, and/or ligamentum flavum help differentiate this disease from rheumatoid arthritis.

Gouty involvement of the spine is distinctly uncommon; however, erosion of the odontoid process and vertebral subluxation has been reported (Kersley, 1950).

Calcium hydroxyapatite crystals have been found to cause calcific tendinitis of the longus colli muscle in the neck (Hall, 1986) and have also been associated with a destructive spondylarthropathy in hemodialysis patients (Kuntz, 1984). The absence of osteophytes, severe narrowing of the intervertebral discs, and deep erosions and geodes of the vertebral end plates are typical findings. Radiologic findings may resemble infectious discitis and disc biopsy may be required for definitive diagnosis. The setting of hemodialysis and a lack of peripheral joint involvement would be helpful clues in differentiating this entity from rheumatoid arthritis.

Amyloidosis has also recently been implicated as a cause of destructive spondyloar-

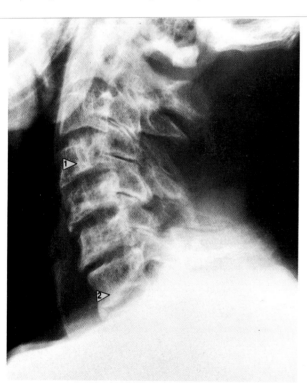

Figure 12.16 Paget's disease. Coarsening of the trabeculae (arrow 1) and expansion of vertebral bodies (arrow 2) are characteristic.

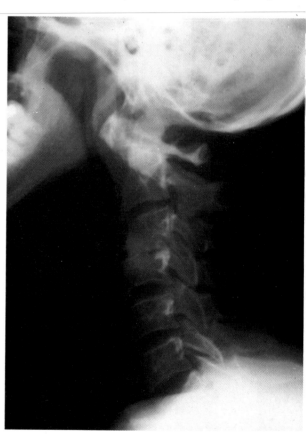

Figure 12.17 Note the marked anterior atlantoaxial subluxation in the neutral lateral view.

thropathy in hemodialysis patients (Bardin, 1986). Radiologic detection in the spine is otherwise uncommon.

Paget's disease may involve the cervical spine leading to cord compression or vertebral collapse. Characteristic features include coarsening of trabeculae, expansion of vertebrae, and condensation of bone along the margins, creating a "picture frame" appearance (Fig. 12.16).

RADIOGRAPHIC FINDINGS

Changes in the rheumatoid spine usually parallel those in the peripheral joints. They are seen most commonly in those patients with advanced disease, but significant radiographic changes may be found in patients with early disease. In fact, in a prospective study of radiologic changes in the cervical spine in rheumatoid arthritis (Winfield, 1981), over 80% of patients with atlantoaxial and subaxial subluxations developed the first evidence of subluxation within two years of diagnosis of the disease.

Anterior atlantoaxial subluxation is the most common type of atlantoaxial subluxation and may be present in up to 25% of patients with rheumatoid arthritis (Matthews, 1969). It is manifested by abnormal separation of the posterior surface of the anterior arch of the atlas and the anterior surface of the odontoid (Fig. 12.17). The normal range for this distance is up to 2.5 to 3.0 mm in adults. Flexion and extension views of the cervical spine usually aid in detection of anterior atlantoaxial subluxation (Fig. 12.18). How-

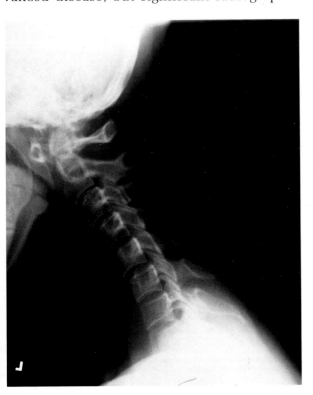
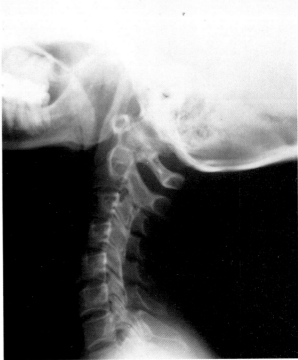

Figure 12.18 Anterior atlantoaxial subluxation is evident only on flexion (*left*) but not on neutral view of the cervical spine (*right*).

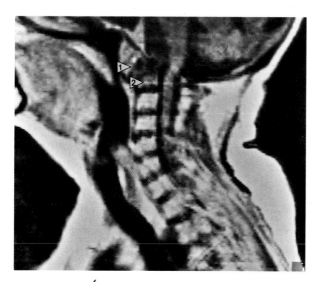

Figure 12.19 MRI study of the cervical spine showing anterior atlantoaxial subluxation (arrow 1) and partial destruction of the body of C-2 (arrow 2).

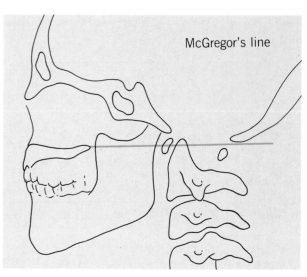

Figure 12.20 McGregor's line extends from the upper surface of posterior edge of the soft palate to the lowest part of occipital curve. Projection of the odontoid greater than 4.5 mm above this line may indicate vertical subluxation.

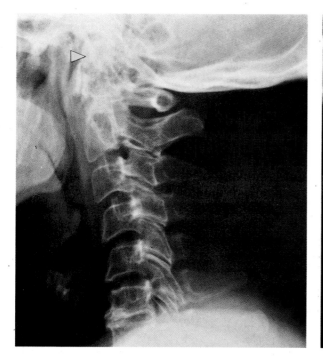

Figure 12.21 Vertical subluxation is seen. The tip of the odontoid extends greater than 4.5 mm above McGregor's line (arrow).

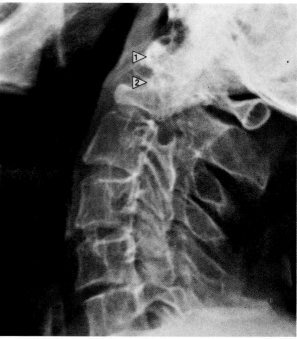

Figure 12.22 Posterior subluxation of C-1 on C-2 (arrow 1) secondary to complete erosion of the odontoid (arrow 2).

ever, occasionally the anatomy may be so distorted due to local destruction that CAT scanning or MRI studies may be necessary to elucidate the presence and degree of subluxation (Fig. 12.19).

Vertical subluxation is less common than anterior, and discrepancies in its reported prevalence may be due to the variety of systems used to measure the degree of invagination (Chamberlain, 1939; McGregor, 1948). McGregor's line, a line drawn from the upper surface of the posterior edge of the soft palate to the most caudal part of the occipital curve, is one of the most frequently used measurements (Fig. 12.20). Any projection of the odontoid greater than 4.5 mm above this line indicates vertical subluxation (Fig. 12.21).

Posterior subluxation is much rarer (Redlund-Johnell, 1984), although the prevalence was found to be 6.7% in one series (Weissman et al, 1982). Extension views may be necessary to demonstrate it (Fig. 12.22). Lateral subluxation is considered to be present when on the frontal view, the lateral masses of C-1 are more than 2 mm lateral to those of C-2 (Fig. 12.23).

Subaxial subluxations have been noted to be present in 7% to 29% of patients with rheumatoid arthritis (Cabot, 1978; Martel and Duff, 1964). Anterior subluxations (Fig. 12.24)

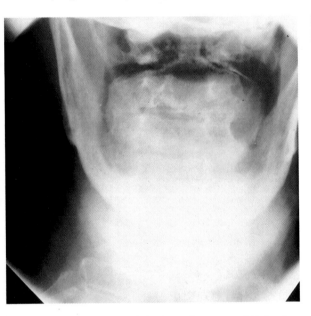

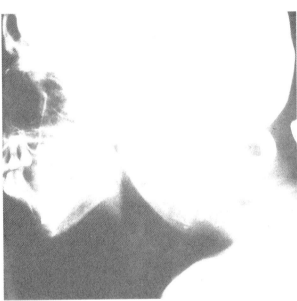

Figure 12.23 Slippage of the lateral masses of C-1 relative to those of C-2 greater than 2 mm is considered lateral subluxation.

Figure 12.24 Severe subluxation is present at C4-5 and milder subluxation present at C6-7 in this patient with subaxial subluxation.

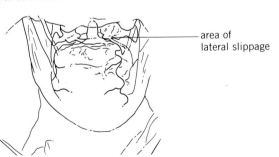

area of lateral slippage

are more frequent than posterior and they are usually mobile, necessitating flexion and extension views to elucidate the degree of subluxation. They are frequently serial and produce a "staircase" appearance (Fig. 12.25).

Discovertebral joint abnormalities in rheumatoid arthritis are characterized by intervertebral disc space narrowing, end plate erosions, and sclerosis with conspicuous absence of osteophyte formation (Fig. 12.26). Apophyseal joints may show joint space narrowing and erosions, usually without reactive sclerosis (Meikle and Wilkinson, 1971). These changes may occasionally lead to fusion of the apophyseal joints (Fig. 12.27) although it is more common in juvenile onset rheumatoid arthritis and the seronegative spondyloarthropathies.

When osteopenia is present, it is related to the chronicity and severity of disease and to the extent of corticosteroid treatment. Likewise, coincidental osteoarthritis and cervical spondylosis may be found in a large number of rheumatoid patients and may sometimes complicate the interpretation of the radiographic picture.

Rheumatoid arthritis rarely involves the dorsal and lumbar spine, either clinically or radiographically. A few reports have noted the presence of destructive lesions of the vertebral bodies, which histologically were composed of granulation tissue resembling rheumatoid nodules (Baggenstoss, 1952). Discovertebral disease with joint space narrowing, subchrondal erosions, and subchrondal sclerosis have also been noted.

Although up to 25% to 30% of rheumatoid arthritis patients may be found to have radiographic abnormalities at their sacroiliac joints (Martel and Duff, 1961; Elhabali et al, 1979), these lesions are rarely symptomatic. They are usually asymmetric and consist of superficial erosions with mild or absent sclerosis (Fig. 12.28).

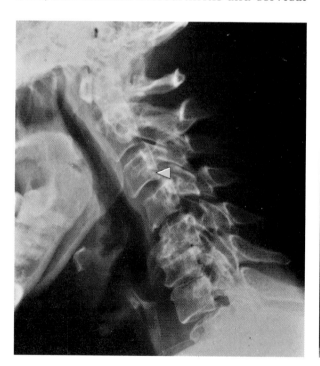 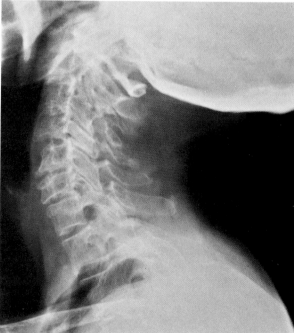

Figure 12.25 Subaxial subluxation at C3-4 (arrow) is most optimally shown on the flexion view (*left*). Extension view is seen on the *right*.

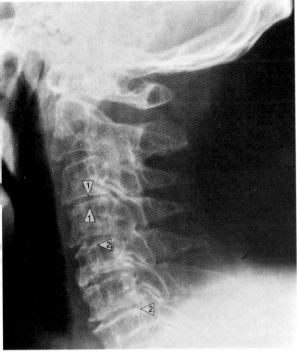

Figure 12.26 In this case of discovertebral disease, there is joint space narrowing at C3-4, C4-5, C5-6 and C6-7. Note the lack of subchondral sclerosis (arrows 1), cortical erosions (arrows 2), and lack of osteophytes.

Figure 12.27 Apophyseal joint fusion is apparent at C2-3.

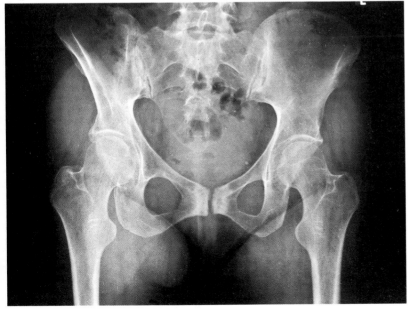

Figure 12.28 Left anterior sacroiliac erosions and joint space narrowing in rheumatoid arthritis.

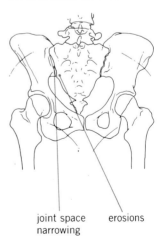

joint space narrowing   erosions

IMPLICATIONS FOR THERAPY

Therapy for rheumatoid involvement of the spine involves both medical therapy, directed at controlling local pain and inflammation, and surgical therapy, when indicated, to halt the progression of joint instability when the integrity of the spinal cord or brain stem is threatened (Fig. 12.29).

A critical component of medical management is patient education. Rheumatoid arthritis is primarily a chronic disorder and patients must often undergo weeks or months of immobilization, traction, physical manipulation, and drug therapy.

Cervical collars may be used to "immobilize" the cervical spine when it is acutely inflamed. Radiographic studies have shown that no type of cervical collar can adequately immobilize the spine in rheumatoid subluxation (Althoff and Goldie, 1980). However collars do help limit motion by providing patients with tactile awareness of the position of their necks, and thus they are able to limit their movement and reduce their pain. For severe subluxation with neurological compromise, only a halo will immobilize the spine sufficiently, pending surgery.

Traction may be useful, either as low-weight (5 lb) continuous traction to immobolize the spine and relieve muscle spasm, or as high-weight (25 lb) intermittent traction to attempt to separate the vertebrae. This latter type may be especially useful for nerve root compression syndromes. Traction should not be attempted in a patient with known subluxation.

Heat, massage, and ultrasound may also be attempted to relieve local inflammation and muscle spasm. Naturally, the patient should be on an adequate nonsteroidal anti-inflammatory drug and, when indicated, a disease-modifying drug.

Surgery to stabilize the cervical spine is usually dictated by the presence of intractable pain or "hard" neurological signs, such as motor weakness, dysfunction of the bowel or bladder, or vertebrobasilar symptoms due to kinking of the vertebral arteries as they pass through the foraminae transversariae. The presence of subluxation by itself is not an indication for surgery since many subluxations are asymptomatic and do not progress (Weissman et al, 1982). The type of surgery depends upon the type of subluxation and the levels involved.

THERAPY FOR RHEUMATOID CERVICAL SPINE DISEASE

MEDICAL			SURGERY
Systemic therapy	**Local physical therapy**	**"Immobilization"**	**Indications:**
Anti-inflammatory drugs and disease-modifying drugs	Heat	Cervical collars	Intractable pain or "hard" neurological signs
	Massage	Contour pillows	
	Ultrasound	Traction (except when subluxation is present)	**Type of surgery:**
	Trigger point injections	Patient education	Anterior fusion
	Stretching exercises		Posterior fusion
			Excision of odontoid (as dictated by anatomical and functional problem)

Figure 12.29   Therapy for rheumatoid cervical spine disease.

REFERENCES

Althoff B, Goldie I: Cervical collars in rheumatoid arthritis subluxation: a radiographic comparison. *Ann Rheum Dis* 1980;39:485–489.

Ansell BM, Kent PA: Radiological changes in juvenile chronic polyarthritis. *Skel Radiol* 1977;1:129–144.

Baggenstoss AH, Bickel NH, Ward LE: Rheumatoid granulomatous nodules as destructive lesions of vertebrae. *J Bone Joint Surg* 1952;34A:601–609.

Ball J: Enthesopathy of rheumatoid and ankylosing spondylitis. *Ann Rheum Dis* 1971;30:213–223.

Bardin, T, Kuntz D, Zingraff J, et al: Synovial amyloidosis and beta 2-microglobulin in patients undergoing long-term hemodialysis. *Arthritis Rheum* (letter) 1986;29:453–454.

Bland JH: Rheumatoid arthritis of the cervical spine. *J Rheumatol* 1974;1:319–342.

Bland JH, David PH: Rheumatoid arthritis of the cervical spine. *Arch Int Med* 1963;112:892–898.

Cabot A, Becker A: The cervical spine in rheumatoid arthritis. *Clin Ortho* 1978;131:130–140.

Chamberlain NE: Basilar invagination (platybasia). *Yale J Biol Med* 1939;11:487–496.

Conlon PW, Markely HE: Rheumatoid arthritis of the cervical spine. *Ann Rheum Dis* 1966;25:120–126.

Elhabali M, et al: Tomographic examination of sacroiliac joints in adult patients with rheumatoid arthritis. *J Rheumatol* 1979;6:417–425.

Hall FM, Docken WP, Hayes WC: Calcific tendonitis of the longus colli: Diagnosis by CT. *AJR* 1986;147:742–743.

Halla JT, Fallahis J, Haroin JG: Non-reducible rotational head tilt and lateral mass collapse. *Arthritis Rheum* 1982;20:1316–1324.

Kamusi T, Munro T, Harth M: Radiological review: The rheumatoid cervical spine. *Sem Arth Rheum* 1985;14:187–195

Kersley GD, Mandel L, Jeffrey MR: Gout: An unusual case with softening and subluxation of the first cervial vertebra and splenomegaly. *Ann Rheum Dis* 1950;9:282–304.

Killebrew K, Gold RH, Sholkoff SD: Psoriatic spondylitis. *Radiology* 1973;108:9–16.

Kuntz D, Naveau B, Bardin T, et al: Destructive spondylarthropathy in hemodialyzed patients: A new syndrome. *Arthritis Rheum* 1984;27:369–374

Latchaw RE, Meyer GW: Reiter's disease with atlanto-axial subluxation. *Radiology* 1978;126:303–304.

Martel W: Pathogenesis of cervical discovertebral destruction in rheumatoid arthritis. *Arthritis Rheum* 1977;20:1217–1225.

Martel W, Duff I: Pelvospondylitis in rheumatoid arthritis. *Radiology* 1961;77:744–755.

Martel W, Duff I, Preston RE, et al: The cervical spine in rheumatoid arthritis: A correlation of radiographic and clinical manifestations. *Arthritis Rheum* 1964;7:326.

Matthews JA: Atlanto-axial subluxation in rheumatoid arthritis. *Ann Rheum Dis* 1969;28:260–265.

McGregor M: The significance of certain measurements of the skull in the diagnosis of basilar impression. *Br J Radiol* 1948;21:171–181.

Meikle JAK, Wilkinson M: Rheumatoid involvement of the cervical spine. *Ann Rheum Dis* 1971;30:154–161.

Redlynd-Johnell I: Posterior atlanto-axial dislocation in rheumatoid arthritis. *Scand J.Rheum* 1984;13:337–341.

Resnick D, Curd J, Shapiro RF, Weisner KB: Radiographic abnormalities of rheumatoid arthritis in patients with diffuse idiopathic skeletal hyperostosis. *Arthritis Rheum* 1978;21:1.5.

Resnick D, Nurayama G, Goergen TG, et al: Clinical, radiographic and pathological abnormalities in calcium pyrophosphate dihydrate deposition disease (CPPD): Pseudogout. *Radiology* 1977;122:1–

Sharp J, Purser D: Spontaneous atlanto-axial dislocation in ankylosing spondylitis and rheumatoid arthritis. *Ann Rheum Dis* 1961;20:47–74.

Weissman BN, Aliabad P, Weinfeld M, et al: Prognostic features of atlantoaxial subluxation in rheumatoid arthritis patients. *Radiology* 1982;144:745–751.

Winfield J, Cooke D, Brook AS, Corbett M: A prospective study of the radiological changes in the cervical spine in early rheumatoid disease. *Ann Rheum Dis* 1981;40:109–114.

CHAPTER 13

THE TEMPORO-MANDIBULAR JOINT

ERIC P. GALL, MD

The involvement of the temporomandibular joint with inflammatory arthritis is not commonly considered by the primary care physician. Rheumatologists and dentists, however, are all too aware of the destructive synovitis that can occur at this joint, although it normally appears with juvenile onset more often than with adult onset rheumatoid arthritis.

The temporomandibular joint (TMJ) is unique in several ways (Friedman et al, 1982) (Fig. 13.1). While virtually all other joints are covered with hyaline cartilage, the articulating surfaces of the TMJ are covered with a nonvascular fibrous tissue and are separated from one another by a fibrous meniscus. The mandible is U-shaped and has articulating condyles at both ends which require the left and right ends of the TMJ to open and close at the same time. A problem on one side will affect the function of the other. Bilateral involvement in rheumatoid arthritis is not unusual. The motion of the joint is both a rotation and an anterior sliding as the jaw opens. Synovium is present as a capsular lining and thus is as susceptible to the inflammatory changes of rheumatoid arthritis as any other joint.

The condylar head is elliptically shaped with a medial-lateral diameter greater than

UNIQUE FEATURES OF THE TEMPOROMANDIBULAR JOINT

Articulating surfaces covered by fibrocartilage instead of hyaline cartilage.

Two bilateral joints must coordinate movements because condyles are connected by mandible.

Capsule lined with synovium.

Fibrocartilagenous disc separates mandibular condyle and temporal bone.

Ball and socket joint slides and normally dislocates during opening of the jaw.

Joints are affected by contact with tooth surfaces.

Friedman, 1982

Figure 13.1 Unique features of the temporomandibular joint.

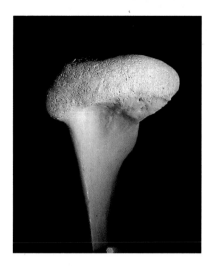

Figure 13.2 The articular condyle of the mandibular bone portion of the TMJ. Note the smooth, round contour in an ovoid shape of the condyle. (Courtesy of Michael Weiss, DDS).

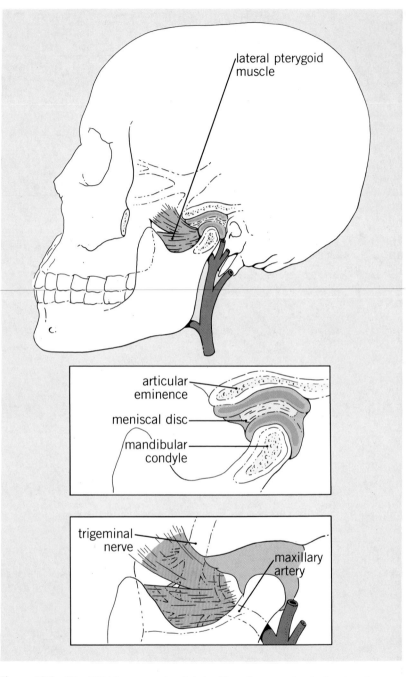

lateral pterygoid muscle

articular eminence

meniscal disc

mandibular condyle

trigeminal nerve

maxillary artery

Figure 13.3 The TMJ is a complex joint with unique anatomic landmarks. This figure denotes the muscles, ligaments, and joint placement. The condyle of the mandible, the articular fossa of the temporal bone, the cartilagenous cover and the meniscus are noted. The meniscus is unique to the TMJ and separates it into a superior and inferior portion. A fibrocartilage covers the joint.

he anteroposterior diameter (Guralnick et al, 1978). The articulating surface is the antero-uperior portion. The meniscal disc is ovoid Fig. 13.2) and separates the mandibular con-lyle from the articular eminence of the tem-oral bone in the glenoid fossa when the jaw s closed. Thus the jaw is separated into an ipper and lower compartment. The capsule s attached to the temporal articular eminence ind the neck of the mandible.

The only muscle attached to the joint is the ateral pterygoid originating from the sphe-ioid and the pterygoid process of the palatine oone and the maxillary tuberosity of the kull. The attachment is to the capsular lig-iment, meniscus, and the condylar neck and read (Messer and Ryan, 1985). The inferior oelly of the muscle contracts on opening, moving the meniscus along with the condyle;

the superior muscle belly contracts in closing the jaw. The joint is innervated by the third division of the fifth nerve (trigeminal) and its blood supply is from the maxillary artery branches (Guralnick et al, 1978) (Fig. 13.3).

JOINT INVOLVEMENT

It is estimated that 30% to 70% of patients with rheumatoid arthritis have involvement of the TMJ (Franks, 1969). Crepitus was present in 63% of these patients while 40% had tenderness on palpation. A visible effusion is rare, although occasionally fluid can be aspirated or is found on operation (Fig. 13.4). Ericson et al (1969) reported pain in the TMJ in 55 out of 65 rheumatoid patients at some time after the onset of the disease.

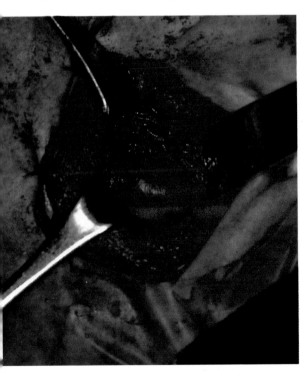

Figure 13.4 Intraoperative view of TMJ of a patient with rheumatoid arthritis. The capsule has not yet been opened and is bulging from an intraarticular effusion. Inflammatory joint fluid was seen when the capsule was opened. (Courtesy of Theodore Kiersch, DDS).

In one of the few prospective studies, Chalmers and Blair (1973) compared 100 consecutive patients with rheumatoid arthritis against a controlled population; 71% of the rheumatoid arthritis patients had pathology in the TMJ versus 41% of control patients. Signs and symptoms included limited range of motion, stiffness, crepitus, and pain (Fig. 13.5). Radiographic changes were common. Blockwood (1963) dissected the TMJ in ten cadavers with extensive rheumatoid arthritis and found significant inflammatory and destructive changes in seven.

TMJ involvement is rarely disabling even in severely crippled adult onset rheumatoid arthritis patients. However, patients complain of pain in chewing and, occasionally, pain at rest. A crackling or clicking sensation may be noted upon joint movement. As the disease progresses, the jaw range of motion may decrease, although usually it is slight. A progressive separation of upper and lower incisors is noted and, with joint resorption, the chin may recede (Fig. 13.6).

PERIARTICULAR INVOLVEMENT

Soft tissue manifestations may include swelling over the TMJ anterior to the ear and muscle spasm with resultant facial pain and/or temporal headache (Marbach, 1976–

Figure 13.5 Comparison of TMJ involvement in arthritic diseases and normal patients.

COMPARISON OF TMJ INVOLVEMENT IN RHEUMATOID AND CONTROL* POPULATIONS

	Control Patients	Rheumatoid Arthritis Patients
TMJ Symptoms	**41%**	**71%**
Limited opening of jaw	3%	23%
Stiffness	1%	14%
Crepitus	18%	40%
Tenderness	8%	17%
Pain on bite	2%	14%
Radiographic changes	**34%**	**79%**
Anterior position	13%	23%
Decreased mobility	9%	27%
Erosions	1%	22%

*100 Control patients: 39 degenerative arthritis; 56 normal

Chalmers and Blair, 1973

77). Earache is not uncommon and must be differentiated from outer or middle ear difficulties. Flexion contractures of the muscles may eventually occur (Marbach and Spiera, 1967). The contractures lead to an inability to open the jaw and to ingest solid foods, leading to a decreased nutritional status.

PHYSICAL EXAMINATION

The physical examination of the TMJ is similar to that of other joints (Fig. 13.7). Inspection alone may reveal telling abnormalities.

Figure 13.6 This patient with rheumatoid arthritis with progressive TMJ involvement is attempting to close her mouth. Displacement of the mandible results in a gradual increase in the opening between the incisors. (Courtesy of Paul Dempsey, MD).

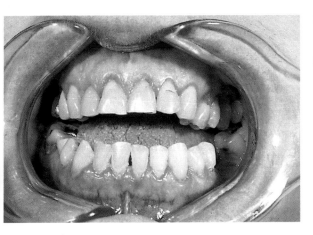

PHYSICAL EXAMINATION OF THE TMJ

Inspection	Range of Motion
Swelling	Interincisor distance with jaw open
Micrognathia	
Malocclusion	Fingers in mouth
Skin and herpetic lesions	Mandibular kinesiograph
Parotid swelling	**Muscle strength**
Palpation	Resist opening jaw
Anterior to tragus	Resist closing jaw
Auditory meatus with anterior pressure with jaw motion	Spasm (palpate resting)
Crepitus Click Pain	**Pain (biting on tongue blade)**
Palpate temporal arteries	**Neck examination for referred pain**

Figure 13.7 Physical examination of the TMJ.

Swelling around the joint anterior to the tragus of the ear may signify an effusion. This must, however, be differentiated from parotid swelling (Fig. 13.8).

With severe resorption of the mandibular head or growth arrest, micrognathia will be present. A receding chin is the most obvious finding in the adult rheumatoid patient with severe TMJ involvement. Malocclusion, particularly an overbite may be evident (Fig. 13.9). In some patients this leads to separation of the incisors even with closed mouth.

Some patients with facial pain similar to that of TMJ involvement can have a neuritis such as that of herpetic infection and the zoster rash should be looked for.

Palpation of the joint anterior to the ear may reveal an effusion in a rare case. Typically there is tenderness directly over the joint. Palpation should continue while the patient opens and closes the mouth (Fig. 13.10). A click may be felt or heard, partic-

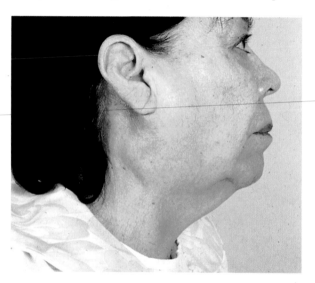

Figure 13.8 Parotid gland swelling in Sjögren's syndrome.

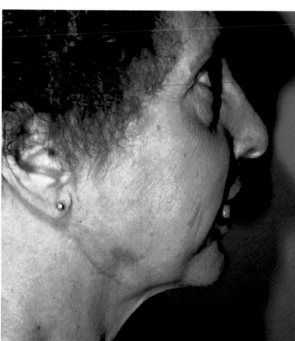

Figure 13.9 Micrognathia in patient with rheumatoid arthritis. Note the overbite and receding chin

larly with meniscal damage or abnormal ubluxation. With loss of cartilagenous cover o the joint, crepitation will occur. Palpation should also be performed by placing the inlex finger in the auditory meatus, and gently pulling anteriorly. This puts the palpating ligit directly in contact with the posterior surface of the TMJ (Figures 13.11 and 13.12).

Range of motion is measured, first by observing the quality and quantity of jaw movement. A stuttering motion as the jaw opens suggests joint pathology. The internal incisor distance can be measured using a ruler from tip to tip of the incisors with the

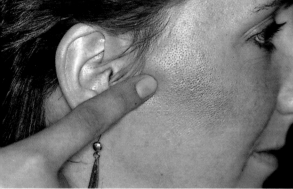

Figure 13.10 Palpation of the TMJ anterior to the tragus of the ear. Patient should open and close mouth during palpation.

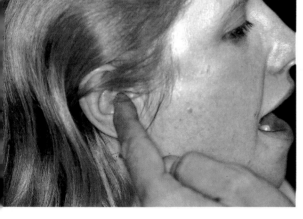

igure 13.11 Finger is placed in the external auditory neatus while patient opens and closes mouth. Palpation of the posterior portion of the TMJ is done during this procedure.

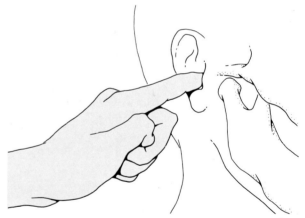

Figure 13.12 The anterior portion of the auditory meatus abuts the condyle of the TMJ.

mouth opened (Fig. 13.13). This is particularly helpful in looking for progressive damage or for any beneficial effects of medication. Bear in mind that the timing of the administration of pain medication and recent chewing or exercise may have an effect on the motion of the jaw. A gross estimation of adequate mouth opening can be done by placing two fingers in the open mouth to assure that there is adequate room for mastication (Fig. 13.14).

Velocity and quality of motion can be measured by using a mandibular kinesiograph (Myo-Tronics Research) (Fig. 13.15). By placing a magnet on the teeth and sensors around the head, jaw motion can be measured and information regarding deviation of the jaw, clicking and interruption of motion and the velocity rate of opening and closing the mouth recorded (Fig. 13.16) (Jankelson, et al, 1975; Jemt, et al, 1979; Jankelson, 1980; Hannam, et al, 1977). The tracing provides a permanent record of joint abnormalities and gives an objective measurement of joint motion. This procedure is usually available from oral surgeons or TMJ specialists.

Muscle strength may be measured by having the examiner forcibly resist the patient's

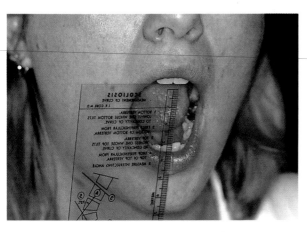

Figure 13.13 Patient opens mouth maximally and the distance between the tips of the incisors is measured with ruler.

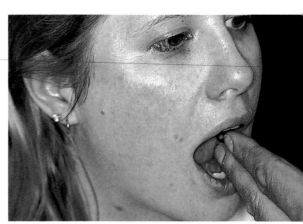

Figure 13.14 To see whether the incisors open enough to allow for the passage of food, insert two fingers in the open mouth.

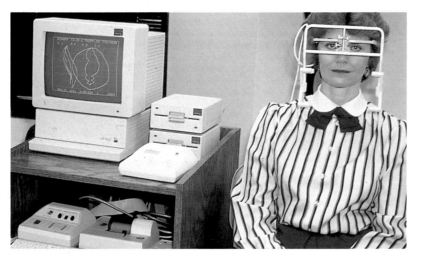

Figure 13.15 The mandibular kinesiograph measures deviation of the jaw during opening and closing, the velocity of movement of the jaw, and any movement abnormalities. A magnet is glued onto the interior portion of the lower jaw on the incisors. An oscilloscope shows a graphic representation of the opening and closing of the mouth and any movement disorders. (© Myo-Tronics Research Inc., Seattle, Wa). (Courtesy of Myo-Tronics).

attempts to open and close the jaw (Fig. 13.17). Strength can be estimated on a scale of 1 to 5, similar to other muscle testing. Pain may be noted during the procedure and the location of such pain may give information regarding its source. Pain may not occur on motion but may occur only with pressure. Synovitis is characterized by resting pain made worse by motion (Solberg, 1986), which may differentiate it from localized inflam-

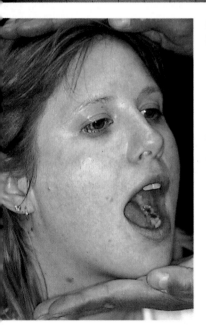

Figure 13.16 The left graph is a velocity curve. The inner curve depicts a normal opening and closing of the mouth and the outside curve the maximum speed of opening and closing of the mouth. The right side of the outside curve denotes normal velocity of opening and is smooth and uninterrupted. Velocity is measured from the midpoint of the curve on opening to the right of the midpoint. An initial increase in velocity is followed by a decrease prior to closing. The left side of the outside curve shows a decreased velocity on closing with an uneven closing motion. The right graph shows a deviation of the jaw to one side on motion. Millimeters of movement from the center line is depicted.

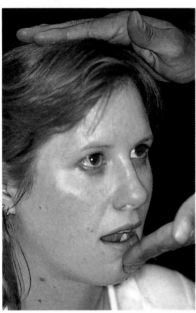

Figure 13.17 Clinician attempts to resist the patient's opening (*left*) and closing (*right*) of the mouth to measure muscle strength.

mation which may be aggravated only by certain motions of the jaw. Diffuse synovitis is aggravated by any motion. Exertional type of pain and chewing pain may be reproduced by having the patient bite on a tongue blade with his molar teeth, which applies pressure to the TMJ. The clinician should ask the patient about any pain from this procedure. The tongue blade can be used on both sides of the mouth to help delineate individual abnormalities. Surrounding structures such as the neck, temporal artery, ear, and mouth should also be examined as possible sources of referred pain or for pain present in these structures which is initially thought to be TMJ pain.

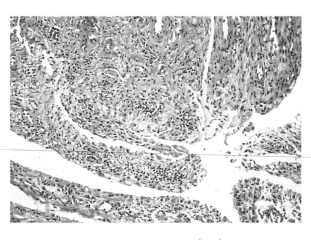

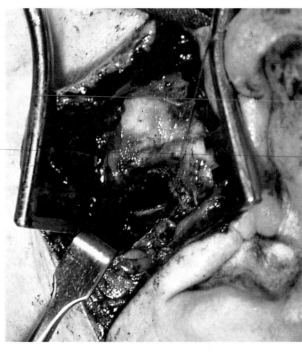

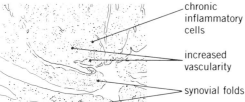

Figure 13.18 Rheumatoid arthritis synovium showing chronic inflammatory infiltrate and increased vascularity with synovial cell lining layer hyperplasia (*left*). Intra- operative view of synovium in a rheumatoid TMJ. Pannus is present. Note destruction of bone and cartilage (*right*). (Courtesy of Paul Dempsey, MD).

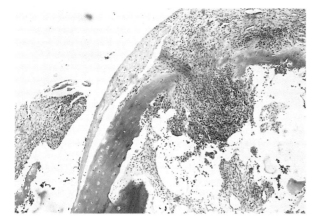

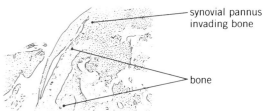

Figure 13.19 Pannus formation with inflamed rheumatoid synovium invading bone and cartilage, causing destruction.

LABORATORY AND RADIOGRAPHIC FINDINGS

Rheumatoid arthritis of the TMJ causes chronic synovial inflammatory changes similar to those of any other joint (Fig. 13.18).

Chronic inflammatory reactions will eventually erode through the cartilage and bone (Fig. 13.19). The inflammation and destruction causes demineralization of the joint and bony erosion (Murphy and Adams, 1981) (Figs. 13.20 and 13.21). Synovial proliferation wraps around the condylar head. Meniscal destruction can occur. The condyle becomes anteriorly displaced with decreased mobility.

Figure 13.20 Radiograph of the TMJ showing erosion, joint space narrowing and decreased bone mass of the mandibular condyle. (Courtesy of Paul Dempsey, MD).

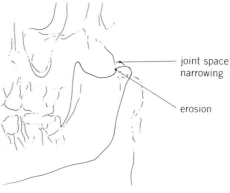

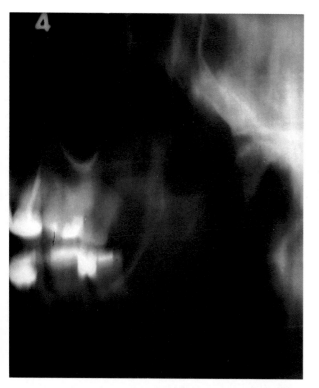

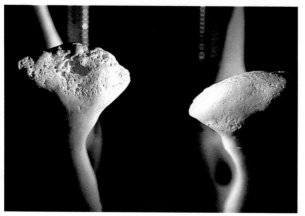

Figure 13.21 Arthritic mandibular condyle on the left shows erosion, flattening and abnormal shape. A normal condyle is seen on the right. (Courtesy of Michael Weiss, DDS).

The mandibular head becomes flattened (Fig. 13.22), and marginal proliferation may occur (Chalmers and Blair, 1973). Remodeling of the temporal fossa may occur (Fig. 13.23) and erosive destructive changes may be seen here (Fig. 13.24). Marked mandibular resorption may occur although it is more commonly seen in juvenile onset rheumatoid arthritis. Loose bodies may also be noted in the joint. Ankylosis is quite rare due to modern disease management. Permanent subluxation of the jaw can lead to decreased mobility and muscle contractures. As the chin recedes, there is an increase in the vertical height of the face; a lisp may occur in speaking (Marbach, 1976–77). With TMJ arthritis bruxism with grinding down of the teeth may occur (Fig. 13.25).

The diagnosis of rheumatoid involvement in the TMJ is usually based on the diagnosis of rheumatoid arthritis by other criteria, implicating the typical involvement of this joint. On occasion joint fluid may be aspirated for diagnostic affirmation by placing a 21 or 22 gauge needle into the joint about 2 cm (one finger's breadth) anterior to the tragus and inferior to the arch (Steinbrocker and Neustadt, 1972). The condyle is readily palpated and the needle is inserted under the usual sterile conditions. Care should be made to avoid the temporal artery and facial nerve (Fig. 13.26). Synovial fluid should be inflammatory for a diagnosis of rheumatoid arthritis. Arthroscopy of the TMJ is now available and tissue may be sampled under direct visualization.

Evaluation of the TMJ is currently done radiographically. The simplest technique is lateral transfacial or transcranial plain films with an angle of the machine to project a clear unobstructed view of the joint (Murphy and Adams, 1981). Reproducibility of such views is a problem. Microfocus magnification technology provides excellent detail and is in common use in specialized medical centers. The Towne projection is particularly helpful

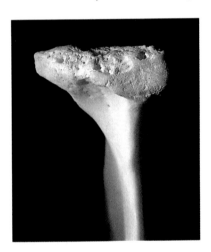

Figure 13.22 Flattening of the mandibular head of patient with inflammatory arthritis. (Courtesy of Michael Weiss, DDS).

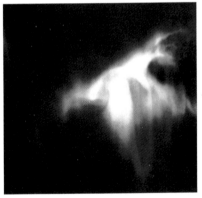

Figure 13.23 Radiographs showing resorption both of the mandibular condyle and remodeling of the temporal fossa (*Left*, closed view; *right*, open view). (Courtesy of Paul Dempsey, DDS).

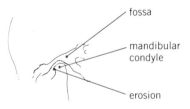
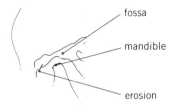

in this technique. Various methods of tomography are used in some medical centers to delineate the detail of the joint. This, however, uses a fair amount of radiation and the image is not always satisfactory. Panoramic radiography gives a survey of the mandible, teeth, and both ends of the TMJ in one projection (Murphy and Adams, 1981). While the detail is not good, the overall view provides important information. Arthrography gives excellent detail of the meniscal structures. CAT scanning by arthrography enhances the ability to find meniscal damage and to describe it accurately. Dynamic studies may be done to look for abnormal motion and to better define changes in anatomy with motion.

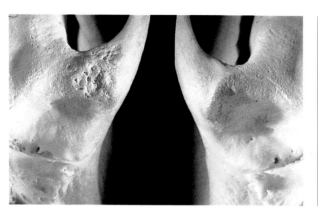

Figure 13.24 The temporal fossa of patient with inflammatory arthritis (on the left) shows erosion. The right side shows a normal fossa. (Courtesy of Michael Weiss, DDS).

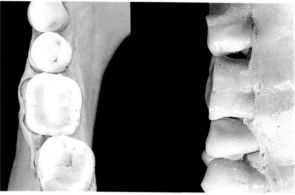

Figure 13.25 Bruxism and grinding down of the teeth occur in patients with TMJ arthritis. (Courtesy of Michael Weiss, DDS).

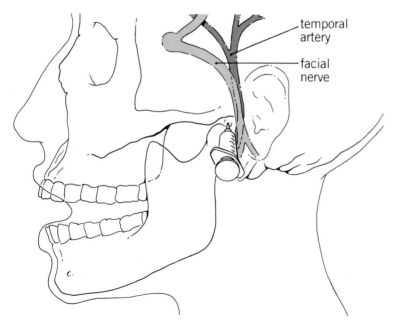

temporal artery

facial nerve

Figure 13.26 Needle in the TMJ for aspiration or injection. Needle is inserted about 1 cm anterior to the tragus of the ear. This procedure should be done by an experienced clinician. Care should be made not to puncture the temporal artery branch or the facial nerve.

DIFFERENTIAL DIAGNOSIS

The differential diagnosis of TMJ abnormalities has been well described by Alderman (1976) (Fig. 13.27). Most inflammatory arthritis is similar to rheumatoid arthritis in its manifestations. The "rheumatoid variants" (spondylitis, psoriasis, Reiter's syndrome) are more likely to produce periosteal new bone and are less likely to be osteopenic if the TMJ is involved. However, there have been many descriptions of severe osteopenia in psoriatic arthritis. Of course, other systemic and joint manifestations of the underlying disease will be present.

Juvenile onset rheumatoid arthritis is particularly severe at the TMJ if the growth plate is destroyed before full development of the mandible. These patients are likely to have severe micrognathia. TMJ involvement is more common in this disease than in adult onset rheumatoid arthritis.

Infection is usually associated with systemic symptoms but in immunosuppressed patients these symptoms may be masked. If TMJ inflammation is markedly more severe than joints in rheumatoid arthritis, aspiration should be done to rule out infection.

Osteoarthritis is common in the TMJ. It does not manifest the inflammatory characteristics of rheumatoid arthritis but causes some of the same end results of mandibular

ALDERMAN CLASSIFICATION OF TMJ DISORDERS (Modified)

EXTRACAPSULAR		INTRACAPSULAR	
Psychophysiologic	**Dental**	**Congenital**	**Trauma**
Tension	Occlusal abnormality	Agenesis	Fracture
Anxiety	Periodontal lesion	Condylar changes	Meniscal tear
Oral habits	Tooth abnormality	**Joint infection**	**Functional**
Iatrogenic	**Infection outside TMJ**	**Arthritis**	Subluxation, dislocation
Misdirected nerve block	**Otologic**	Rheumatoid arthritis	Meniscal
Mandibular displacement under anesthesia	Otitis media	Juvenile arthritis	Hypermobility/ankylosis
	Otitis externa	Osteoarthritis	**Neoplastic**
Traumatic (without fracture)	**Neoplastic**	"Psoriatic arthritis" and rheumatoid variants	
	Parotid		
	Nasopharyngeal		(Alderman, 1976)

Figure 13.27 Alderman classification of TMJ disorders (modified).

condylar flattening, crepitation, and decreased motion. Unilateral involvement is not uncommon in this disease.

TMJ dysfunction syndrome is a disease associated with stress, malocclusions, muscle tension and frequent psychologic problems. The pain may be confused with arthritis and appropriate diagnostic tests for these underlying problems should be performed. The muscles of mastication for these patients are frequently tense.

IMPLICATIONS FOR THERAPY

The medical treatment for rheumatoid arthritis of the TMJ is the same as for rheumatoid arthritis of other joints. Physicans may feel more comfortable in managing the TMJ with the help of a competent rheumatologist, oral surgeon, and orthodontist. Severe micrognathia is unsightly and may warrant reconstructive procedures (Fig. 13.28). Local injection of small amounts of depot steroids into the TMJ is sometimes helpful for inflammation and pain. The dentist may wish to use bite blocks in order to decrease reduced or limited motion of the jaw. Local heat to the area, stretch exercises and muscle relaxants may be helpful. With the help of a dentist, judicious and slow lowering of the molar teeth to bring the incisors anteriorly closer may be done (Marbach, 1976–77). Orthodontic correction is helpful but should ideally be done after the disease has been controlled medically. In some cases arthroscopic debridement of the joint may now be attempted through a tiny fiber optic arthroscope. Rarely TMJ arthroplasty may be done by an experienced surgeon (Kent, 1983).

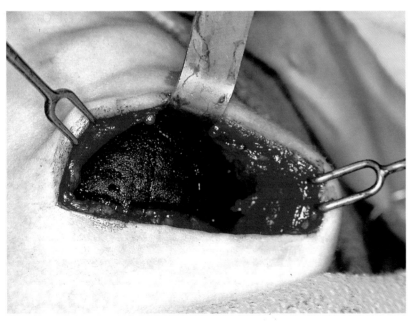 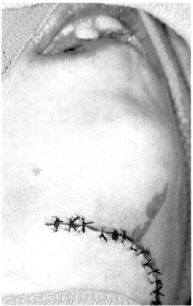

Figure 13.28 Prosthesis placed in receding chin of patient with inflammatory arthritis (*left*). Postoperative view shows normal contour to the chin (*right*).

REFERENCES

Alderman MM: Disorders of the temporomandibular joint and related structures: Rationale for diagnosis, etiology, management. *Alpha Omegon* December 1976;12.

Blockwood HJJ: Arthritis of the mandibular joint. *British Dent J* 1963;115:317–326.

Chalmers IM, Blair GS: Rheumatoid arthritis of the temporomandibular joint. *QJ Med* 1973;42:369–386.

Ericson S, Lundberg M: Alterations in the temporomandibular joint at various stages of rheumatoid arthritis. *Acta Rheum Scand* 1967;13:257–274.

Franks TS: Temporomandibular joints in adult rheumatoid arthritis. *Ann Rheum Dis* 1969;28:139–145.

Friedman MH, Weisberg J, Agus B: Diagnosis and treatment of inflammation of the temporomandibular joint. *Semin Arthritis Rheum* 1982;12:44–51.

Guralnick W, Kaban LB, Merrim RG: Temporomandibular joint afflictions. *N Engl J Med* 1978; 299:123–129.

Hannam AG, Scott JD, DeCou RE: A computer based system for the simultaneous measurement of muscle activity and joint movement during mastication in man. *Arch Oral Biol* 1977;22:18–23.

Jankelson B: Measurement of the mandibular kinesograph: A computerized study. *J Prosthet Dent* 1980;44:656–666.

Jankelson O, Swain CW, Crane PF, Radke JC: Kinesiographic instrumentation: A new technology. *J Am Dent Assoc* 1975;90:434–440.

Jemt T, Karlsson S, Hedegard B: Mandibular movements of young adults recorded by intraorally placed light emitting diodes. *J Prosthet Dent* 1979; 42:669–673.

Kent JN, Misiek DJ, Akin RK etal: Temporomandibular joint condylar prosthesis. *J Oral Maxillofacial Surg* 1983; 41:245-254.

Marbach JJ: Arthritis of the temporomandibular joints and facial pain. *Bull Rheum Dis* 1976–77; 27:918–921.

Marbach JJ, Spiera H: Rheumatoid arthritis of the temporomandibular joints. *Ann Rheum Dis* 1967; 26:538–543.

Messer EJ, Ryan DE: Painful temporal mandibular joint, in McCarty DJ: *Arthritis and Allied Conditions,* ed 10. Philadelphia, Lea & Febiger, 1985, pp 1262–1270.

Murphy WA, Adams RJ: The temporomandibular joint, in Resnick D and Newarjama G: *Diagnosis of Bone and Joint Disorders.* Philadelphia, WB Saunders, 1981, pp 3061–3101.

Solberg WK: Temporomandibular disorders: Management of problems associated with inflammation, chronic hypermobility and deformity. *British Dent J* 1986;16:421–428.

Steinbrocker O, Neustadt DH: *Aspiration and Injection Theory in Arthritis and Musculoskeletal Disorders.* Hagerstown, Md, Harper & Row, 1972.

3

SYSTEMIC FEATURES, COMPLICATIONS, AND MANAGEMENT

Initial diagnosis and management of rheumatoid arthritis frequently focus on the joint disease. However, from onset, rheumatoid arthritis is a systemic disease and the systemic features often assume increasing importance as the disease progresses. This Section reviews the systemic aspects that are directly related to the disease process, and the complications that occur less directly as a result of having rheumatoid arthritis. Management can be extremely complex and proper care requires frequent and thorough reevaluation of the entire patient and not just of the joints. Physical and pharmacologic treatment is still surprisingly imprecise. Current management measures, as well as a philosophy of an approach to care are discussed. Only with better understanding of the pathogenesis of the disease will a definitive, detailed plan for treatment be possible.

CHAPTER 14

SYSTEMIC FEATURES OF RHEUMATOID ARTHRITIS

ERIC P. GALL, MD AND H. RALPH SCHUMACHER Jr, MD

A dramatic feature of rheumatoid arthritis is its systemic nature. Fatigue, myalgia, and anemia are prominent features. This chapter will address a number of the other aspects of the systemic nature of the disease, which can offer important clues to diagnosis, possibly hold implications for pathogenesis, and can serve as potential sources of diagnostic confusion. They may also require special consideration in management. As noted elsewhere, systemic features in general correlate with more severe articular disease, but there are exceptions. For instance, some patients will have prominent subcutaneous rheumatoid nodules with little residual arthritis (rheumatoid nodulosis); in patients who develop Felty's syndrome, arthritis may have been severe but often improves with the appearance of neutropenia.

GENERAL SYSTEMIC FEATURES OF RHEUMATOID ARTHRITIS

Although specific systemic complications are described in this chapter, rheumatoid arthritis has many more vaguely described generalized features. Patients with significant disease invariably report not only specific joint discomfort and swelling, but also such nonspecific symptoms as malaise, morning stiffness, muscle soreness, fever, and anemia. Generalized weakness, shoddy adenopathy, and low-grade febrile episodes often occur. In addition to the actual joint findings, muscular and periarticular tenderness are not unusual.

At onset of the disease, about 30% of patients complain of fatigue, 26% of weight loss, 19% of muscle pain, and 13% of sweating (Empire Rheumatism Council, 1950). Stiffness, particularly in the morning, is a common manifestation of all inflammatory arthritis. It tends to correlate with joint activity and may be the patient's predominant complaint. This stiffness typically lasts an hour or more after arising, and in a severely ill patient it may last all day. To support the diagnosis of rheumatoid arthritis, morning stiffness should last at least 30 minutes. Shorter periods of stiffness may be associated with noninflammatory arthritis. A similar phenomenon, joint gelling, occurs following periods of inactivity such as reading, watching television or driving significant distances.

Nonspecific, low-grade fever is common. This fever may be persistent in patients with active seropositive disease and be associated with weight loss and fatigue. Interleukin-1 is

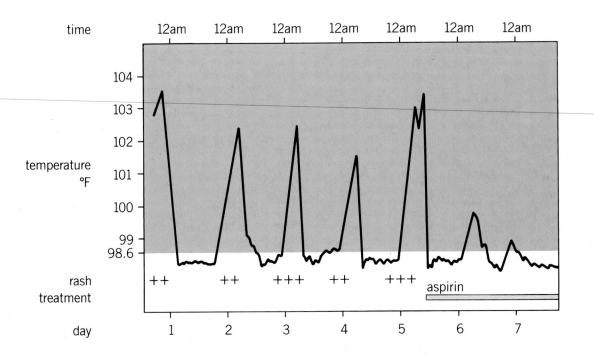

Figure 14.1 Fever curve of a patient with juvenile rheumatoid arthritis or adult onset Still's disease. The fever, frequently accompanied by a rash, typically spikes once or twice daily, generally at night (vesperal fever), and returns to normal throughout the day. Fever responds to treatment with high-dose aspirin, other nonsteroidal anti-inflammatory agents, or to corticosteroid therapy.

present in significant amounts in the inflammatory exudate of joints. This monokine is known to provoke a febrile response in inflammatory states. Other acute phase reactants are elevated in the serum and lead to an increased sedimentation rate and nonspecific systemic symptoms.

In patients with an acute explosive course of rheumatoid arthritis, high fevers up to 104°F may be seen (Shapiro et al, 1985). Since patients with rheumatoid arthritis are subject to bacterial infection, a careful evaluation of the fever is essential. Determining the etiology of the fever can be difficult, often leading to lengthy, expensive workups, hospitalization, and fruitless trials of antibiotics. After such screening is complete, the rheumatoid arthritis should be treated aggressively to alleviate fever and other symptoms. Septic arthritis is suggested if a single joint is more inflamed than other joints. However,

some patients with septic arthritis superimposed on active rheumatoid disease are unable to mount a febrile response because of systemic medications (NSAIDs, steroids) and neutrophil abnormalities secondary to immune complex ingestion. Dramatic febrile episodes are seen more often in adult onset Still's disease. The febrile curve typically occurs at night; it spikes once or twice daily (Fig. 14.1). It may be associated with a fine, pink evanescent rash that fades with the febrile episode (Fig. 14.2). The rash may be brought out by a hot bath.

Lymphadenopathy may occur in 30% of patients with active rheumatoid arthritis (Short et al, 1957). A controlled study showed significant axillary, epitrochlear, and inguinal adenopathy in patients with rheumatoid arthritis (Robertson et al, 1968). Lymphadenopathy has been found to occur more often in patients with seropositive, ac-

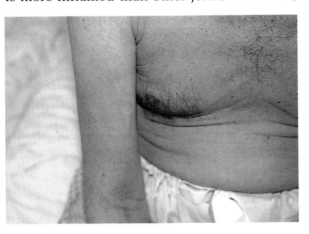 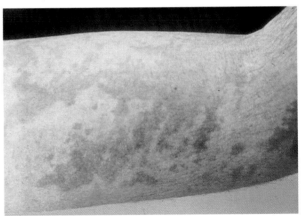

Figure 14.2 Very faint, typical salmon-colored maculopapular rash on the arm and chest of a patient with adult onset Still's disease (*left*). This rash comes and goes with the fever and is difficult to see. Close-up view of salmon-colored evanescent maculopapular rash in juvenile rheumatoid arthritis (*right*). This rash shows the Koebner's phenomenon, with extension in the area of scratching.

tive disease. The lymph nodes show follicular hyperplasia, which may simulate malignant follicular lymphoma (Nasanchuk et al, 1969; Motulsky et al, 1952) (Fig. 14.3). Since the incidence of lymphoma in rheumatoid patients may be higher than that in the normal population, biopsy of the affected nodes may be necessary (Hurd, 1979).

In addition to Felty's syndrome (described later) anemia is common in patients with rheumatoid arthritis (Fig. 14.4). Ineffective marrow production in chronic inflammatory states (etiology unknown) and the loss of iron through gastrointestinal bleeding, iron sequestration, and ineffective iron metabolism, as well as numerous other factors, are involved (Hurd, 1979). A remarkable amount of synovial iron sequestration may occur (Fig. 14.5). When the hemoglobin level drops below 10g%, iron depletion is a clinical concern, and symptoms of iron deficiency fre-

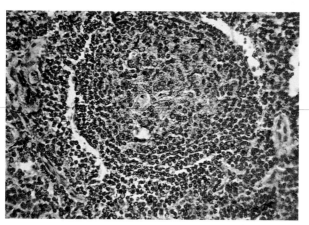

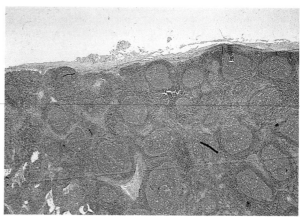

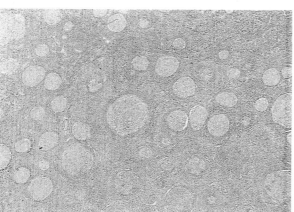

Figure 14.3 Lymphoid follicle, the site of active lymphoid proliferation, in a normal lymph node (*top left*). Patients with inflammatory conditions such as rheumatoid arthritis frequently have marked follicular hyperplasia with abnormal numbers of reactive lymphoid nodules (*top, right*). A patient with follicular lymphoma has varying sites of lymphoid follicles with abnormal cells (*bottom, left*). Differentiation of this from follicular hyperplasia requires expert pathologic analysis.

quent; at these levels, treatment may be indicated.

Muscle weakness and atrophy are common in rheumatoid arthritis (Hurd, 1979). Cellular infiltrates may be seen on biopsy, in addition to fiber degeneration (Steiner et al, 1946), which may be the result of disuse atrophy and lymphokine-induced muscle damage (Johnson, Fink, and Ziff, 1972). Control of the underlying, rheumatoid arthritis, adequate nutrition, and exercise help restore muscle strength.

Generalized rheumatoid arthritis is associated with similarly generalized systemic signs and symptoms. Attention to systemic problems often permits patients to feel better and thus to tolerate better the joint manifestations of their disease.

CAUSES OF ANEMIA IN RHEUMATOID ARTHRITIS

Anemia of chronic disease
normocytic normochromic
microcytic normochromic

Blood loss
gastric ulcer, NSAIDs
microcytic, hypochromic

Iron sequestration in diseased synovium

Defective iron absorption

Plasma volume expansion

Hemolysis

Ineffective marrow production

Figure 14.4 The causes of anemia in rheumatoid arthritis are multiple, and when anemia is present, a careful analysis of the patient is required to determine the reasons for its occurence.

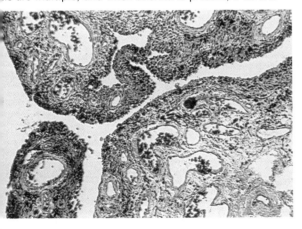 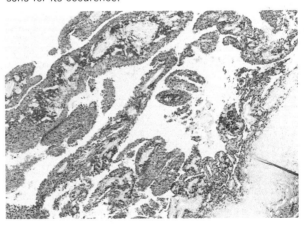

Figure 14.5 Inflammatory synovitis with obvious hemosiderin deposition in the synovium (*left*). The brownish granules are the remnants of hemosiderin, deposited by blood escaping from fragile vessels in inflammatory arthritis (H&E). Blue coloring indicates large amounts of hemosiderin deposition in inflammatory synovium (*right*) (Gomori's stain).

RHEUMATOID NODULES

Necrotizing granulomas, which are often seen in subcutaneous tissue, are a characteristic but by no means invariable feature of rheumatoid arthritis. They can help in establishing the diagnosis, especially when they are confirmed histologically, but they are not unique to rheumatoid arthritis, and only infrequently create clinically significant problems. The etiology of rheumatoid nodule formation is not fully established and is an important area for continued investigation.

Incidence

Rheumatoid nodules are said to occur in approximately 20% to 25% of patients with definite or classic rheumatoid arthritis in the United States. In a recent report from West Virginia, nodules, or a history of nodules, were found in 70% of 238 patients (Bathon et al, 1985). They appear to be less common in Chinese people (Chen et al, 1986; Moran et al, 1986) and in some other non-whites. Reasons for these discrepancies may provide clues to genetic, dietary, and other factors in the pathogenesis of these nodules.

Nodules have been reported to be more common in men (Lewis et al, 1980), with incidences up to 85% (Bathon et al, 1985), and in one study they were seen in 75% of patients with Felty's syndrome (Sienknecht et al, 1977). Nodules generally are associated with more severe articular and systemic disease and high titers of rheumatoid factor.

Rheumatoid nodules, however, can occur and even be massive in patients with little or no detectable synovitis or with only palindromic arthritis. This condition, which has been termed rheumatoid nodulosis, can occur in both children and adults. Such nodules may be associated with large bone cysts and may sometimes be clinically confused with gout or xanthomas (Wisnieski and Askari

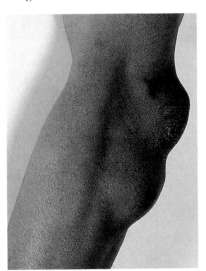

Figure 14.6 Rheumatoid nodules classically occur on the extensor surface of the forearm.

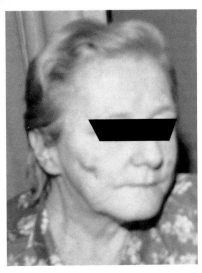

Figure 14.7 This patient developed nodules over the maxillae, apparently from resting her head on her hand over a long period of time.

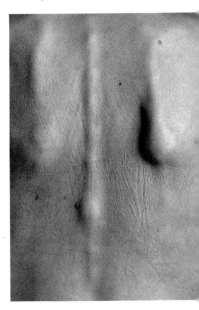

Figure 14.8 Rheumatoid nodules are seen along the spine and over the scapula in this thin, bedridden patient.

1981). Some associated bone cysts have been shown to contain rheumatoid granulomas (Morales-Piga et al, 1986). Rarely, classical rheumatoid arthritis can evolve after years of rheumatoid nodulosis.

Clinical Features

Rheumatoid nodules typically appear on the extensor surface of the forearm below the elbow (Fig. 14.6) and are presumably associated with mild, repetitive irritation. Many other common locations for nodules are also sites of local pressure. "Pump bumps" are rheumatoid nodules thought to be caused by shoes rubbing at the Achilles tendons. Nodules on the bridge of the nose may be related to eye glass use, and nodules have even occurred where fatigued patients rest their hands against their cheeks (Fig. 14.7). Bedridden patients often develop occipital nodules or a chain of nodules along their spinous process (Fig. 14.8); wheelchair patients can develop nodules on their buttocks. However, nodules often occur near joints without any obvious relation to local pressure (Fig. 14.9).

Subcutaneous nodules can be single or multiple, freely movable or fixed, barely palpable or several centimeters in diameter; most are firm. Small areas of skin necrosis can appear over superficial nodules (Fig. 14.10); and in some patients, vasculitis-like skin lesions can be seen over some nodules (Fig. 14.11). Whether this is a factor in nodule necrosis is not clear.

Figure 14.9 Large rheumatoid nodules can overlie joints even at sites with no history of repetitive pressure.

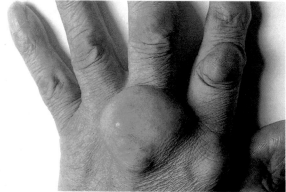

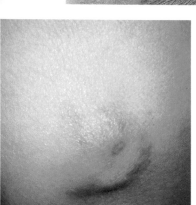

Figure 14.10 A small area of necrosis is healing over this buttock nodule.

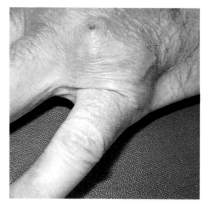

Figure 14.11 Vasculitis-like lesions may be seen overlying nodules.

Rheumatoid nodules also develop in the viscera. Pleural nodules commonly accompany rheumatoid pleural effusions. Pulmonary parenchymal nodules also occur, but even when subcutaneous nodules are present, biopsy is needed to exclude malignancy. Large conglomerate pulmonary rheumatoid nodules are seen in coal miners (Caplan's syndrome) (Fig. 14.12). Parenchymal nodules can cavitate or cause pneumothorax. Pulmonary nodules may rarely antedate demonstrable joint disease (Nüsslein et al, 1987).

Nodules in the heart are found coincidentally at autopsy, but valvular nodules rarely cause valvular insufficiency. Involvement of the conduction system can lead to arrhythmias, which may require the implantation of a pacemaker.

Dural nodules can cause cord compression and extradural nodules can compress spinal roots (Jackson et al, 1984). Vocal cord nodules can be one cause of hoarseness in patients with rheumatoid arthritis, but cricoarytenoid synovitis is a more common cause. Scleral nodules may lead to perforating scleromalacia.

Although rheumatoid nodules are considered so important that, upon histologic confirmation, they provide two of the ARA criteria for the diagnosis of rheumatoid arthritis, they are not completely pathognomonic. Nodules that are virtually identical histologically can be seen in systemic lupus erythematosus (SLE) (Hahn et al, 1970), mixed connective tissue disease or other collagen diseases, acute rheumatic fever, juvenile rheumatoid arthritis, and hypogammaglobulinemia (Barnett et al, 1970). Most such nodules tend to be smaller, and have less extensive necrosis and less regular pallisading than those of rheumatoid arthritis (Bywaters, 1979).

Granuloma annulare, a benign cutaneous and subcutaneous lesion with similar histology, is unrelated to rheumatoid arthritis. A tissue reaction similar to that of a rheumatoid nodule has been reported at a corticosteroid injection site (Balogh, 1986), and the nodules of chronic caseating infections may also be difficult to distinguish from rheumatoid nodules. Nodules histologically identical to rheumatoid nodules have been reported in

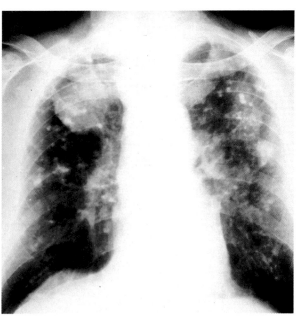

Figure 14.12 Massive conglomerate nodules are typical of Caplan's syndrome.

prostate tissue from 11 patients with second transurethral resections. None of these patients had other features of rheumatoid arthritis. Although classic nodules in a typical location can favor the diagnosis of rheumatoid arthritis, they must be recognized as not unique to rheumatoid arthritis (Pieterse et al, 1984).

Pathogenesis and Therapy

Rheumatoid nodules have been thought to be caused by vasculitis; recent reviews of many biopsies, however, do not substantiate this, since vasculitis is rarely found at the margins of even early nodules (Rasker and Kuipers, 1983). The classic, three-layered structure of central necrosis, surrounded by pallisaded histiocytes and then chronic inflammatory cells, is well known (see Chapter 4.)

Nodules can contain a considerable amount of lipid, and large foamy macrophages and cholesterol crystals can be seen in the nodule margin and in the necrotic center (Fig. 14.13). Also, release of cholesterol and other lipids from nodules into bursae can cause milky bursal effusions (Taccari and Teodori, 1984).

When there is a question about what is causing the arthritis and/or the nodules (Fig. 14.14), a nodule can be aspirated and examined for urate crystals. If none are found, a surgical excisional biopsy may demonstrate characteristic rheumatoid nodule features or

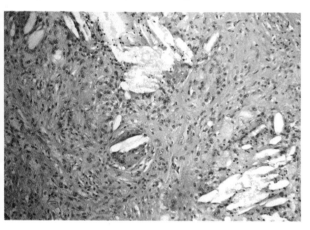

Figure 14.13 Clear clefts in this nodule result from sites where lipid crystals were dissolved during fixation (H&E).

CAUSES OF NONRHEUMATOID NODULES AND ARTHRITIS

Behçet's disease	Amyloidosis
Whipple's disease	Gout
Fibroblastic rheumatism	Multicentric reticulohistiocytosis
Histoplasmosis	
Hemochromatosis	Lupus profundus
Ehlers-Danlos syndrome	Malignancy primary metastatic
Hypereosinophilic syndrome	Sebaceous cysts
Mycoplasma infection	Ganglions
Pancreatic disease	Weber-Christian syndrome
Calcinosis	
Sarcoidosis	Farber's disease

Figure 14.14 Causes of nonrheumatoid nodules.

another cause of the nodule. Almost all patients with rheumatoid nodules have rheumatoid factor detectable by the serum latex fixation test (Kaye et al, 1984).

No drug consistently alters rheumatoid nodules; improvement as the arthritis abates is not predictable. Even when the synovitis of rheumatoid arthritis responds to a second-line drug, nodules may persist.

Intralesional injections with depot corticosteroids occasionally appear to help, but they may be followed by persistent drainage or infection. Protection against irritation by padding or a change in use of affected area may allow nodules to decrease, and ulcerated or draining lesions to heal. Huge nodules or nodules that cause severe cosmetic problems can be excised surgically. Nodules may be expected to recur if disease activity persists.

Although generally felt to be associated with more highly expressed joint and systemic disease, nodules do not indicate a worse functional or radiographic prognosis (Bathon et al, 1985).

RHEUMATOID VASCULITIS

Disease of the extra-articular vessels can be an important feature of rheumatoid disease. Presenting in at least three distinct subsets, the incidence of rheumatoid vasculitis is variously estimated, depending on whether one or all three subset patterns are included. The most common vascular disease is the relatively bland obliterative endoarteritis that

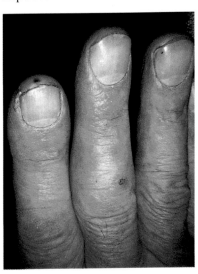

Figure 14.15 Bland fingertip nailbed and mild phalangeal vasculitic lesions are common, as seen here in a case of chronic rheumatoid disease.

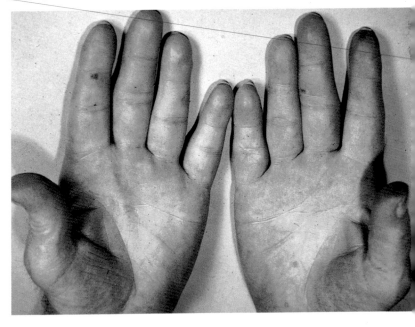

Figure 14.16 Bland vasculitis lesions are seen on the palms.

occludes small vessels and produces painless infarcts in nailbeds and paronychial areas. Leukocytoclastic vasculitis of cutaneous venules produces palpable purpura. Thirdly, necrotizing arteritis of both small- and medium-sized vessels is very similar to idiopathic polyarteritis lesions. Fortunately, this last, potentially devastating type is uncommon, occurring in no more than 1% of patients. Severe arteritis often occurs along with other extra-articular features in patients with high titers of rheumatoid factor, but it has also been reported as the first manifestation of rheumatoid arthritis (Gray and Poppo, 1983). Arthritis need not be especially active for vasculitis to occur.

Clinical Features

The three subsets of rheumatoid vascular disease have very different clinical presen-

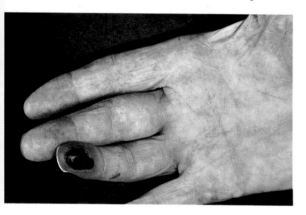

tations. Bland obliterative arteritis most often presents as small, dark nontender infarctions in the fingers. Most lesions are around the nails (Fig. 14.15), but some are more proximal (Fig. 14.16). It is proposed that lesions occur at the nailfolds because of vascular blanching during pressure grip (Edwards, 1980). These lesions are more often seen in men who work with their hands than in men who do not; other effects of occupational trauma occasionally may be difficult to distinguish. Similar tiny vasculitic lesions can overlie joints or appear on the surface of rheumatoid nodules, often appearing in crops and healing without tissue loss. Rarely, similar lesions are associated with ischemic fingertips (Fig. 14.17); it may not be clear whether the process is the same or if a large-vessel necrotizing arteritis is also present. In contrast to the digital ischemia seen in systemic sclerosis, this is usually not accompanied by Raynaud's

Figure 14.17 Fingertip ischemia in rheumatoid vasculitis.

phenomenon. Typically only one or two digits are involved. This vascular disease does not seem to correlate well with the presence of synovial inflammation.

Leukocytoclastic vasculitis is less common, occurs much more often on the legs, and presents with characteristic, palpable purpura (Fig. 14.18) or, less often, urticaria. These lesions can cause pruritis or a sensation of burning but usually heal without ulceration or significant scarring.

The feared complication of rheumatoid arthritis is larger-vessel necrotizing vasculitis. This often occurs concomitantly with other extra-articular features of highly expressed disease, including episcleritis, scleromalacia, or serosis. The joint disease need not be especially active.

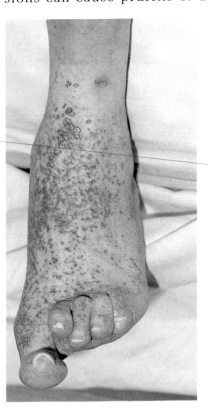

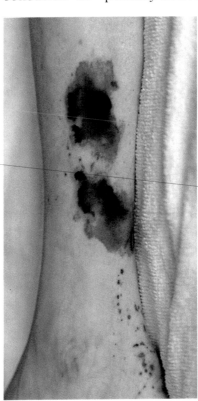

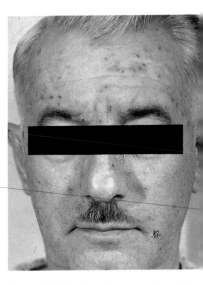

Figure 14.20 A cutaneous rheumatoid vasculitis in a male is developing along with mononeuritis multiplex.

Figure 14.18 Palpable purpura typical of leukocytoclastic vasculitis are seen in a patient with rheumatoid arthritis.

Figure 14.19 Acute hemorrhagic necrotizing skin lesions, as seen in rheumatoid arteritis.

Pathogenetic mechanisms are not clearly established for any type of vasculitis, although a role for circulating immune complexes has been suggested. Patients are often febrile at the onset of vasculitis, with temperatures up to 104° or 105°; there is frequently a sudden appearance of sensorimotor neuropathy, with a patchy "mononeuritis multiplex" distribution. Painful deep necrotizing skin lesions (Fig. 14.19) can ulcerate, and ulcers are typically seen along the shin. Digital gangrene can occur and visceral vasculitis can cause infarctions at various sites. A more indolent, limited disease also occurs. Other less dramatic skin lesions can appear at the same time (Fig. 14.20); facial lesions have occasionally become scarring and granulomatous (White et al, 1986). Severe vasculitis appears to be more common in men.

Arteritis infrequently can cause intestinal infarction (Adler et al, 1962), myocardial infarction (Voyles et al, 1980), or central nervous system vasculitis. Cerebral vasculitis, although reported (Watson et al, 1977), is extremely rare, and documentation has understandably been difficult in suspected cases. Amyloid in cerebral vessels can be a factor in cerebral vascular disease (Mandybur, 1979), whereas dural nodules (Jackson et al, 1984) and pachymeningitis (Markenson et al, 1979) can produce neurologic signs that must be distinguished from actual vasculitis. Renal vasculitis is rare (Burry, 1971), and as with any infrequent finding, the possibility of another coincidental disease must always be considered. Avascular necrosis has rarely been attributed to rheumatoid vasculitis (Shupak et al, 1983).

Many other causes of vasculitis can coexist with rheumatoid disease or can be associated with an arthritis that might be confused with rheumatoid arthritis. For example, bullous vasculitic lesions are more common in SLE (Fig. 14.21). Wegener's syndrome can present

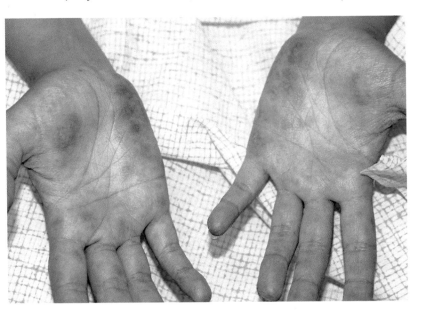

Figure 14.21 Bullae on the palms seen here are due to SLE vasculitis.

with a mild arthritis along with a destructive midline, pulmonary, and renal granulomatous vasculitis (Fig. 14.22). Because this type of arthritis improves dramatically with cyclophosphamide therapy, the differential diagnosis is important. A rare cutaneous vasculitis termed erythema elevatum diutinum (Schumacher et al, 1977) is also associated with arthritis (Fig. 14.23).

Laboratory Findings

Polymorphonuclear leukocytosis is common and eosinophilia may occur. Worsening anemia is often seen in severe vasculitis. Hyperviscosity complicating the rheumatoid arthritis may occasionally contribute to vascular disease (Silberman, 1986).

Serum complement levels are usually elevated or normal, except in some patients with necrotizing arteritis. Immune complexes can often be detected and are felt to be important in the pathogenesis of this serious disease. Some recent studies suggest that measurement of serum products of endothelial or platelet injury, such as factor VIII or alkaline ribonuclease, may be used to determine the severity of the vasculitis (Oribe et al, 1986).

Vasculitis can be suspected on the basis of the clinical and laboratory picture but should be confirmed by biopsy. If sites for biopsy are not clinically obvious, rectal mucosal suction biopsy (Tribe et al, 1981) or muscle biopsy can be helpful. Vessel wall necrosis and fibrinoid infiltration must be present to confirm a diagnosis of necrotizing arteritis (see Chapter 4). Perivascular infiltrates should not be overinterpreted as vasculitis. Intense infiltration of capillary or venule walls with neutrophils and nuclear debris from necrotic cells (leukocytoclastic vasculitis) is less serious, as noted above.

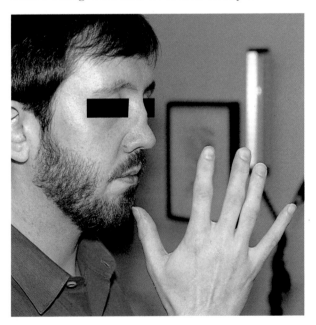

Figure 14.22 This patient with the necrotizing granulomatous vasculitis of Wegener's syndrome has destruction of nasal cartilage and polyarthritis in the hands that might be mistaken for rheumatoid arthritis.

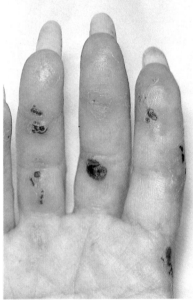

Figure 14.23 Erythema elevatum diutinum is a rare type of cutaneous vasculitis with very painful, indurated crusted lesions seen mostly on the hands and feet.

Therapy

The mild vascular disease commonly manifested by nailfold infarcts does not require any new therapy. Many patients continue with intermittently appearing distal cutaneous infarcts for years or for the duration of their disease without developing a more severe vasculitis.

Leukocytoclastic vasculitis with widespread cutaneous palpable purpura or urticaria usually is helped by a course of moderate-dose adrenocorticosteriods (20 to 40 mg of prednisone daily). It is also important to consider whether this vasculitis might be a reaction to some drug, which might be discontinued to resolve the vasculitis.

Polyarteritis-like systemic necrotizing vasculitis is the most devastating vascular disease and the most difficult to manage. As it is an uncommon feature of rheumatoid disease, no controlled therapeutic trials are available as a guide to management. Scott et al (1981b) found a 30% five-year mortality in rheumatoid patients who had multiple sites of necrotizing vasculitis.

The tendency to spontaneous remissions and exacerbations makes evaluation of therapy difficult. It also suggests that very toxic drugs should be used only in the clearly active, progressive stage of the disease. Clinical improvement in severe vasculitis has been reported to coincide with cyclophosphamide use, so this drug is often suggested to treat severe necrotizing arteritis (Abel et al, 1980).

Other proposed treatments have included penicillamine administration (Jaffe, 1970) and plasmapheresis (Scott et al, 1981a; Winkelstein et al, 1984). Neuropathy associated with vasculitis seems to resolve very slowly at best under any treatment, although skin ulcers usually heal.

Corticosteroid therapy is controversial, with some authors suggesting that steroids actually predispose to vasculitis while others increase the dose or start the patient on high-dose steroids. We personally prefer to taper off steroids, if tolerated, when patients develop vasculitis while already receiving medium- or high-dose therapy. Although we occasionally do start high-dose steroids in patients who have not previously received steroids, it is not clear how often this is helpful.

FELTY'S SYNDROME

The association of deforming arthritis typical of rheumatoid arthritis with splenomegaly and leukopenia was reported by Felty in 1924. Although it occurs in fewer than 1% of patients with rheumatoid arthritis, it is important because of the differential diagnosis (Fig. 14.24) and because of its pathogenic and therapeutic implications. As will be described, it is probably best to consider this a clinical syndrome, with different mecha-

Figure 14.24 Causes of splenomegaly and/or leukopenia

SOME CAUSES OF SPLENOMEGALY AND/OR LEUKOPENIA WITH RHEUMATOID ARTHRITIS OR OTHER ARTHRITIS

Systemic lupus erythematosus	Amyloidosis
Drug-induced leukopenia	Leukemia or lymphoma
Viral or other infection	Subacute bacterial endocarditis
	Aplastic anemia

nisms predominating in different patients. An enlarged spleen does not account for all the leukopenia seen in Felty's syndrome.

Felty's syndrome occurs in adults with rheumatoid arthritis of all ages. More women than men are affected, and in reports in which race is specified, virtually all cases have been in whites (Termini et al, 1979). A familial tendency to develop Felty's syndrome has been reported (Blendis et al, 1976). Increased mortality, related mostly to infection, has also been reported.

Clinical Features

Arthritis almost always antedates the other clinical features of Felty's syndrome (in one series by 1 to 39 years) (Spivak, 1977). It is severe in most patients, although there may be little actual joint inflammation in some patients when their neutropenia is detected. Other systemic features are common (Fig. 14.25). Leg ulcers, most often around the ankles (Fig. 14.26), occasional skin pigmentation, and lymphadenopathy can complicate

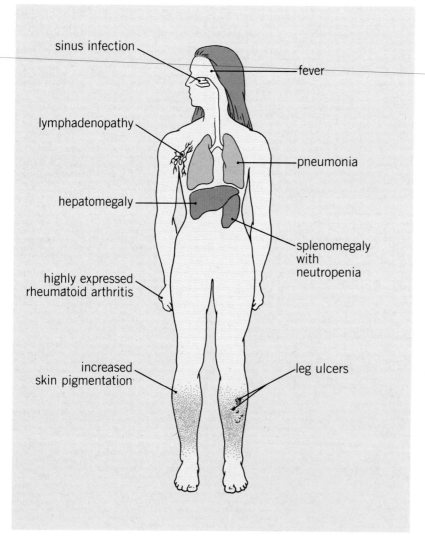

Figure 14.25 Some features of Felty's syndrome.

sinus infection

fever

lymphadenopathy

pneumonia

hepatomegaly

splenomegaly with neutropenia

highly expressed rheumatoid arthritis

increased skin pigmentation

leg ulcers

Felty's syndrome (Barnes et al, 1971). Leg ulcers often show little inflammatory reaction; vasculitis at the ulcer margin is uncommon.

Infection is the main concern but does not invariably occur despite a very low neutrophil count. Gram-positive infections are especially common, with skin, pulmonary, and oral sinus or nasopharngeal sites being the most frequent. Some fevers are not explained by any infection but require thorough evaluation.

Spleen size can vary widely, from the less common spleen that is not detectably involved to the truly massive spleen that extends into the pelvis. The most common finding is a firm spleen, palpable 2 to 4 cm below the costal margin. Such spleens are generally not tender. Rarely there is splenic rupture (Granirer et al, 1958). Hepatomegaly can also occur. Up to 50% of patients can have elevated serum alkaline phosphatase or transaminase levels. Nodular regenerative hyperplasia of the liver, with nodular expansion and fibrosis around the portal veins, can occur (Termini et al, 1979), whereas other patients have isolated portal fibrosis. Portal hypertension with further enlargement of the spleen occasionally results (Klofkorn et al, 1976). There may also be esophageal varices.

Pathogenesis

As noted above, different factors seem to be important in the neutropenia seen in different patients. Figure 14.27 lists some of the mechanisms involved in the production of

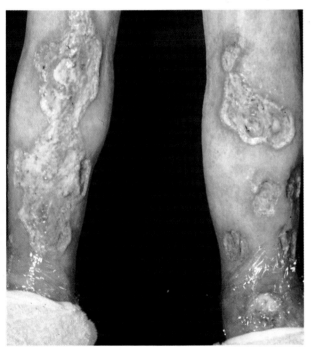

Figure 14.26 Unusually extensive leg ulcers in a patient with Felty's syndrome and vasculitis.

MECHANISMS INVOLVED IN THE PRODUCTION OF NEUTROPENIA IN FELTY'S SYNDROME

Margination of neutrophils in the enlarged spleen.

Removal or destruction of neutrophils by splenic reticuloendothelial cells.

Decreased granulopoiesis induced by humoral or cellular factors from the spleen.

Autoimmune activity against circulating leukocytes.

Figure 14.27 Neutropenia in Felty's syndrome.

neutropenia (Gupta et al, 1975). Neutrophil function is often abnormal, and defects in chemotactic, phagocytic, killing, or other neutrophil function may be more important than the absolute leukocyte count in determining if infection will occur. Splenomegaly does not seem to be essential to the other features of the syndrome, and neutropenia can recur after splenectomy (Logue et al, 1981).

Although increased IgG can be found on the surface of neutrophils in patients with Felty's syndrome, this finding is not unique to this syndrome, and many patients with such bound IgG do not develop neutropenia. This suggests that several combinations of factors may be involved in the pathogenesis of this syndrome.

Pathology

The leukopenia in Felty's syndrome is predominantly a selective neutropenia, and criteria for leukopenia have varied in different series. Most patients have total white blood cell counts of less than 2500/mm^3. Immature circulating cells are not seen and, if they are detected, a hematologic malignancy should be considered. Toxic effects of drugs or coexistence with SLE (in which lymphopenia is more common) should be considered in differential diagnosis. A subset of patients with rheumatoid-like polyarthritis and neutropenia with increased large granular lymphocytes has been described (Wallis et al, 1985). Thrombocytopenia is seen in about 40% of cases but is usually mild. Anemia, seen in most patients, is usually consistent with the anemia of chronic disease. Some reticulocytosis appears to reflect erythrocyte destruction. The bone marrow most often shows a moderate hypercellularity, with few mature neutrophils. In some marrows, however, mature granulocytes are increased in number. Less often there is a distinctly hypocellular marrow, possibly due to marrow-suppressing factors, and circulating neutrophils have been described as having immunocomplex-like inclusions that may affect their function (Fig. 14.28). High levels of IgG neutrophil-binding

Figure 14.28 Granular inclusions stain darkly with immunoperoxidase to label IgG in a neutrophil from a patient with Felty's syndrome. (Electron micrograph).

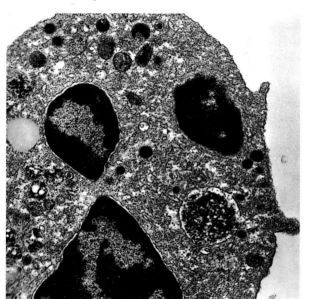

activity have been seen in Felty's syndrome and seem to be associated with depressed superoxide generation (Davis et al, 1987).

Splenic tissue in Felty's syndrome typically shows follicular, histiocyte, and vascular endothelial hyperplasia. Erythrophagocytosis is also observed in some cases.

Therapy

Remissions and cyclic variations in neutropenia occur spontaneously in some patients, and most neutropenic patients without infections do not need treatment.

Despite some natural hesitancy to use it in patients with neutropenia, gold has frequently helped correct the neutropenia (Percy, 1981). This is usually the initial drug of choice when treatment is needed. Splenomegaly can decrease and other features of the rheumatoid arthritis can improve. Penicillamine, cyclophosphamide methotrexate, and high-dose corticosteroids decrease neutropenia in some patients. The latter three drugs are more risky, because they can lower resistance to infection. Lithium can increase neutrophil counts, at least temporarily, but apparently does not alter the course of the disease. Since recent studies suggest that lithium can actually stimulate granulopoiesis (Levine and Toback, 1987), some authors use it early in the treatment of neutropenia.

Splenectomy can correct the neutropenia, generally within hours. This may help with the handling of difficult active infections, but long-term results are unpredictable. The incidence of infections sometimes declines after splenectomy even when the neutropenia is not altered (Barnes, 1971; Moore, 1971). Recurrent infections continued in 26% to 60% of patients after splenectomy and neutrophil counts fell again after splenectomy in about one quarter of the patients (Goldberg and Pinals, 1980). There is also a recognized incidence of overwhelming sepsis following splenectomy for any reason, so splenectomy is a calculated risk. The danger of pneumococcal sepsis can be decreased by vaccination before splenectomy.

CARDIAC MANIFESTATIONS

Rheumatic fever and rheumatoid arthritis have often been confused, and nineteenth century and early twentieth century reports of cardiac disease in rheumatoid arthritis are inaccurate. Bywaters (1950) and Sokoloff (1953) designated "rheumatoid heart disease" as a distinct pathologic entity. It is estimated that 30% to 50% of patients with rheumatoid arthritis have cardiac involvement (Pizarello and Goldberg, 1985); most lesions, however, are asymptomatic and are found in less than 10% of patients premortem. Any area of the heart can be involved (Fig. 14.29), including the pericardium, the myocardium, cardiac vessels, the conducting system, and valves. None of the symptoms is specific to rheumatoid involvement in the heart, so other causes of signs and symptoms must be sought. Cardiac involvement is more common in active seropositive disease.

The most sensitive diagnostic tool used to determine cardiac involvement with rheumatoid arthritis is the echocardiogram (Bacon and Gibson, 1974; Nomier et al, 1973; Shorn et al, 1976). In patients with classic rheumatoid arthritis, 47% had pericardial abnormalities, and 30% demonstrated valvular problems (Nomier et al, 1973). Bacon and Gibson (1974) found pericardial effusion in 34% of patients with rheumatoid arthritis and in 50% of patients with rheumatoid nodules. A radiographic study of 309 patients with rheumatoid arthritis demonstrated cardiac and aortic enlargement in significantly more arthritic patients than controls (Jurik et al, 1984).

Pericardial Involvement

Pericarditis is the most common cardiac manifestation of rheumatoid arthritis. Necropsy studies have shown an incidence of 11% to 50% involvement in rheumatoid arthritis (Pizarello and Goldberg, 1985). A prospective echocardiographic search revealed posterior effusion not detected by chest radiographs or electrocardiograms in 44% of a small series of rheumatoid arthritis patients (Prakash et al, 1973). Most of these patients had had rheumatoid disease for a long time (8 to 27 years). Large effusions can also be seen (Fig. 14.30).

Postmortem studies can reveal a fibrous adhesive pericarditis (Fig. 14.31). The fluid, which may be yellow or hemorrhagic (Fig.

Figure 14.29 Incidence of cardiac lesions in rheumatoid arthritis in clinical and autopsy studies.

INCIDENCE OF CARDIAC LESIONS IN RHEUMATOID ARTHRITIS

LESION	NECROPSY SERIES	CLINICAL SERIES
Pericarditis	11% to 50%	1.6% to 2.4%
Myocarditis		
Focal, nonspecific	4% to 30%	Rare
Diffuse, necrotizing	Rare	Rare
Granulomatous	3% to 5%	Rare
Amyloid	Rare	Rare
Conductive pathway disease	Unknown	8% to 10%
Coronary arteritis	15% to 20%	Rare
Valvular disease	6% to 62%	Rare
Any cardiac disease	30% to 62%	1.6% to 10%

Pizarello and Goldberg, 1985

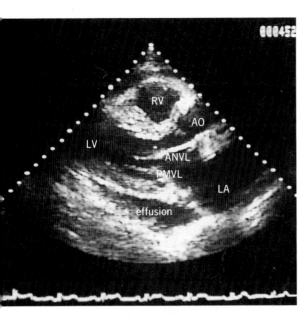

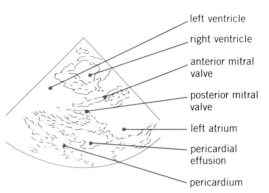

Figure 14.30 Echocardiogram in a patient with rheumatoid arthritis showing a large pericardial effusion.

left ventricle
right ventricle
anterior mitral valve
posterior mitral valve
left atrium
pericardial effusion
pericardium

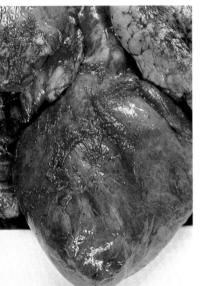

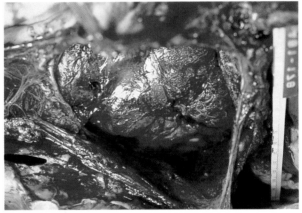

Figure 14.31 A "bread and butter," fibrinous pericarditis typical of that seen in rheumatoid arthritis (*left*). Note the thick fibrin on the cardiac surface. Fibrinous pericarditis with pericardium stripped away with difficulty on an autopsy specimen (*right*). Note the reflected pericardium and the underlying heart with marked fibrin deposition over the cardiac surface. (Courtesy of Samuel Paplanus MD)

14.32), is an exudate with inflammatory cells and elevated protein and LDH levels (Pizarello and Goldberg, 1985). Cholesterol crystals may be seen in chronic effusions (Fig. 14.33) (Cohen and Canoso, 1976). Complement titers (C3, C4, CH50) are usually decreased due to the presence of immunocomplexes, and rheumatoid factor titers are elevated (Ball et al, 1975). Reduced glucose levels are found even in the absence of infection. The majority of patients are seropositive for rheumatoid factor, with significant titers and sedimentation rates also elevated.

The incidence of pericarditis seen clinically is far less than that determined at autopsy. Patients with symptomatic disease often will complain of left-sided and precordial chest pain (Franco et al, 1972), which is sometimes pleuritic. Symptoms of congestive heart failure may be present in some individuals, particularly if constrictive disease is present or other cardiac structures are involved. Constrictive pericarditis and cardiac tamponade can produce severe dyspnea, peripheral edema, and signs of compromised cardiac contractility (Thadani et al, 1975). Most patients with symptomatic complica-

tions have rheumatoid nodules.

Physical examination reveals a friction rub in some patients. In one series, 59% of patients with known pericarditis had distended jugular veins, elevated venous pressure, liver enlargement, and moist rales (Franco et al, 1972), while concomitant pleural effusions are not unusual. Patients may run low-grade fevers. No pathognomic findings suggest a rheumatoid origin for pericarditis over other causes for this disorder.

Radiographs may show cardiac enlargement in patients with extensive effusions (Fig. 14.34). The echocardiogram, as noted, is a far more sensitive procedure (Comess et al, 1982). Loculated fluid and fibrous strands can be demonstrated, and on occasion, loculation can cause a mass effect leading to outflow obstruction (Goldman et al, 1978). In such cases, cardiac catheterization may be needed to delineate a structural abnormality that may be causing symptoms (Fig. 14.35).

Treatment of mild symptoms requires only aspirin or nonsteroidal anti-inflammatory drugs, such as indomethacin. In more severe cases, systemic corticosteroids such as prednisone (20 to 60 mg daily) may be administered. Intrapericardial injection of depot ster-

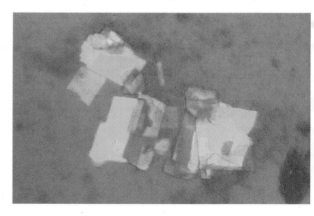

Figure 14.32 Hemorrhagic fluid removed during pericardiocentesis. Brownish blood-tinged pericardial fluid was filled with cholesterol crystals.

Figure 14.33 Using polarizing microscope with first-order red compensator, a pericardial effusion from patient with rheumatoid pericarditis reveals typical cholesterol crystals, which are square or rectangular, stacked and often missing one corner.

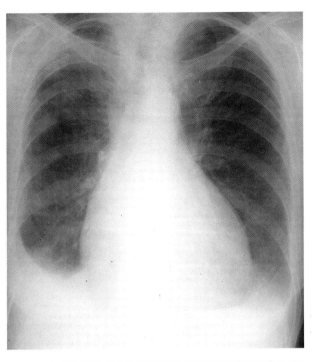

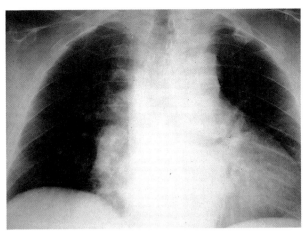

Figure 14.34 A patient with rheumatoid arthritis had mild to moderate pericardial effusion (*left*). There is an increase in the cardiac silhouette and a straightening of the left ventricular border. A pleural effusion on the right side is also seen. A large pericardial effusion in patient with rheumatoid pericarditis is seen on the *right*. The heart is boot-shaped and occupies almost three quarters of the diameter of the chest wall.

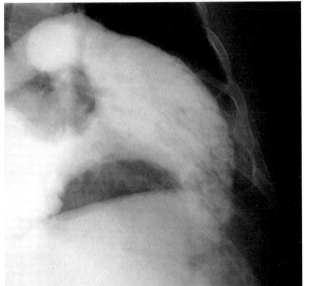

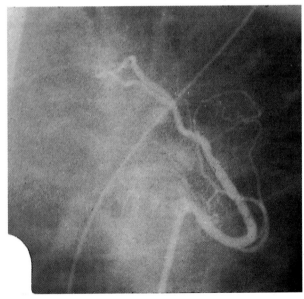

Figure 14.35 Cardiac catherterization. Ventriculogram of patient with loculated pericardial effusion. There is deformity of the right ventricle and pressure on the tricuspid valve (*left*). Coronary arteriogram of same patient demonstrates that the right coronary artery is displaced by the effusion. Preoperative anatomic delineation of these lesions led to a successful pericardial window.

oids has been successful in some cases (Scharf et al, 1976). Surgical pericardectomy, while difficult, may be lifesaving in constrictive disease (Burney et al, 1979). Pericardiocentesis may relieve restrictive disease and provide diagnostic information to aid in ruling out other causes of the pericarditis, such as tuberculosis or viral infection.

Myocardial Disease

The heart muscle itself can be affected indirectly through vascular and valvular derangements caused by rheumatoid arthritis, or directly through myocarditis, nodule formation, or conduction abnormalities. Amyloid infiltration can lead to congestive heart failure and cardiomegaly (Fig. 14.36). Nonspecific myocarditis may be demonstrated histologically in 4% to 30% of rheumatoid arthritis patients at autopsy (Pizarello and Goldberg, 1985). Such patients had cardiomegaly and chronic inflammatory cell infiltrates.

The pathologic picture is identical to idiopathic myocarditis but rarely is symptomatic, and EKGs and clinical studies are usually normal. Granulomatous myocarditis is very rare (Bonfiglio and Atwater, 1969); diffuse, more severe myocarditis, however, can lead to chamber dilatation and cardiac failure. Echocardiography reveals ventricular wall dysfunction in patients with signs of severe congestive failure. Early treatment with cardiac drugs, anticoagulants (if thrombi are present), and diuretics is requisite. Arrythmias and conduction disturbances should be appropriately addressed. Systemic corticosteroids are sometimes used.

Conduction abnormalities can be caused by rheumatoid nodules in cardiac tissue (Ojeda et al, 1986). Antibodies to conducting tissues have been demonstrated in some patients with rheumatoid arthritis (Villecco et al, 1983), many of whom (35%) have bundle branch blocks by EKG. Of the patients with right bundle branch block and rheumatoid arthritis, 76% will have these antibodies, whereas this finding is rare in patients with bundle branch blocks without rheumatoid arthritis (1 in 42 patients). Nodules that interfere with conduction are very rare.

Coronary Artery Disease

The incidence of small vessel coronary arteritis is 15% to 20% at autopsy of patients with rheumatoid arthritis (Pizarello and Goldberg, 1985). Severe necrotizing arteritis may occur in patients with polyarteritis-like disease complicating the rheumatoid arthritis (Fig. 14.37). In such patients, myocardial infarction may occur, although this is only seen at autopsy (Voyles et al, 1980). There is no way to differentiate coronary artery vasculitis from atheromatous disease during life. It had been thought that coronary artery athrosclerotic disease would be less frequent in rheumatoid patients than in other patients because of their long-term salicylate ingestion, but this has not turned out to be true (Davis and Engleman, 1974).

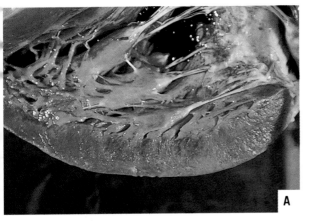

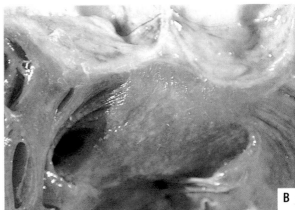

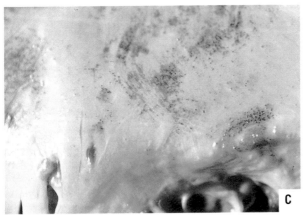

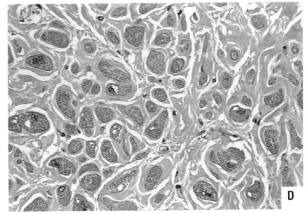

Figure 14.36 Cardiac amyloidosis in a patient with rheumatoid arthritis. The pale yellow coloring of the ventricle is due to the amyloid deposition (**A**). Yellow nodular discoloration of endocardium (**B**) is due to amyloid deposi-tion. Endocardial amyloid deposits stain brown with io-dine (**C**). Cardiac muscle tissue section stained bright purple in the area of amyloid deposition in patient with cardiac amyloidosis (**D**) (crystal violet stain).

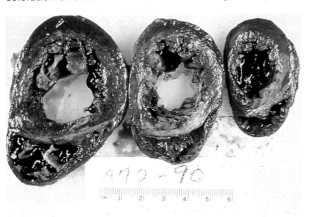

Figure 14.37 Myocardial infarction due to coronary arteritis. Arteritis similar to that seen in polyarteritis rarely causes necrotizing lesions in the coronary arteries. However, in this patient there was complete occlusion of the coronary artery, leading to myocardial infarction and death.

Valvular Disease

Valvular abnormalities are found in 30% to 40% of patients with rheumatoid arthritis (Pizarello and Goldberg, 1985). All four valves may be involved and the frequency parallels that of rheumatic fever. Mitral valvular disease is the most common problem; either stenosis or insufficiency may occur, with the latter occurring more often. Similar lesions can occur on aortic valve and nodular and inflammatory changes may be seen (Fig. 14.38). In extreme cases, aneurysmal dilatation of the aorta secondary to aortitis can occur causing aortic rupture (Fig. 14.39). Granulomatous tissue lesions similar to rheumatoid nodules may be found on pathologic examination of cardiac valves (Fig. 14.40). Such lesions are rarely symptomatic. In some cases, a progressive valvular insufficiency may require surgical valve replacement (Flores et al, 1984). Otherwise, medical management appropriate to the cardiac symptoms is in order.

PULMONARY ABNORMALITIES

Many pulmonary manifestations of rheumatoid arthritis can involve the lung parenchyma, the vasculature, the airways, and the pleura (Fig. 14.41). Drugs can also cause pulmonary abnormalities. The incidence of pulmonary involvement in rheumatoid arthritis is unknown, but Hyland et al (1983) were able to correlate physical and radiographic findings with lung pathology.

Pulmonary complications are more severe in older males, patients with other marked systemic features, with HLA-DR3 or HLA-DR4 genotypes, with α-1-antitrypsin deficiency, with occupational or other exposure to pulmonary toxins, and for those taking immunosuppressive medication (Gordon et al, 1985).

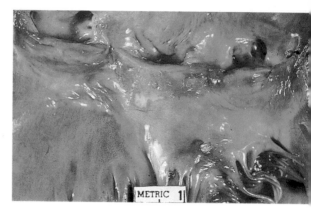

Figure 14.38 Aortitis with nodular inflammation of the aortic valve in a patient with rheumatoid arthritis. This lesion can lead to aortic valvular insufficiency.

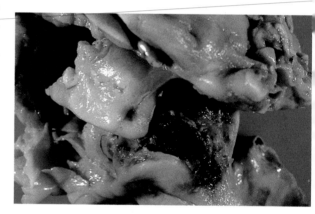

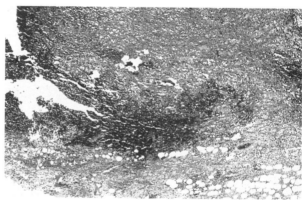

Figure 14.39 Postmortem specimen (*top*) is from a rheumatoid arthritis patient with aortitis and aortic aneurysm. Death was caused by aortic rupture. Microscopic section (*bottom*) shows aneurysmal dilatation and hemorrhage into the wall of the aorta (H&E).

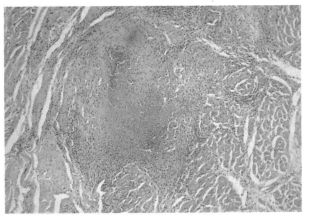

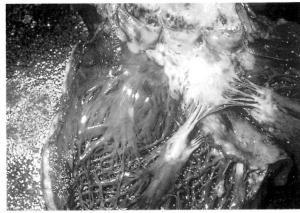

Figure 14.40 Typical rheumatoid granuloma occurring within the myocardium at the aortic root is seen in this postmortem specimen (*left*) (H&E, × 80). Intraoperative view of heart, showing aortic valve and mitral valve chordea tendinae (*right*). Rheumatoid nodules are seen at the base of the aortic valve cusps and in the tips of the papillary muscles. (Courtesy of PA Dieppe, MD)

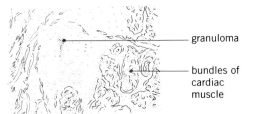

granuloma

bundles of cardiac muscle

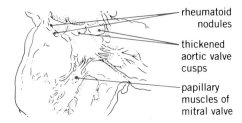

rheumatoid nodules

thickened aortic valve cusps

papillary muscles of mitral valve

LUNG INVOLVEMENT IN RHEUMATOID ARTHRITIS

Parenchymal disease
Interstitial fibrosis

Interstitial pneumonitis

Pulmonary nodules (with or without cavitation)

Caplan's syndrome

Bullous disease

Amyloidosis

Infection

Neoplasm

Airway
Restrictive lung disease (chest wall)

Bronchiolitis

Sleep apnea

Obstructive airway disease

Pleura
Pleural effusion

Pleuritis and nodules

Drug Induced

Vasculature
Pulmonary hypertension

Pulmonary hemorrhage (hemosiderosis)

Vasculitis

Figure 14.41 Lung involvement in rheumatoid arthritis.

Pleuritis

Pleural involvement is a common manifestation of rheumatoid arthritis (Walker and Wright, 1968). Although some authors feel that pleural effusions are no more common in rheumatoid arthritis patients than in other patients, the nature of the pleural exudate suggests that it is caused by the disease. The incidence of pleural effusion is 0.6% of rheumatoid arthritis patients (Jurik et al, 1982). Chest radiographs suggest the presence of a pleural effusion, which then can be confirmed in a decubitus view (Fig. 14.42). Ultrasonography also can confirm the presence of fluid. Characteristic findings in pleural fluid analysis for rheumatoid arthritis are listed in Figure 14.43.

Pleural effusion may be asymptomatic or may appear with the typical symptoms of pleurisy, such as chest pain and fever. Physical examination will reveal dullness at the base, decreased breath sounds, and in some cases, a pleural friction rub.

The most reliable diagnostic features differentiating rheumatoid pleural effusion from other pleural effusions include low pH and low glucose and low C_4 levels. The presence of rheumatoid factor is not much help in this diagnostic analysis (Pettersson et al, 1982). The fluid is typically an exudate with a white blood cell count below 5000/mm³, usually with mononuclear cells present. Cholesterol crystals may be seen in long-standing effusions. Immune complexes with rheumatoid factor deplete complement, particularly C_4 (Gordon et al, 1985). Rheumatoid factor levels parallel those seen in serum and may be positive in patients with such other diseases as tuberculosis, chronic infection, and idiopathic pulmonary fibrosis. Glucose levels may be extraordinarily low (on occasion, not measurable), which is unusual in other diseases, with the exception of tuberculosis, mesothelioma, and rarely, severe bacterial infection. The glucose defect is thought to be

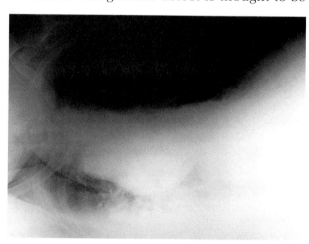

Figure 14.42 Radiograph of patient with rheumatoid pleuritis (*left*). A small pleural effusion is present. Note the blunting of the posterior sulcus. Decubitus view of another patient with rheumatoid arthritis and pleural effusion (*right*) shows the layering of a small amount of pleural effusion on the lower side (right chest). A small amount of pulmonary fibrosis is also present.

due in part to defective transport across the pleura (Bankhurst and Rowe, 1980). Other markers of rheumatoid pleural effusions are similar to those seen in other inflammatory pleural exudates.

Cytologic examination may help differentiate underlying malignancy, with pleural biopsy giving a higher yield of positive findings for infectious or malignant diseases. Biopsy is nonspecific for rheumatoid arthritis, however

CHARACTERISTICS OF PLEURAL EFFUSION: RHEUMATOID ARTHRITIS v OTHER DISEASES

	PROTEIN (G%)	GLUCOSE MMOL/D	PH (MEAN)	LACTIC DEHYDROGENASE (μ/L)	C3 (G%)	C4 (G%)	RHEUM FACTOR
Rheumatoid arthritis	5.3	1±	7.13	2,343	.39	.04	Similar to serum
SLE	5.0	4.5±**	7.29	414	.59	.13****	Similar to serum
Tuberculosis	4.9	3.8±*	7.31*	717*	1.08*	.47*	Similar to serum
Malignancy	4.5±	5.0±*	7.37*	569**	1.05*	.40*	0
Empyema	6.9±	0.1±	6.89***	18,138	.61	.21**	0
Pneumonia	4.7±	4.4±**	7.28	745	1.12*	.41*	0
Congestive heart failure	2.5±*	5.6±*	7.40*	170*	.85****	.33*	0
Nonspecific effusion	4.7±	4.9±*	7.33**	573	1.09*	.42*	0

* P ≤ .001 rheumatoid arthritis, United States
** P ≤ .005 rheumatoid arthritis, United States
*** P ≤ .01 rheumatoid arthritis, United States
**** P ≤ .025

Figure 14.43 Characteristics of pleural effusions. Mean values are given.

(Fig. 14.44). Rarely, constrictive pleuritis or a large effusion may compromise pulmonary function. Characterizing the pleural fluid to rule out infection or neoplasm is indicated before instituting treatment for rheumatoid pleuritis.

The treatment involves an attempt to control the underlying rheumatoid arthritis. Depending on the severity of the pleural involvement, nonsteroidal anti-inflammatory drugs with or without systemic corticosteroids, may control pleuritis. Mild asymptomatic cases may require no treatment. Intrapleural steroids may be of some use in selected patients (Gordon et al, 1985). Surgical decortication is rarely performed (Yarbrough et al, 1975). In one series, rheumatoid pleuritis was described as occurring an average of 13 years after the onset of disease and resolved on an average of 14 months after onset (Faurschou et al, 1985).

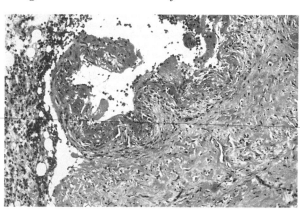

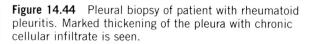

Figure 14.44 Pleural biopsy of patient with rheumatoid pleuritis. Marked thickening of the pleura with chronic cellular infiltrate is seen.

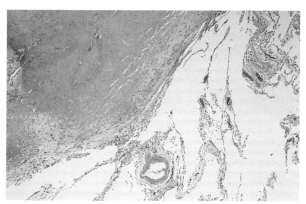

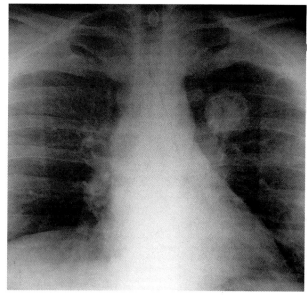

Figure 14.45 Pulmonary biopsy of a nodule shows typical rheumatoid nodule within the lung parenchyma (*left*). The amorphous staining material surrounded by a cellular capsule is a rheumatoid nodule. Normal lung parenchymal tissue surrounds the nodule. (H&E) (Courtesy of Anna Graham, MD). Solitary pulmonary nodule (*left*) is seen on chest radiograph in the left upper lobe. The nodule is large, well circumscribed and cannot be differentiated by radiography alone from infection or neoplasm.

Pulmonary Nodules

Pulmonary rheumatoid nodules are not uncommon in rheumatoid arthritis. They may be solitary or multiple (Fig. 14.45). They may appear in the absence of other parenchymal disease or in association with pulmonary fibrosis or pleural effusion (Fig. 14.46). Although usually sharply demarcated, they may be radiographically indistinguishable from neoplasms or infection. The decision to perform a biopsy is often difficult; just because an earlier nodule was rheumatoid in origin does not mean that subsequent nodules might not be more ominous. Rheumatology, pulmonary, radiology, and thoracic surgical consultation, with joint decision-making, is often helpful. To complicate matters, rheu-

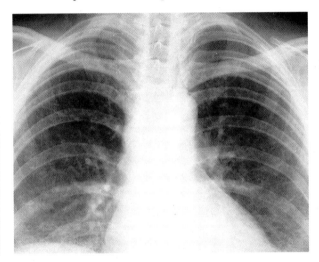

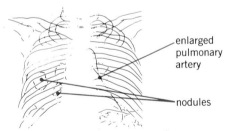

Figure 14.46 Patient with rheumatoid arthritis had mild pulmonary fibrosis, and a solitary pulmonary nodule on the right side (*left*). The nodule is located close to the pleural surface, has a somewhat irregular outline, and could be confused with a malignant or infectious nodule.

Pulmonary fibrosis with multiple tiny pulmonary nodules (*right*). Not all pulmonary nodules are large and disseminated rheumatoid granulomas can look very much like those seen in miliary tuberculosis. In this patient the small nodular infiltrates are due to rheumatoid granuloma.

matoid nodules may cavitate (Fig. 14.47), further simulating tuberculosis or fungal infection, as well as neoplasm.

Many nodules are discovered incidentally on routine chest radiographs. They are usually seen in seropositive, active, classic rheumatoid arthritis patients with a high titer of rheumatoid factors. Most patients are male and have rheumatoid nodules on their extremities as well (Fig. 14.48). Pulmonary nodules are usually subpleural, vary in diameter from 1 mm to several centimeters, and often occur in the upper portion of the lung (Gordon et al, 1985). Serial chest radiographs to evaluate changes can be helpful. Rarely, pulmonary rheumatoid nodules may be the initial manifestation of rheumatoid arthritis

or they may appear without evidence of joint disease (Hull and Mathews, 1982; Eraut et al, 1978; Walters and Ojeda, 1986).

Workup initially should include sputum for culture and cytology; review of previous chest radiographs; and if necessary, bronchoscopy with biopsy, brushings, or bronchoalveolar lavage. Fine needle aspiration or open biopsy may be needed for a definitive diagnosis. Adjunctive workup, such as skin tests and serum complement fixation test for fungi, may be helpful.

Most rheumatoid pulmonary nodules do not require treatment. Excision should be considered for very large cavitary nodules with secondary infection or hemoptysis.

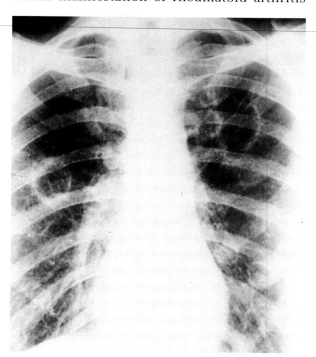
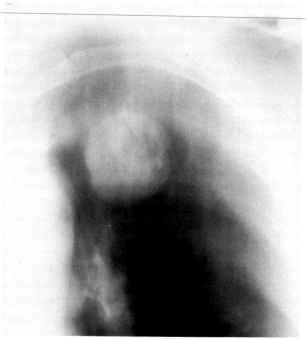

Figure 14.47 Cavitary pulmonary nodules in rheumatoid arthritis on radiograph (*left*) (From Revised Clinical Slide Collection on Rheumatic Diseases, © 1981. Used by permission of American Rheumatism Assn.). Tomography of a solitary nodule shows cavitation (*right*). Cavitation of a pulmonary nodule can occur in rheumatoid arthritis but can also occur with neoplasm and infection. Bronchoscopy and/or biopsy is required. (Courtesy of James Standen, MD).

Caplan's Syndrome

Caplan, in 1953, reported severe pulmonary fibrosis in 90% of 51 coal miners with rheumatoid arthritis in the United Kingdom and in only 30% of other miners. He noted that this fibrosis was complicated by the presence of pulmonary nodules in a number of patients (Fig. 14.49). Other researchers have verified his findings (Petry, 1954). Patients with pneumoconiosis and pulmonary fibrosis from other causes frequently have positive rheumatoid factors in the absence of arthritis; however, in one American study of 100 coal miners with rheumatoid arthritis, 43 had no pneumoconiosis, 40 had mild, 16 had moderate, and 1 had severe disease (Benedek et al, 1976). Three patients presented with all the criteria for Caplan's syndrome. These data are similar to the data for the nonrheumatoid population and do not agree with European data. There is no adequate treatment for this syndrome.

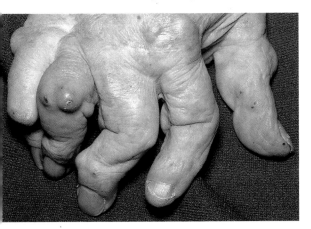

Figure 14.48 Multiple rheumatoid nodules are seen on the hand of a patient with rheumatoid arthritis and a pulmonary nodule.

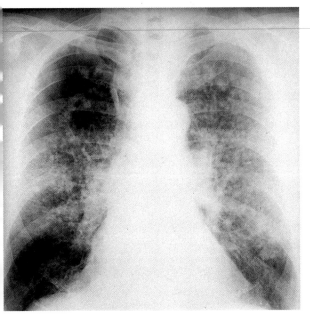

Figure 14.49 A patient with exposure to coal dust exhibits severe pulmonary fibrosis and nodule formation (Caplan's syndrome).

Pulmonary Fibrosis

Pulmonary fibrosis begins with a basilar interstitial infiltrate that may spread and involve the entire lung (Fig. 14.50). It is caused by a chronic lymphocytic and monocytic infiltrate in the pulmonary interstitium, with

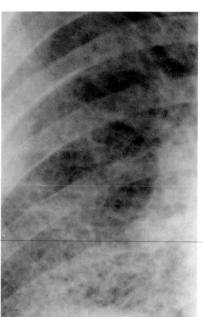

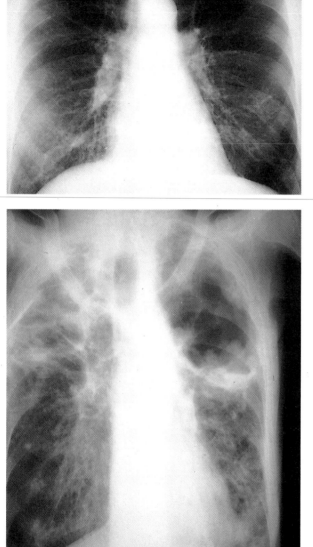

Figure 14.50 A patient with pulmonary fibrosis and rheumatoid arthritis has a mild increase in interstitial fibrosis at the base of the lung (*top left*). In more advanced pulmonary fibrosis, there is marked interstitial fibrosis throughout the lung. The fibrosis is more dense at the base of the lung (*top, right*). Severe pulmonary fibrosis in a patient with rheumatoid arthritis (*bottom, left*). There is marked fibrosis throughout the lung, with large bullae.

desquamation of large mononuclear cells, which eventually leads to fibrosis (Gordon et al, 1985). In its extreme form, there is a rapidly advancing bronchiolitis obliterans with progressive pulmonary insufficiency, cor pulmonale, and death (Fig. 14.51). The disease is present mainly in strongly seropositive patients with systemic nodular disease; most are males (Tomasi et al, 1962). Most of these patients show immunologic abnormalities, including antinuclear factors and immune complexes (Cerventes-Perez et al, 1980; Erhardt et al, 1979). A few patients with pulmonary fibrosis and rheumatoid arthritis develop "cystic honeycombing" (Fig. 14.52). Pulmonary function tests in patients without obvious pulmonary fibrosis may still be abnormal (Geddes et al, 1979). Spirometry in

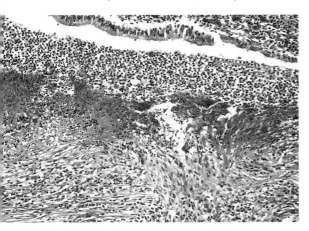

Figure 14.51 Postmortem microscopic section from a patient who has severe bronchiolitis obliterans. There is marked chronic inflammatory exudate and breakdown of the bronchial wall. The infiltrate has a granulomatous appearance. (H & E).

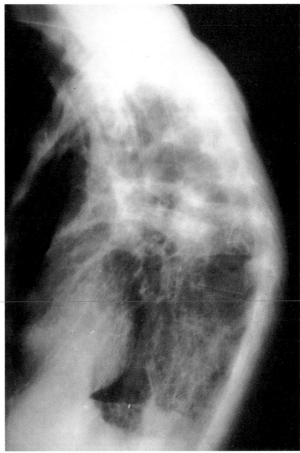

Figure 14.52 Severe pulmonary fibrosis shows honeycombing with large portions of lung destroyed (lateral view).

100 patients with rheumatoid arthritis and in 84 age-, sex-, and smoking-matched controls demonstrated significantly decreased parameters in the rheumatoid arthritis population; 32 patients had airway obstruction (Fig. 14.53). Rarely patients with long-standing fibrosis will develop the so-called scar tumor, which is adenocarcinoma of the lung.

The symptoms of pulmonary fibrosis include dyspnea on exertion and, later, at rest, fatigue, and a nonproductive cough. Chest crackles and decreased breath sounds are heard on auscultation, and clubbing of the fingers may be seen (Fig. 14.54).

Open lung biopsy or transbronchial biopsy will reveal chronic inflammation (Fig. 14.55).

AIRWAY OBSTRUCTION IN RHEUMATOID ARTHRITIS

	FORCED EXPIRATION VOLUME (1 sec) (FEV$_1$)	FORCED VITAL CAPACITY (FVC)	FEV/FVC%	MAXIMUM MIDEXPIRATION FLOW RATE (L/dec)
Smokers: rheumatoid arthritis	2.05* ±0.11	2.91 ±0.15	71.6 ±1.3	1.59 ±0.14
Smokers: control	2.51 ±0.10	3.25 ±0.13	78.8 ±1.3	2.37 ±0.12
P <	0.01	**	0.001	0.001
Nonsmokers: rheumatoid arthritis	2.11 ±0.12	2.61 ±0.12	77.7 ±1.3	2.03 ±0.15
Nonsmokers: control	2.61 ±0.12	3.35 ±0.17	78.6 ±1.2	2.61 ±0.13
P <	0.01	0.01	**	0.01
Total: rheumatoid arthritis	2.09 ±0.08	2.77 ±0.10	77.7 ±1.0	1.80 ±0.10
Total control	2.56 ±0.08	3.30 ±0.10	78.7 ±0.9	2.48 ±0.09
Total P <	.001	.001	0.02	0.001

*± = standard error
** = not significant

Geddes et al, 1979

Figure 14.53 Airway obstruction in rheumatoid arthritis.

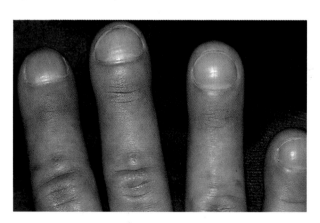

Figure 14.54 Swelling of the distal digits with soft tissue in the base of the nails is present ("clubbing") in this patient with pulmonary fibrosis.

In active disease, bronchioalveolar lavage may show neutrophils as well as immunoglobulins (Greening, 1982) or more lymphocytic- and macrophage-laden lavage material (Fig. 14.56). Patients with the former type of exudate are more likely to respond to drug therapy.

Treatment with steroids and cytoxic agents may give symptomatic relief but rarely alters the long-term course of this progressive disease. Treatment with routine bronchodilators and other respiratory agents may help.

An acute allergic interstitial pneumonitis has been reported with several drugs, including gold, penicillamine, methotrexate, and some of the nonsteroidal, anti-inflam-

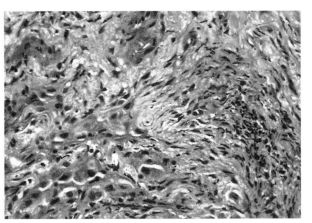 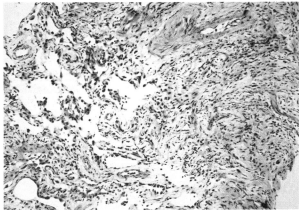

Figure 14.55 Pulmonary specimen from a lung biopsy of patient with progressive pulmonary fibrosis (*left*). There are inflammatory cells and active fibrosis formation (H&E). Trichrome stain in a patient with fibrosing alveolitis (*right*). The trichrome stain shows the marked fibrosis (green).

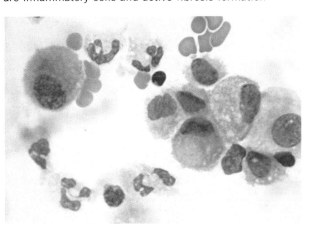

Figure 14.56 A cytologic preparation of lavage material from a patient with rheumatoid arthritis and fibrosing alveolitis. Normally there are very few neutrophils and less than 10% lymphocytes. In this patient there is a marked increase in the number of neutrophils suggesting active fibrosing alveolitis. There would be an increase in lymphocytes if more of a granulomatous inflammation were occurring. (Wright's stain). (Courtesy of Robert Barbee, MD and Mary J. Hicks, MD)

matory agents (Fig. 14.57) Most cases of pneumonitis respond to withdrawal of the drug, and corticosteroids usually help reverse the disease. In some patients, however, progressive fibrosis and pulmonary insufficiency will occur. Goodpasture's syndrome has been reported with penicillamine therapy.

Obstructive sleep apnea has been reported with microagnathia in rheumatoid arthritis (Davies and Iber, 1983). Upper airway obstruction is discussed later in this chapter under cricoarytenoid arthritis.

Pulmonary hypertension can occur with or without pulmonary fibrosis (Asherson et al, 1985), and fibrosis, pulmonary embolic disease, and unknown factors may be involved in its pathogenesis. It should be noted that angiography, or cardiac catheterization, carries a high risk of arrythmia in pulmonary fibrosis patients.

Pulmonary arteritis may lead to pulmonary hemorrhage with hemoptysis or hypertension. Lymphocytic vessel wall infiltration occurs in subacute disease, as may necrotizing arteritis with fibrinoid degeneration (Asherson, 1985) (Fig. 14.58). Necrotizing arteritis can lead to severe pulmonary insufficiency and is frequently associated with systemic vasculitis.

Infection

Patients with rheumatoid arthritis, particularly those on immunosuppressive drugs, are more susceptible to bacterial and nosocomial infections, although mucociliary clearance is normal (Sutton et al, 1982). Empyema occurs in patients with nodular or pleural pulmo-

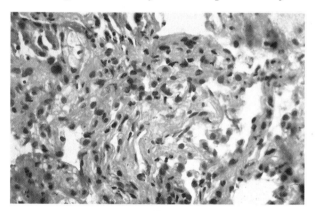

Figure 14.57 Acute inflammatory infiltrate with early fibrosis is seen in a patient on methotrexate therapy. Fibrosing alveolitis can occur secondary to this drug treatment (H&E).

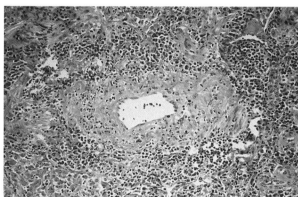

Figure 14.58 Necrotizing vasculitis of the lung in a patient with rheumatoid arthritis. Large vessel with thickened wall and inflammatory infiltrate is surrounded by inflammation in the lung parenchyma (H&E). (Courtesy of Anna Graham, MD).

nary disease or in rheumatoid arthritis patients without such risk factors (Dieppe, 1975). Bronchitis, tuberculosis, and bacterial pneumonia are seen most commonly in men with rheumatoid arthritis (Walker and Wright, 1968). Pulmonary infection preceding the onset of rheumatoid arthritis has often been reported (Gordon et al, 1985), but its etiologic significance is unclear.

GASTROINTESTINAL AND LIVER INVOLVEMENT

Intestinal involvement in rheumatoid arthritis is unusual. However, peptic ulceration secondary to NSAID treatment is common (Fig. 14.59); dyspepsia is seen in 15% of patients on NSAIDs (Gibberd, 1966). Upper gastrointestinal radiographs were performed in 140 consecutive patients with rheumatoid arthritis regardless of symptoms; endoscopy was performed in 66 of these. Gastric ulceration was found in 12 and duodenal ulcer in 27 (ulcer incidence, 30%) (Sun et al, 1974).

Lactose intolerance and malabsorption have been reported in some patients (Petterson et al, 1970; Dyer et al, 1971). Inflammatory infiltrates of the lamina propria with loss of superficial epithelium in bowel biopsies of rheumatoid arthritis patients suggest some chronic inflammatory process (Marcolongo et al, 1979), although most patients are asymptomatic. Bowel infarction with vasculitis can occur rarely in the patient with systemic medium-sized vessel necrotizing vasculitis (Fig. 14.60). Postprandial abdominal angina may precede frank infarction. Barium studies show "thumb printing," suggesting arterial

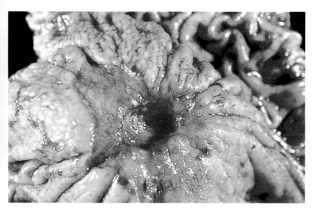

Figure 14.59 A large gastric ulcer is surrounded by inflamed gastric mucosa and edema.

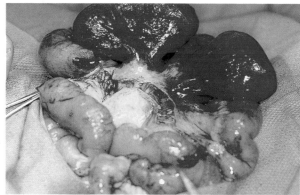

Figure 14.60 This intraoperative view shows acute small bowel infarction.

insufficiency (Figs. 14.61 and 14.62). Arteriography or exploratory surgery gives a definite diagnosis. Early surgical intervention is necessary in cases of frank infarction. Medical treatment can include corticosteroids and/or cytotoxic agents.

Amyloid involvement in the gut is usually asymptomatic but may lead to diarrhea or malabsorption (Hollingsworth, 1968). Confirmation is by rectal biopsy (Fig. 14.63).

Hepatic disease in rheumatoid arthritis has been said to improve joint symptoms (Still, 1987; Hench, 1940). Still has noted that "catarrhal jaundice [appears] to be followed by the improvement of joint symptoms." There is no evidence that it alters disease course.

Drug-induced liver disease in rheumatoid arthritis may be dose or time related. Similarly, the reaction may be sporadic or idiosyncratic; thus, the onset of liver problems is unpredictable (Gottlieb and Gray, 1983).

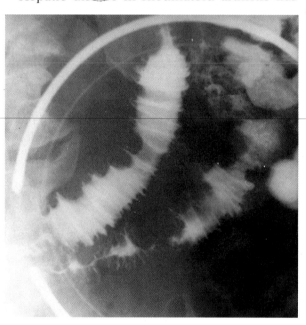 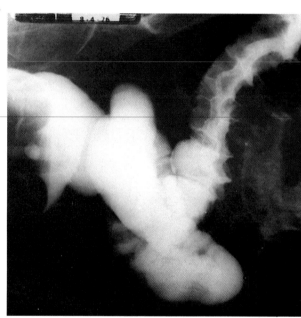

Figure 14.61 Small bowel vasculitis produces an ischemic bowel as seen on a contrast GI study (*left*). Typical "thumb printing" is seen with loss of substance of the bowel wall in a well-delineated distribution. Barium enema shows ischemic vasculitis (*right*). Ischemic colon shows "thumb printing" with sharply marginated imprinting of the edematous bowel wall. Note the narrow stream of barium through this portion of the ischemic bowel. (Courtesy of Tim Hunter, MD)

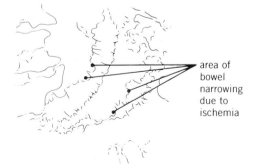

area of bowel narrowing due to ischemia

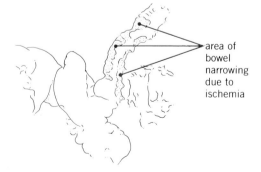

area of bowel narrowing due to ischemia

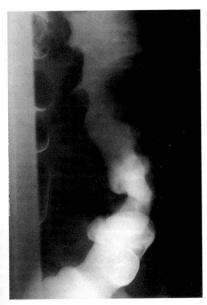

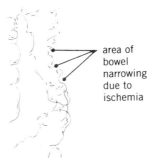

Figure 14.62 Close-up view of a barium study shows vasculitis and ischemic bowel. Large "thumb printing" is seen in the bowel wall. (Courtesy of Tim Hunter, MD)

area of
bowel
narrowing
due to
ischemia

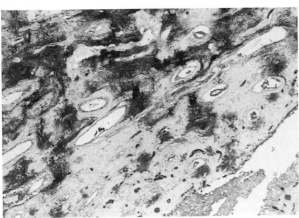

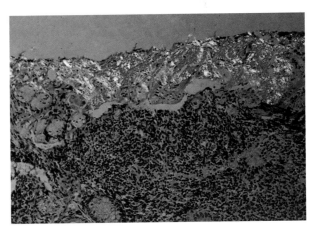

Figure 14.63 Bright purple stain shows amyloid deposition in specimen (*left*). (crystal violet stain). Rectal biopsy with amyloid deposition stained with Congo red under polarized light (*right*). Note the apple green birefringence of the polarized amyloid.

Hepatitis, cholestasis, and vasculitis are all seen (Fig. 14.64).

Salicylates have been implicated as the cause of abnormal hepatic enzyme levels, particularly in juvenile onset arthritis and SLE as well as in adult rheumatoid disease, but parenchymal changes are minimal (Saltzman et al, 1976). Cholestatic hepatitis following gold therapy is rare (Fig. 14.65) and rapidly resolves upon cessation of therapy. Penicillamine has been shown to reversibly elevate hepatic enzymes in 6% of treated cases (Rosenbaum et al, 1980).

Methotrexate has recently been considered to be a possible cause of hepatitis and cirrhosis. The danger has probably been overstated, since these conditions usually are seen in patients with high-dose or frequent dosing patterns (an obsolete regimen) and in patients drinking significant amounts of alcohol (Boh et al, 1986). Nonetheless, patients taking methotrexate are screened for liver function and liver biopsy may be recommended for some patients taking more than 1500 mg of the drug. Individuals taking corticosteroid drugs are susceptible to fatty changes in the liver (Tucker, 1982) (Fig. 14.66).

Nonspecific elevations of hepatic enzymes in rheumatoid arthritis are mild and frequent (Weinblatt et al, 1982); most of these patients, however, are on drug therapy. Histologically, Kupffer cell hyperplasia and periportal mononuclear cell infiltrate are seen in the liver (Dietrichson et al, 1976). Granulomatous hepatitis not related to drug therapy has been rarely reported (Roberts and Coblyn, 1983), and no other cause could be found for these abnormalities.

Patients with Sjögren's syndrome are found to have a higher incidence of hepatomegaly

HEPATOTOXIC POTENTIAL OF SOME DRUGS USED TO TREAT RHEUMATOID ARTHRITIS

	Hepatocellular necrosis	Cholestasis	Granulomatous hepatitis	Fibrosis	Cirrhosis
NSAIDs	+	+	+ *		
Gold	+	+			
Penicillamine	+	+			
Methotrexate	+	+		+	+
Azoathioprine	+	+		+	
Cyclophosphamide	+				

* with phenylbutazone

modified from Gottlieb and Gray, 1983

Figure 14.64 Hepatotoxic potential of some drugs used to treat rheumatoid arthritis.

and splenomegaly, as well as abnormal liver function tests and antimitochondrial and smooth muscle antibodies (Webb et al, 1975). Nodular regenerative hyperplasia of the liver has been reported in Felty's syndrome (Blen-dis et al, 1974; Cohen et al, 1982). Diffuse nodularity and, in contradistinction to cirrhosis, minimal fibrosis are seen in this syndrome. Portal hypertension, with esophageal varices with bleeding, also occurs.

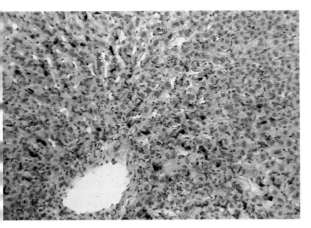

Figure 14.65 A drug-induced cholestatic hepatitis. Marked cholestasis and inflammatory infiltrate is seen in liver biopsy section. This is typical of many types of drug-induced cholestasis in rheumatoid arthritis and other diseases.

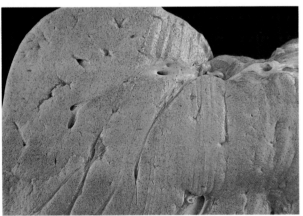

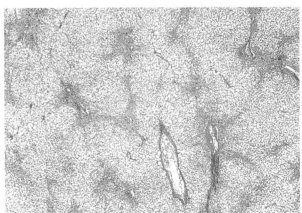

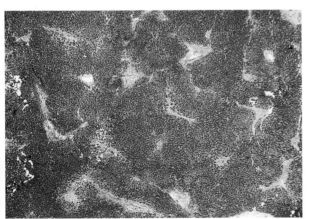

Figure 14.66 Massive fatty deposition in liver (*top, left*) can be due to drug ingestion (such as corticosteroids) or toxins (such as alcohol). Massive fatty infiltration is seen in a microsection of liver tissue (*top, right*) (H&E). Cells are ballooned with fatty globules, which are white, giving a starry sky appearance. Fatty globules stained red with fat stain can be seen in a grossly fatty liver (*bottom, left*).

RENAL MANIFESTATIONS

Renal disease is not thought of as a frequent manifestation of rheumatoid arthritis. Yet some reports in the older literature dispute this premise (Lawson and McLean, 1966). There are multiple potential mechanisms of renal abnormalities in rheumatoid arthritis (Fig. 14.67). Bulger et al (1968) looked carefully at 42 patients with known rheumatoid arthritis and found renal abnormalities in 22, 16 of whom had decreased creatinine clearance (52 to 79 mL/min). Eleven patients had interstitial nephritis, and two had glomerular disease; the other patients were unclassified. In 1965, Brun et al performed 32 renal biopsies on rheumatoid arthritis patients. Nine patients had interstitial nephritis, four amyloidosis, and one glomerularnephritis. The latter patient also had a systemic necrotizing arteritis. More recent studies have shown mesangial proliferation and mild functional abnormalities in patients with rheumatoid arthritis, with a slightly increased matrix and/or hypercellularity (Salomon et al, 1974; Helin et al, 1986) (Fig. 14.68). Immunoflourescent abnormalities and electron microscopic deposits were also seen, as were proteinuria and slightly abnormal cells in the urine. It should be noted that all these patients with rheumatoid arthritis have been treated with a variety of antirheumatic drugs, many of which can cause renal abnormalities.

Aspirin and other nonsteroidal agents can block prostaglandin synthesis, and in patients with underlying renal insufficiency, this can decrease renal blood flow and can cause renal dysfunction. Severe renal failure and death can occur if the drug is not discontinued. Drugs that do not inhibit prostaglandins, blocking drugs (nonacetylated salicylates), and drugs (eg, sulindac) that are converted by renal parenchyma to an inert metabolite probably do not produce renal failure (Clive and Staff, 1984). Any anti-inflammatory drug may cause an allergic interstitial nephritis. This may be associated with malaise, fatigue, low-grade fever, pyuria, eosinophilia, and eosinophiluria. Both drug-related syndromes

RENAL INVOLVEMENT IN RHEUMATOID ARTHRITIS

Drug induced
NSAIDs
Prostaglandin blockade
Interstitial nephritis (allergic)
Renal tubular acidosis
Papillary necrosis (with phenacetin)
Gold
Penicillamine
Immune complex
Goodpasture's syndrome
SLE

Amyloidosis

Sjögren's syndrome
Renal tubular acidosis

Vasculitis with polyarteritis

Infection
Cystitis
Pyelonephritis

Overlap with other collagen/vascular diseases

Mesangial glomerulonephritis

Figure 14.67 Renal involvement in rheumatoid arthritis.

are reversed upon prompt discontinuation of the agent. Renal tubular acidosis with hyperkalemia has been described in association with NSAIDs. Analgesic abuse, particularly with a mixture of aspirin and phenacetin, has been associated with papillary renal necrosis and kidney failure (Fig. 14.69). Long-term, high-dose aspirin therapy has not been associated with permanent renal disease (Gall, 1982).

Gold and penicillamine have both been associated with immunocomplex glomerulonephritis, renal failure, proteinuria, and, particularly for penicillamine, the nephrotic syndrome. Penicillamine rarely produces antiglomerular basement membrane antibody and nephrosis (Goodpasture's syndrome) (Fig. 14.70). These abnormalities are reversed upon discontinuation of the drugs, although the proteinuria may be prolonged.

Secondary amyloidosis can cause proteinuria, renal failure, and enlarged kidneys. Renal biopsy, although diagnostic, can cause severe bleeding. The diagnosis is often supported by finding amyloid deposits with Congo red stain on renal, subcutaneous fat,

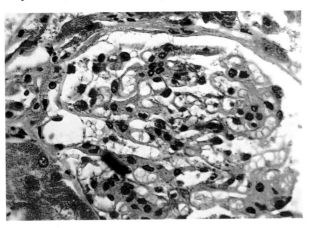

Figure 14.68 Mild mesangial proliferative glomerulonephritis can be seen in rheumatoid arthritis. There is a slight increase of cellularity in the glomerulus particularly in the mesangial area. The rest of the biopsy is normal. (Courtesy of Anna Graham, MD)

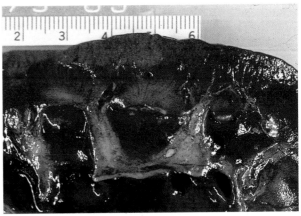

Figure 14.69 Section of kidney shows marked papillary necrosis. Whitish necrotic tissue at the base of the renal papilla is characteristic and causes renal failure. Identical lesions are caused by diabetes and by analgesic-induced nephropathy. (Courtesy of Samuel Paplanus, MD)

Figure 14.70 This kidney biopsy shows the typical cresenteric glomerulonephritis of Goodpasture's syndrome. Immunoflourescent staining would show a typical antiglomerular basement membrane pattern. Penicillamine therapy in rheumatoid arthritis can cause this histologic picture (H&E). (Courtesy of Anna Graham, MD)

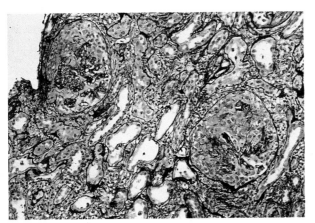

rectal, or gingival biopsy (Fig. 14.71). No treatment is available.

Other causes of renal disease include renal tubular acidosis associated with lymphocytic infiltrate in Sjögren's syndrome, necrotizing tubular acidosis associated with lymphocytic infiltrate in Sjögren's syndrome, necrotizing vasculitis involving the kidney (Fig. 14.72), and bacterial infection.

SJÖGREN'S SYNDROME

Sjögren's syndrome is described as a triad of dry eyes (keratoconjunctivitis sicca), dry mouth (xerostomia), and connective tissue disease in one half to three quarters of cases (Fig. 14.73). The connective tissue disease is most often rheumatoid arthritis; arthritis or arthralgia is present at some time in almost all cases of Sjögren's syndrome (Adachi et al, 1985). When collagen disease is present, the disorder is said to be secondary Sjögren's syndrome; when there is no accompanying disease, the disorder is described as primary. Historically, many authors have described features of this syndrome, including Leber in 1882, who recognized dry eyes with "filamentary keratitis," and Hadden (1888), who demonstrated the association between dry eyes and dry mouth. Mikulicz in 1888 de-

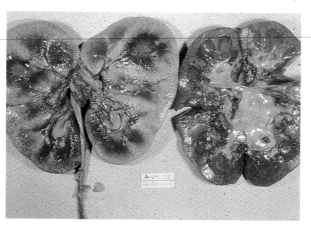

Figure 14.71 Renal amyloid deposition secondary to rheumatoid arthritis. The kidneys on the left have a pale cortex and are enlarged due to amyloid deposition in the cortical tissue (*left*). A relatively normal kidney appears

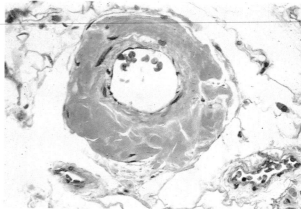

on the right. Amyloid deposition in medium-sized vessel wall is seen in histologic specimen (*right*). Amorphous purple stain is present in tissue and reveals thickening of the vessel wall. (Gentian violet stain).

Figure 14.72 Acute hemorrhagic, necrotizing vasculitis of the glomerulus is seen in a kidney section. (H&E).

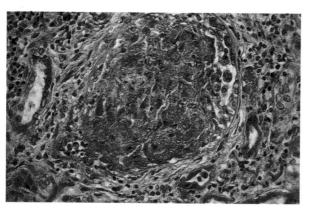

scribed the glandular lymphocytic infiltrate associated with the disease. Although arthritis had been described previously, Sjögren, a Swedish ophthalmologist, published a large monograph covering 19 of his own patients in 1933. Thirteen of these patients had arthritis. He felt the entity was a systemic disease and presented compelling evidence for this over the ensuing 19 years, by which time

he had collected 80 patients and published many papers (Adachi et al, 1985). Bloch and colleagues (1965) studied 62 Sjögren's syndrome patients, finding 30 with definite and two with probable rheumatoid arthritis. Others have reported similar rates. The rheumatologist, however, is more likely to see rheumatoid arthritis patients with this syndrome than are other practitioners.

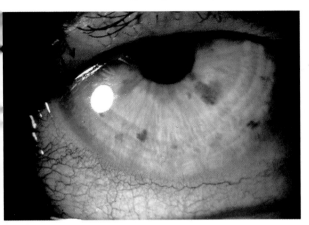 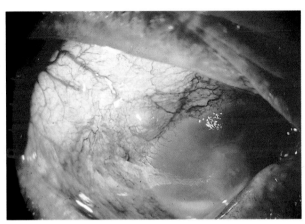

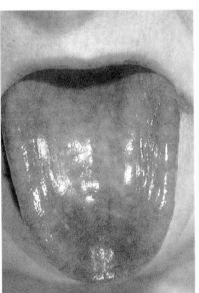

Figure 14.73 Mild dry eye syndrome (*top, left*). Conjunctival redness with some small punctate red stains from the rose bengal stain on the iris very close to the cornea. The brownish stains in the iris are congenital. Severe dry eye syndrome (*top, right*). Marked scleral and conjunctival injection with one small nodular mass from the scleritis. This patient has a corneal ulcer. Parotid enlargement and dry tongue with mucosal atrophy (*bottom, left*) occur with Sjögren's syndrome. (Courtesy of PA Dieppe, MD)

Similar lymphoid infiltrates, with consequent immunologic mediated tissue damage and secretory dysfunction, may also involve organs other than the lacrimal gland and the salivary gland (Fig. 14.74).

Pathogenesis/Pathology

The lesion in Sjögren's syndrome is characterized by lymphoid infiltration of the involved tissue, defined in salivary gland biop-

SYSTEMIC FEATURES OF SJÖGREN'S SYNDROME

Sicca syndrome
Salivary gland dysfunction
Dry mouth
Parotid enlargement
Dental caries

Lacrimal gland dysfunction
Dry eyes
Keratitis
Corneal ulceration

Vaginal infiltration
Atrophic vaginitis

Connective tissue disease
Rheumatoid arthritis
Nonspecific arthritis/arthralgia
SLE
Progressive systemic sclerosis
Polymyositis
Necrotizing vasculitis

Hypergammaglobulinemic purpura

Hyperviscosity syndrome

Pseudolymphoma/lymphoma

Cryoglobulemia (macroglobulinemia)

Renal tubular acidosis (distal type I)

Hepatosplenomegaly

Neuropathy

Chronic pulmonary disease

Gastrointestinal disorders
Dysphagia
Pancreatitis

Figure 14.74 Systemic features of Sjögren's syndrome.

sies as one lymphocytic focus per 4 mm² of tissue (deWilde et al, 1986). A focus consists of 50 or more lymphocytes and histiocytes, usually with a few peripheral plasma cells (Fig. 14.75). The ductal epithelium is displaced and ductal cells may proliferate to form characteristic myoepithelial islets in up to 40% of parotid glands biopsied (Bloch et al, 1965) (Fig. 14.76). Both T cells and B cells are present and immunoglobulin is synthesized locally (Talal et al, 1974). Since a number of autoimmune phenomena are seen in this primarily glandular focused disease, it has been termed "autoimmune exocrinopathy" (Strand and Talal, 1980).

Sjögren's syndrome associated with rheu-matoid arthritis tends to be associated with the HLA-Dw4 tissue type; primary Sjögren's syndrome is more often associated with histocompatibility antigens as seen in SLE, HLA-B8, and HLA-Dw3 (Fye et al, 1978; Moutsopoulos et al, 1979). There is a decrease in natural killer (NK) cells, which may be a factor in progression to malignant lymphoma (Talal, 1985).

About 50% of patients will have a polyclonal elevation of gammaglobulin, which, in some cases, will lead to the hyperviscosity syndrome. Benign monoclonal spikes, particularly of IgM, are common, and mixed cryoglobulinemia may be seen. Over 90% of patients have significant elevations (greater

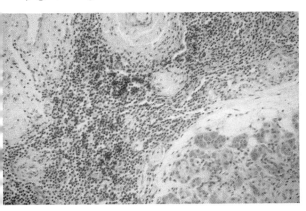

Figure 14.75 Histologic appearance of one of the minor salivary glands in the sicca syndrome showing lymphocytic infiltration and glandular destruction (H&E). (Courtesy of PA Dieppe, MD)

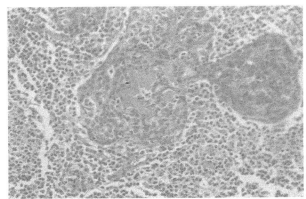

Figure 14.76 Parotid gland biopsy from patient with Sjögren's syndrome, showing marked round cell infiltrate of the parenchyma. The lumen of the salivary ducts is blocked with eosinophilic deposits of inspissated secretions and the linings of the ducts are hyperplastic and also infiltrated with round cells. Ductal changes are called epimyoepithelial islands (H&E). (Courtesy of Samuel Paplanus, MD).

than 1:80) of latex rheumatoid factors. Antinuclear factors (either homogeneous or speckled) are seen in 70% of Sjögren's syndrome patients and low titers of antibodies to native DNA may be found. Specific antibodies to salivary ductal epithelium are seen in about one half of patients (MacSween et al, 1967). Antibodies to SSB (La) are seen in 50% to 70% of patients with primary Sjögren's syndrome and rheumatoid arthritis precipitate (RAP), an antibody to the Epstein-Barr virus related-antigen RANA, is seen in Sjögren's syndrome with rheumatoid arthritis (Talal, 1985). Beta-2-microglobulin is secreted in the saliva and is quantitatively related to the amount of lymphoid infiltrate of the salivary gland (Michalski et al, 1975).

Diagnosis/Clinical Features

Sjögren's syndrome is diagnosed on the basis of the clinical features of the sicca syndrome and the associated collagen disease, if any. It may be confirmed with clinical and laboratory tests, including biopsy of minor salivary glands, if necessary.

The onset of the disease may be sudden, with rapid progression, but more often is insidious. Patients complain of a foreign body sensation in their eyes, burning, lack of tearing (although increased watering may be noted at first), redness and itchiness, photosensitivity, and pain (Adachi et al, 1985).

The most common sign is photophobia. The eyes appear dry and occasionally red, and punctate corneal pits are seen (Fig. 14.77). The diagnosis of keratoconjunctivitis sicca is confirmed by a Schirmer test, corneal staining with fluorescein or rose bengal, and/or a slit-lamp examination. In the Schirmer test (Fig. 14.78), a strip of Whatman #41 filter paper is placed in the conjunctival sac for 5 minutes. The paper is then removed, and the amount of tearing absorbed from the point outside the lid is determined. Fifteen millimeters or more is normal; less than 5 mm is diagnostic of the sicca syndrome; and between 5 and 15 mm is indeterminate.

When the eye is stained with 1% rose bengal (ocular preparation) or fluorescein, the stain will normally disappear after a few minutes. Residual stain reveals ulceration of the bulbar conjunctival or corneal tissue (Fig. 14.79). Slit-lamp examination reveals corneal

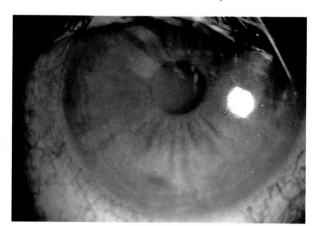

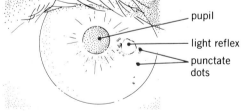

Figure 14.77 Small punctate corneal dots reveal superficial damage caused by dry eye syndrome. They can be seen by looking carefully at the superficial surface of the eye over the iris particularly around the light reflection. Note the mild conjuntival injection in this patient.

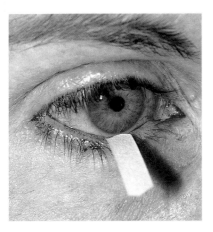 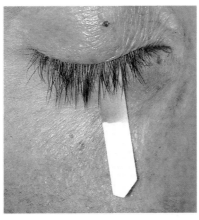 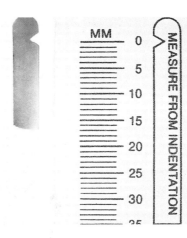

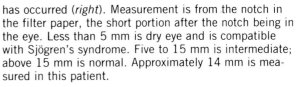

Figure 14.78 The Schirmer test is done to document dry eyes in Sjögren's syndrome and related diseases. A strip of # 41 Whatman filter paper is placed over the lower lid (*left*) and the eye is closed for 5 minutes. Here rose bengal stain has been placed in the eye to make the tearing more obvious on the filter paper (*middle*). The filter paper is measured to see the amount of tearing that has occurred (*right*). Measurement is from the notch in the filter paper, the short portion after the notch being in the eye. Less than 5 mm is dry eye and is compatible with Sjögren's syndrome. Five to 15 mm is intermediate; above 15 mm is normal. Approximately 14 mm is measured in this patient.

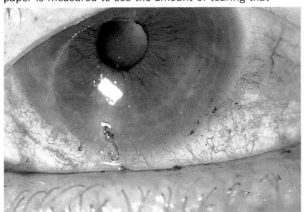

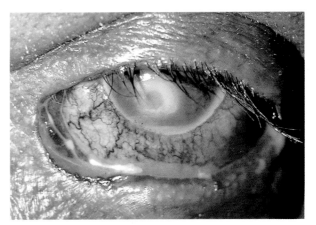

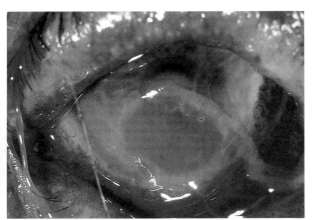

Figure 14.79 Filamentary keratitis in a patient with rheumatoid arthritis and Sjögren's syndrome. The eye has been stained with fluorescein and rose bengal. Filamentous debris is seen (*top left*). Intermediate corneal ulceration is seen in another patient (*top right*), with the eye also stained with fluorescein and rose bengal. Conjunctival and scleral injection is seen. Severe corneal ulceration (*bottom left*) in marked conjunctival injection and hemorrhage surrounding the ulcer.

debris with attached epithelial filaments (filamentary keratitis) (Fig. 14.80).

Xerostomia may be more difficult to detect. Parotid enlargement may be more apparent (Fig. 14.81) and other salivary glands may also hypertrophy. Hypertrophic glands often recur and may be tender; a rapid fluctuation in symptoms and size is common. Parotid swelling is often bilateral. The tongue, in severe cases, is red and dry and the lips may be parched. Severe dental caries and gingivitis follow. Parotid gland biopsy reveals typical infiltrates (described previously), but biopsy of minor salivary glands is the preferred method, with small tissue samples taken from the inner portion of the lip (Fig. 14.82).

Salivary volume may be determined by various techniques, and although it is seldom used, sialography shows ductal ectasia (Rubin and Holt, 1957) (Fig. 14.83). Scintography with ^{99m}Tc-pertechnetate measures uptake, concentration, and excretion of material. Treatment of xerostomia with a variety of artificial salivas and careful dental care is helpful.

Other findings in patients with Sjögren's syndrome include lymphadenopathy (pseudolymphoma or lymphoma), hypergammaglobulinemic purpura, and findings related to other organ infiltration, as previously noted. Of 136 patients followed for a mean of 8 years, 10 had B cell neoplasms, 3 had Wal-

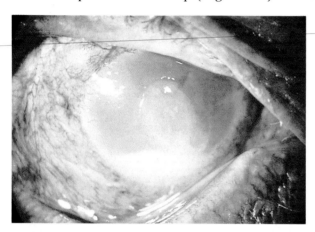

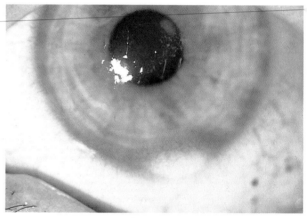

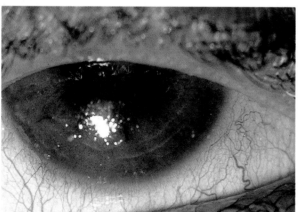

Figure 14.80 Severe loss of corneal tissue due to dry eyes is seen with a secondary infection, hypopyon and corneal ulceration (*top left*). Note a layer of pus in the anterior chamber. The surrounding ocular tissues are severely injected. In an unstained eye, filamentous debris can be seen (*top right*). The lower portion of the iris has an incidental thermoid scar. A denuded area of cornea is caused by dry eye syndrome (*bottom left*).

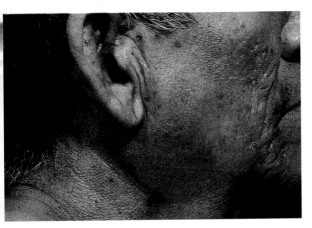

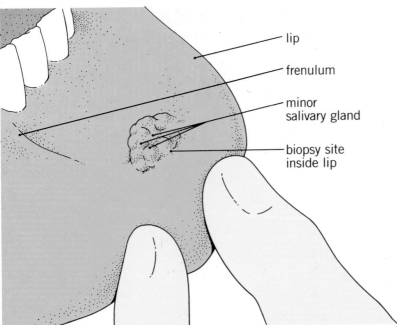

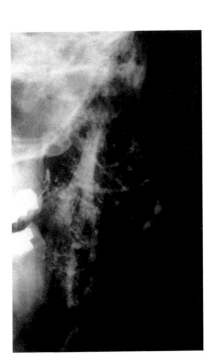

Figure 14.81 Parotid enlargement patient with Sjögren's syndrome. Note the bulging of the parotid gland anterior to the ear.

lip

frenulum

minor salivary gland

biopsy site inside lip

Figure 14.82 Lip biopsy. Under local anesthesia, a small portion of tissue is removed at the vermillion border. Granular material in the biopsy should contain minor salivary glands for histologic study.

Figure 14.83 Injection of the parotid duct shows abnormal nodular dilation of these ducts.

denstrom's macroglobulinemia, and 7 had nonHodgkin's lymphoma (Kassen et al, 1978). This is 44 times the expected incidence of such diseases. Myelomas and other gammopathies have also been reported (Fig. 14.84).

Treatment

Treatment is usually symptomatic. Eye problems are treated with methylcellulose tears several times a day, hydroxypropyl cellulose ophthalmic inserts and nighttime ointments. Topical steroids are not recommended, since they cause corneal thinning. Oral problems respond to artificial saliva with either methylcellulose or glycerin, sugar-free hard candy, and careful dental care. Only rarely are corticosteroids or cytotoxic agents used, and then only in severe or life-threatening conditions. Organ involvement is treated appropriately (ie, correction of renal tubular acidosis).

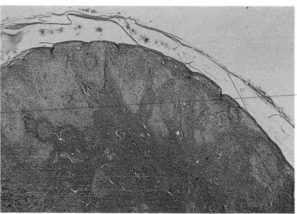

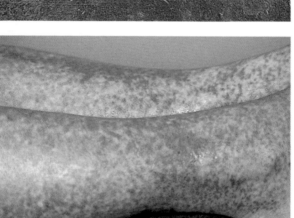

Figure 14.84 Reactive hyperplasia accompanying lymph node proliferation with multiple new follicles shows very active nodular degeneration (*top left*), similar to that seen in the pseudolymphoma syndrome. Lymph node with malignant lymphoma (*top, right*) contains a monotonous infiltration of abnormal lymphoid cells. Multiple palpable purpura is associated with hypergammaglobulinemia (*bottom, left*). There can be other causes of this condition, but rheumatoid arthritis with systemic involvement, such as Sjögren's syndrome or SLE, is often the culprit.

OCULAR INVOLVEMENT

Eye problems are not unusual in rheumatoid arthritis. Iritis and iridocyclitis, common in the juvenile onset form of the disease (Fig. 14.85), are no more common in adult onset rheumatoid arthritis than in the general population. However, dry eyes, scleritis, and episcleritis occur frequently (Kimura et al, 1967). The ocular manifestations of rheumatoid arthritis are listed in Figure 14.86. As with many extra-articular problems, these manifestations tend to be seen more in patients with severe disease expression and in with exacerbation of joint problems. Patients with eye involvement have a greater mortality than age-matched controls (McGavin et al, 1976).

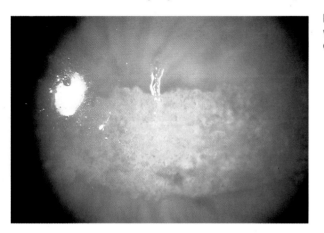

Figure 14.85 Calcification over the cornea of a patient with juvenile onset rheumatoid arthritis.Chronic iridocyclitis causes calcium deposition and a band keratopathy.

Figure 14.86 Ocular manifestations of rheumatoid arthritis.

OCULAR MANIFESTATIONS OF RHEUMATOID ARTHRITIS

Scleritis
Anterior
Diffuse
Nodular
Necrotizing
Scleromalacia

Posterior

Episcleritis
Simple
Nodular

Keratoconjunctivitis sicca

Keratitis

Keratolysis

Motility disorders (2° to vasculitis)

Changes 2° to drugs
NSAIDs
Gold
Antimalarial drugs
Steroids

Burke, 1985

The eye is commonly involved in other rheumatic syndromes (Fig. 14.87).

It is important to know the anatomy of the eye to better understand some of the ocular manifestations of rheumatoid arthritis (Fig. 14.88). The eye itself is encased in the sclera, which is primarily collagen and theoretically a harbor for immune complexes similar to the

OCULAR PROBLEMS IN ARTHRITIC CONDITIONS

	Rheumatoid arthritis	Juvenile onset rheumatoid arthritis	SLE	Spondylitis	Reiter's syndrome
Sicca	+	−	+	−	−
Episcleritis/ Scleritis	+	−	±	−	−
Vasculitis (retinal)	+	−	+	−	−
Muscle disorders	± (2° to nodules)	−	+ (2° to vasculitis)	−	−
Anterior uveitis/iritis					
Acute	−	±	−	+	+
Chronic	−	+ +	−	−	−
Conjunctivitis	−	−	−	−	+
Drug reactions	+	+	+	+	+
Infections	+	+	+	+	+

Key:
± = possible but unusual
+ = occurs
− = not associated
+ + = common

modified from Fox et al, 1985

Figure 14.87 Ocular problems in arthritis.

cartilagenous layer of joints. The anteriormost portion, the cornea, is transparent. A thin transparent covering to the sclera, the episclera, is continuous with the conjunctiva. A vascular layer beneath the sclera, the choroid, provides nutrients to the eye. The innermost layer, the retina, contains light sensory cells as well as vascular channels. The iris contracts over the lens to control the amount of light reaching the posterior portion of the eye. The surface of the eye is bathed by fluid secreted by the lacrimal glands. Aqueous humor is present in the anterior chamber of the eye, and a jelly-like vitreous material fills the posterior chamber.

Analogies have been drawn between the synovial membrane surrounding the avascular cartilage and the vascular choroid and the retina surrounding the avascular vitreous and collagenous sclera (Tessler, 1985). Joint fluid and vitreous humor both contain hyaluronic acid and both manifest inflammatory changes in the same rheumatic diseases.

Anatomic similarities may explain some of these coincidences. Major ocular abnormalities will be described. Keratoconjunctivitis sicca, the most common ocular problem in rheumatoid arthritis, is described under Sjögren's syndrome, because other organs are involved in addition to the eye.

Scleritis

The sclera is a collagenous tissue of mesodermal origin (Tessler, 1985). It differs from the iris in that the latter organ also contains neuroectodermal tissue. Any inflammatory change in this layer of the eye is called scleritis and occurs in slightly less than 1% of all rheumatoid arthritis patients (McGavin et al, 1976). Thirty percent of patients with scleritis, however, have rheumatoid arthritis (Watson and Hazelman, 1976). The symptoms of scleritis include deep aching and increased tearing, but lesions may occa-

Figure 14.88 Anatomic structure of the eye.

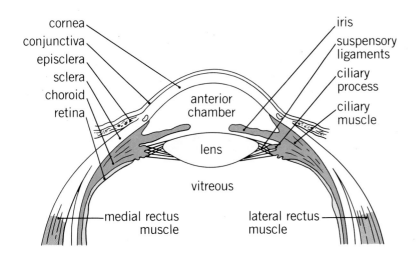

cornea
conjunctiva
episclera
sclera
choroid
retina

iris
suspensory ligaments
ciliary process
ciliary muscle

anterior chamber

lens

vitreous

medial rectus muscle

lateral rectus muscle

sionally be asymptomatic. These symptoms may be the initial manifestation of rheumatoid disease (Fig. 14.89).

Histologically, lesions in scleritis resemble rheumatoid nodules and occur more frequently in patients with such nodules (Fox et al, 1985). Scleritis is classified as focal, diffuse, or nodular (Tessler, 1985).

Figure 14.89 Scleritis. Congestion and inflammation of the scleral layers is seen in rheumatoid scleritis.

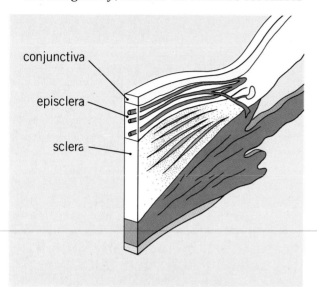

conjunctiva

episclera

sclera

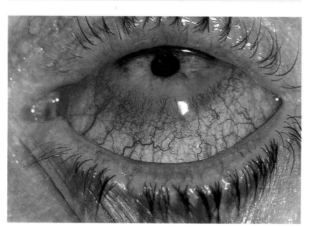

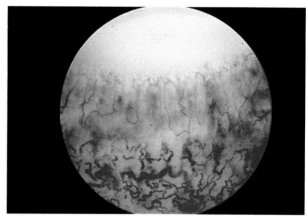

Figure 14.90 Diffuse scleritis of the eye showing injection of the scleral and overlying episcleral vessels (*left*). The scleral vessels are deeper and larger than the episcleral vessels. (Courtesy William Mathers, MD). Vascular engorgement in a patient with diffuse scleritis leading to a corneal ulcer (*right*).

On physical examination, the eye is tender to palpation. The overlying conjunctiva may be engorged (Fig.. 14.90), but phenylephrine hydrochloride drops clear this lesion to reveal underlying violaceous episcleral vessels (Fig. 14.91). Although tearing may increase, the thick discharge, which is seen in conjunctivitis and which crusts at night, is not seen (Fig. 14.92). Since the uveal vessels underlie the sclera, a secondary uveitis may occur. Nodular lesions eventually erode the sclera, with perforation of underlying ocular

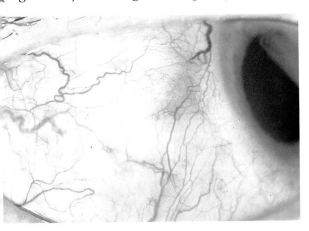

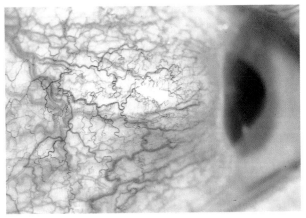

Figure 14.91 Episcleral and scleral injection of eye in a patient with rheumatoid arthritis. (*Left*) The deep episcleral vessels are tortuous, large, and have a bluer cast than the superficial narrow episcleral vessels which are secondarily affected. More severe episcleral injection was present but cleared with topical phenylephrine. Scleritis with overlying episcleritis (*right*). Large tortuous bluish scleral vessels are easily seen with overlying episcleral secondary injection. This patient has active rheumatoid scleritis. (Courtesy of William Mathers, MD)

Figure 14.92 Crusting of the lids in a patient with conjunctivitis. This is not seen in rheumatoid arthritis patients except in the presence of secondary infection.

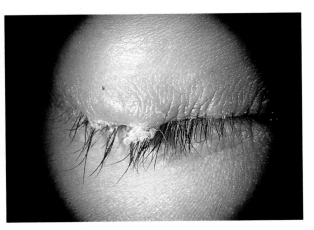

material (scleromalacia perforans) (Figs. 14.93 and 14.94). A broad blue discoloration often appears before actual perforation occurs (Fig. 14.95). This diffuse thinning is termed scleromalacia (Fig. 14.96).

Most of the scleral inflammation in rheumatoid arthritis is anterior, but posterior changes can lead to choroiditis (Fig. 14.97)

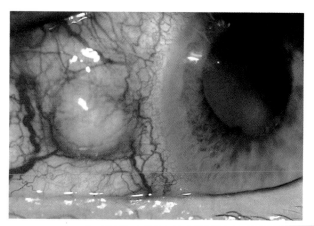

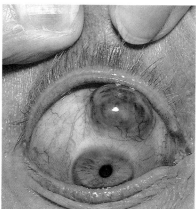

Figure 14.93 Nodular scleritis. Large yellow nodule is present in the sclera with large scleral vessel injection and secondary episcleritis in this patient with rheumatoid arthritis. (Courtesy of William Mathers, MD)

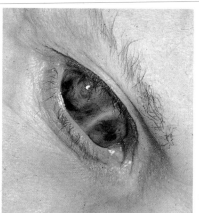

Figure 14.94 Severe scleromalacia perforans causes blindness.

Figure 14.95 Scleromalacia perforans (anterior view). Scleritis and episcleritis has caused thinning of the sclera with performation of the underlying uveal tract, resulting in bluish discoloration and nodules (*left*). Lateral view (*right*) shows anterior bulging.

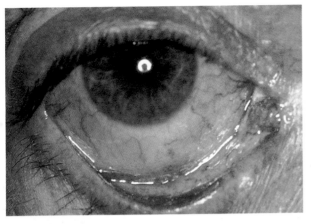

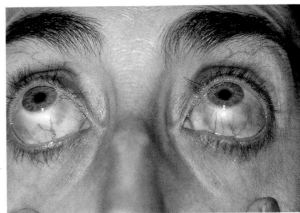

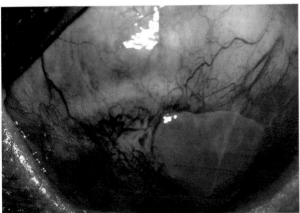

Figure 14.96 Moderate scleromalacia without perforation shows bluish color of the sclera, due to thinning. A mild to moderate amount of inflammation is seen in the scleral vessels (*top left*). More advanced scleromalacia without perforation (*top right*) causes a deep blue tinge in the sclera surrounding the cornea. Another patient is blind secondary to scleromalacia with perforation (*bottom left*). The deep bluish scleromalacia is obviously present. The yellowish tissue is granulation tissue overlying the eye secondary to the perforation and attempted self repair.

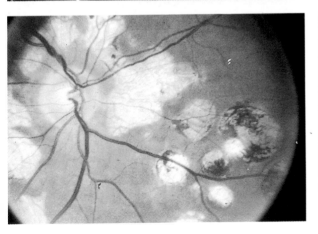

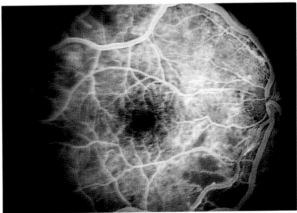

Figure 14.97 Diffuse choroiditis with vascular involvement (*left*) occurs rarely in rheumatoid arthritis. Fluorescein angiogram of patient with choroidal vasculitis and choroiditis (*right*). Angiogram shows diffuse abnormalities of the choroidal vessels with fluorescein leaking into the posterior eye. Severe active vasculitis is present.

and retinal detachment (Fig. 14.98) and, eventually, to blindness.

The most severe type of scleritis is the necrotizing variety. Thirty percent of patients with this type are dead in five years (Watson and Hazelman, 1976). The melting cornea syndrome (keratolysis) is an emergent condition with rapid deterioration of the eye and blindness (Fig. 14.99). This disorder requires prompt, aggressive ophthalmologic treatment, often with systemic cytotoxic agents (Foster

et al, 1984). Some ophthalmologists feel that the time-honored treatment of ocular inflammation with topical steroids may cause scleral thinning and predispose the eye to the more serious complication of perforation. Similarly, orbital steroid injections, which were used frequently in the past, may cause scleral thinning. Nonsteroidal, anti-inflammatory drugs may be a useful therapy in mild inflammation. Secondary infections of the eye may be devastating and require appropriate treatment with anti-

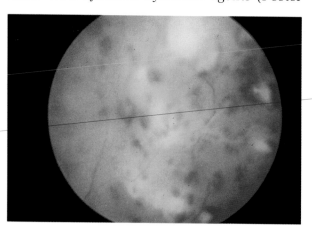
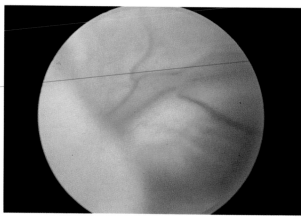

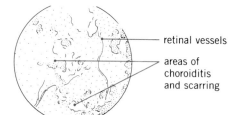
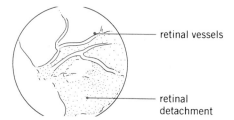

Figure 14.98 Retinal detachment caused by uveal vasculitis (*left*). The lifted retina is typical in posterior scleral inflammation (*right*). The vessels in this specimen are normal in appearance but the fuzzy retinal detachment is the same as that of posterior vessel inflammation.

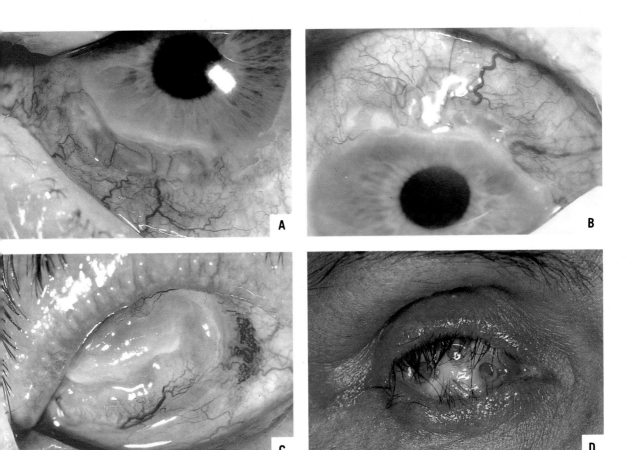

Figure 14.99 A patient has active scleritis with injected scleral vessels and a peripheral corneal melting syndrome obviously seen about the iris (**A**). Another patient has continued scleritis with tortuous vessels (**B**). The scleral melt is present at the edge of the iris; however, there is repair and scar tissue seen around the sclera. In cases of severe corneal melt syndrome blindness results, secondary to active scleritis and overlying scar tissue (**C**). The eye has been destroyed despite aggressive treatment (**D**).

biotics (Fig. 14.100). Glaucoma may complicate scleritis in 10% to 22% of cases (McGavin et al, 1976) (Fig. 14.101).

Episcleritis

The episclera is a layer of loose connective tissues which lies between the conjunctiva and sclera. Inflammation of this layer is often localized, evanescent, asymptomatic, and less serious than that of the sclera (Tessler, 1985) (Fig. 14.102). Bilateral involvement is seen in 50% of patients (McGavin et al, 1976) (Fig. 14.103).

Vascular engorgement of the episclera results in a redness, in contrast to the dark blue of scleritis (Watson and Hayreh, 1976). Simple episcleritis is associated with edema and yellow opacities (Fig. 14.104). In nodula

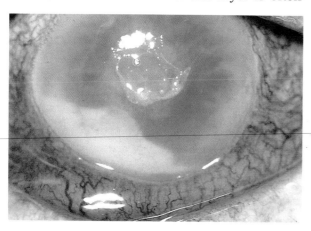

Figure 14.100 Corneal melt syndrome with secondary bacterial infection. The patient has active scleritis which is diffuse and easily seen throughout the eye, with increased vasculature. There is a bacterial keratitis and en-

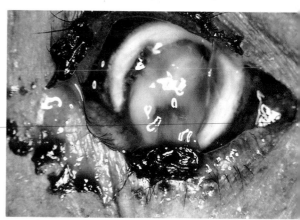

dophthalmitis. Pus is seen in the anterior chamber (*left*). Bacterial infection of the eye leads to severe corneal damage (*right*).

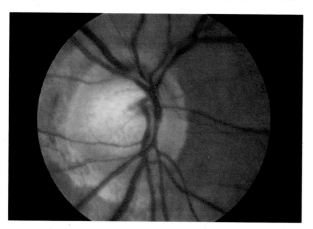

Figure 14.101 Typical glaucoma with deep indentation of the optic nerve and disc. Glaucoma may complicate both scleritis and iritis with scarring and synechia.

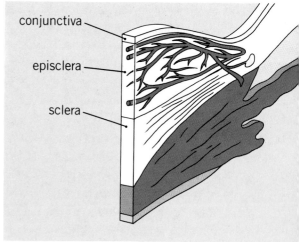

Figure 14.102 Episcleritis, showing inflammation and prominent vascular engorgement.

disease, nodules are confined to the episcleral layer. Often no treatment is needed, or brief therapy with local steroids will suffice. Recurrence is seen in over 60% of patients (Watson and Hayreh, 1976). An ophthalmologic examination is needed, nonetheless, to determine the possible coexistence of other ocular problems. The differences between episcleritis and scleritis are outlined in Figure 14.105 (Jayson and Jones, 1971).

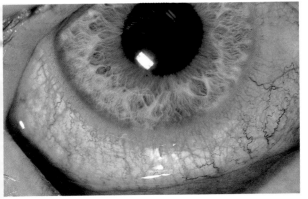

Figure 14.103 Diffuse episcleritial injection is seen throughout the eye of this patient with rheumatoid arthritis.

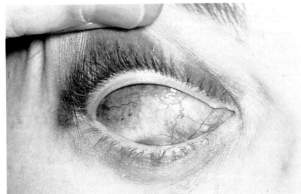

Figure 14.104 This patient has active episcleritis with yellowish coloration. The episcleral vessels are easily seen.

CLINICAL DIFFERENTIATION OF EPISCLERITIS AND SCLERITIS

CHARACTERISTICS	EPISCLERITIS	SCLERITIS
Course	Acute; resolves quickly (weeks)	Acute or insidious; may last 1 to 2 years
Symptoms	Slight discomfort, no visual change	Severe pain; blurred vision
Types	Simple, nodular	Simple; diffuse; nodular; necrotizing
Signs	Episcleral vascular injection; superficial, moveable nodules; no corneal involvement	Deep and superficial vessels involved; deep fixed nodules; cornea may be involved
Outcome	No residual	Scleromalacia; perforation

modified from Jayson and Jones, 1971

Figure 14.105 Clinical differentiation of episcleritis and scleritis.

Eye Movement Disorders

Rheumatoid nodules in the tendons of ocular muscles may interfere with eye movement. These nodules require systemic treatment of the rheumatoid disease and, occasionally, more aggressive local treatment. Symptoms include diplopia and painful eye movement.

Vasculitis in rheumatoid arthritis as in polyarteritis may involve the central nervous system and cause local cranial nerve palsy with movement disorders (Fig. 14.106). Cortical blindness has been described with such vasculitis.

Drug Reactions

Antirheumatic medication may be toxic to the eye. Nonsteroidal, anti-inflammatory drugs have been implicated in ocular toxicity but in many cases this has not been substantiated (Burke, 1985). Indomethacin deposits are poorly documented. Other nonsteroidal drugs may rarely be associated with local eye irritation, blurred vision, changes in color vision, refractive error, optic neuritis, amblyopia, and other problems. However, none of these problems has been definitively proven to be drug-related.

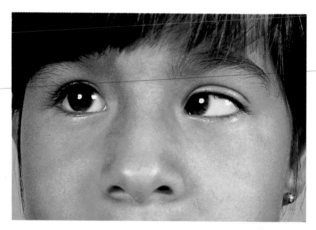

Figure 14.106 Movement disorders of the eye can occur in rheumatoid arthritis due either to nodules forming on the ocular muscle or to vasculitis, causing paralysis of the muscle on gaze.

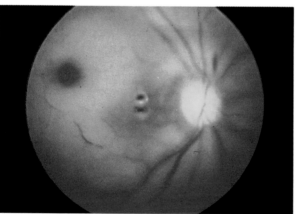

Figure 14.107 Chloroquine retinopathy can cause a bull's-eye maculopathy in its late stages very similar to that seen in polyarteritis nodosum. This is caused by light-induced damage and has a central red area surrounded by clear area of retinal damage.

When gold therapy is prolonged over many years, patients develop corneal deposits of gold (chrysiasis), which are diffuse and may be reversible. Of gold therapy patients, 40% to 75% have been shown to have minimal asymptomatic gold deposition visible in the eye (Burke, 1985). Conjunctival and other ocular inflammation may be secondary to allergic drug reactions.

Antimalarial ocular side effects have been the most heralded of the drug reactions. With modern management, this problem can be minimized. Hydroxychloroquine appears to be less toxic than its parent drug, chloroquine. Reversible corneal deposition of this drug may occur (see Chapter 15). Toxic reactions in the posterior eye are more serious and can cause macular pigmentation and light-induced retinopathy, with an end-stage bull's eye maculopathy (Fig. 14.107). Loss of color vision and of central visual fields may be irreversible and progressive even after discontinuation of drug therapy (Fig. 14.108). Patients should receive minimal antimalarial drug dosages (400 mg or less of hydroxychloroquine per day), and a careful ophthalmologic examination should be performed every six months. This should include central visual fields (done with a red test object), as well as careful fundoscopic and slit-lamp ex-

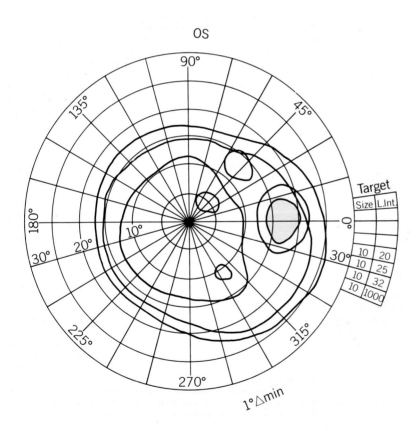

Figure 14.108 Schematic of visual field. Field defects (scotoma) are usually seen in the central area (cones) and are revealed only by testing central visual fields in contradistinction to peripheral fields. Sensitivity is increased by using a red test object.

aminations (Fig. 14.109). Central visual field determinations may be performed with an Amsler grid. These follow-up examinations can detect toxicity at an early enough time so that it can often be reversed by discontinuation of the drug.

Chronic oral corticosteroids lead to posterior subcapsular cataracts in 33% of patients on steroids, in contrast to 3% to 4% of rheumatoid patients not taking the drug (Burke, 1985) (Fig. 14.110). Glaucoma can also be exacerbated by drug-caused fluid shifts. The complications of topical corticosteroid applications have been noted previously. Ocular infections, like other infections, are more common in immunosuppressed patients.

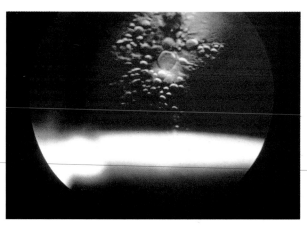 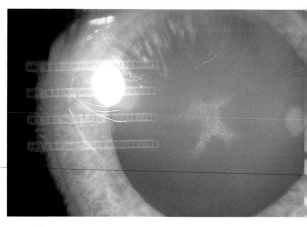

Figure 14.109 Slit-lamp examination showing posterior subcapsular cataract in patient on chronic corticosteroid therapy (*left*). A cataract in the lens has occurred in another patient on chronic steroid therapy (*right*).

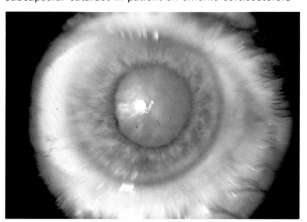 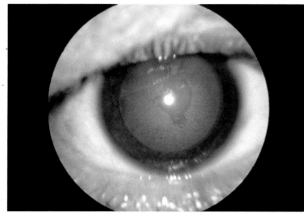

Figure 14.110 Prominent cataract in a patient with rheumatoid arthritis on chronic steroid therapy (*left*). A true posterior subcapsular cataract from a patient with rheumatoid arthritis on corticosteroids (*right*). Note the clouding of the cornea and the obvious opacity in the pupil. (Courtesy William Mather, MD)

NEUROPATHIES

Peripheral neuropathies can complicate rheumatoid arthritis by a number of different mechanisms (Good et al, 1965; Peyronnard et al, 1982). Sensory or motor neuropathies can be distal and symmetric or can occur in the pattern of mononeuritis multiplex when associated with vasculitis. Isolated compression neuropathies can be caused by soft tissue swelling or bony deformities. Drugs, such as gold, may induce peripheral neuropathies (Schlumpf et al, 1983). Antimalarials and nonsteroidal agents can also occasionally cause neuropathies.

Whether autonomic neuropathy contributes to common vasomotor changes in the hands is not clear (Edmonds et al, 1979). Secondary amyloid formation could possibly be a factor in autonomic neuropathy.

Clinical Appearance

Neuropathies are common in rheumatoid arthritis, with various studies suggesting an incidence of noncompressive neuropathies of 1.2% to 9.8% (Hart and Golding, 1960). Mild distal sensory impairment in which the mechanism is unclear is most common. A variety of neurologic problems may occur more frequently in rheumatoid arthritis patients with Sjögren's syndrome.

Common compressive neuropathies are the carpal tunnel syndrome and the tarsal tunnel syndrome. These and other compressive neuropathies are described in this book by their anatomic site. Less common entrapment neuropathies include that of the posterior interosseous nerve at the elbow, which causes an extensor paralysis of all digits (Chang et al, 1972). Occipital neuropathy results from C1–2 spinal disease.

Nerve conduction studies can help confirm clinical suspicions about sites of nerve compression. Such studies can also help identify such problems as root involvement, which is only rarely related to rheumatoid pachymeningitis or dural nodules; it is much more often due to coincidental disease.

Diagnosis

Laboratory tests are of limited value but may be helpful, as described above, in confirming a diagnosis of vasculitis.

Sural nerve biopsy is an excellent way to demonstrate vasculitis in patients with clinical involvement of that nerve (Conn et al, 1972). In patients with proven vasculitis or with rheumatoid arthritis and Sjögren's syndrome, nerve biopsies typically show axonal neuropathy. In many cases, necrotizing arteritis of the vasa nervorum is found (Fig. 14.111), although a focal mild vasculitis may be missed (Peyronnard et al, 1982; Kim and Collins, 1981).

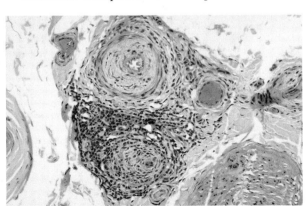

Figure 14.111 Perineural vessel from sural nerve biopsy shows vasculitis with inflammatory infiltrate and thickening of vessel wall. This is a necrotizing vasculitis. (H&E).

Therapy

The identification of a diffuse neuropathy requires that readily reversible causes, such as the administration of certain drugs or coincidental disease, first be considered. Compression neuropathies can be treated by local splinting, injections, or surgical decompression. Mononeuritis multiplex requires the same management as for necrotizing vasculitis.

Mild, symmetric, peripheral neuropathy is usually benign and generally requires no treatment other than a consideration of treatable unrelated causes. Reassurance that neuropathy frequently persists but in a more tolerable form is often helpful.

It has been suggested that neuropathies occur more frequently since the advent of steroid therapy, but this is not well substantiated. High-dose steroids or a rapid withdrawal of steroids can have central nervous system effects, however.

MUSCLE INVOLVEMENT

Rheumatoid arthritis can affect muscles in a variety of ways. Eighty percent of patients have been said to have some evidence of muscle weakness, and incompletely ex-

plained myalgias are very common during early disease. Later, atrophy can occur adjacent to inflamed, painful, and underused joints (Fig. 14.112), and tendon ruptures and neuropathies can cause local atrophy. Corticosteroid therapy also can produce a proximal myopathy, and contribute to atrophy. Penicilliamine can cause a polymyositis (Schrader et al, 1972) or myasthenia gravis (Russell and Lindstrom, 1978), and antimalarials can induce a vacuolar myopathy or neuromyopathy (Hughes et al, 1971; Estes et al, 1987). Generalized cachexia can occur during severe multisystem complications. Rheumatoid disease itself can involve muscles with lymphocytic infiltrates or with vasculitis directly. There may be a slightly increased risk of myasthenia gravis in patients with rheumatoid arthritis.

Clinical Appearance

Many of the above muscular complications with rheumatoid arthritis are readily evident clinically. Many workers agree that generalized muscle weakness appears to be out of proportion to that produced by local problems. Halla et al (1984) noted weakness in several settings in rheumatoid patients, some in patients with active arthritis and some in patients with only slight synovitis but persistently elevated sedimentation rates.

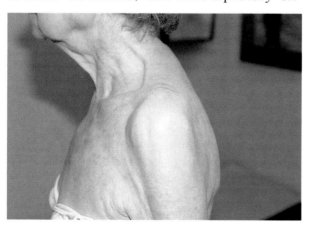

Figure 14.112 Muscle atrophy around the shoulder in this patient with chronic rheumatoid arthritis is probably mutifactorial.

Significant weakness in the quadriceps muscle, but not in the hamstring muscles of rheumatoid patients, compared to age-matched normals, has been noted, even at a time of mild disease activity and virtual remission of knee synovitis (Hsieh et al, 1987). This incompletely explained weakness is more proximal than distal. Although it may be associated with some histologic fingings (Halla et al, 1984), direct correlation with the histopathology is not established. Hand weakness usually is more clearly related to joint disease or neuropathy.

Electromyographic findings in rheumatoid muscles vary and often have not been correlated with biopsies and long-term followup. Most patients without overt myopathy have only a few nonspecific changes (Halla et al 1984; Moritz 1963; Mueller and Mead, 1952), and this finding can help exclude some muscle diseases.

Diagnosis

Creatine kinase and other muscle enzyme serum levels are not usually elevated in rheumatoid arthritis, even with muscle weakness caused by a variety of conditions. Creatine kinase can be elevated by intramuscular injections or vigorous exertion, but this elevation should also suggest more overt muscle involvement, such as vasculitis in the muscle, the uncommon rheumatoid necrotizing myositis (Halla et al, 1984), an "overlap syndrome" with other collagen disease, and myositis or drug-induced muscle disease, as with penicillamine (Petersen et al, 1978) or chloroquine. Corticosteroid myopathy does not elevate creatine kinase—this often helps in the differential diagnosis.

Nodular infiltrates, mostly consisting of lymphocytes and other mononuclear cells, are common in rheumatoid muscles. Although Sokoloff et al (1950) found such infiltrates in 56% of patients with rheumatoid arthritis, they also noted infiltrates in 23% of muscle biopsies from normal subjects; the occurrence of nodular infiltrates could not be correlated with clinical muscle disease. Halla et al (1984) did note some muscle necrosis in a few biopsies, which seemed to occur more often in the infrequently seen patient with otherwise unexplained increased creatine kinase levels and more severe muscle weakness. More recently, atrophy of type II, or fast twitch, low aerobic capacity muscle fibers, in contrast to type I endurance fibers, has been reported. Recent isokinetic muscle testing supported this, showing better retention of endurance in rheumatoid quadriceps muscles (Hsieh et al, 1987). However, type II muscle fiber atrophy is a nonspecific finding seen in many chronic diseases.

More specific muscle findings can include the occasional demonstration of rheumatoid vasculitis, polymyositis due to penicillamine with muscle degeneration and regeneration, and a dramatic vacuolization of muscle in antimalarial myopathy (Whisnant et al, 1963).

Therapy

The common muscle weakness in rheumatoid disease seems to be a part of the general process, does not alone affect prognosis, and is best managed by usual methods of disease control. Throughout the disease, general conditioning and systematic use of all muscles must be attended to. Isometric exercise can yield excellent results in patients with painful joints. Immobilization, when required, should be for as short a period as possible.

A recent study (Hsieh et al, 1987) supported the greater need for exercise of the quadriceps muscle, rather than the hamstring, muscles. Corticosteroid doses should be minimized except in the rare patient with overt inflammatory polymyositis or vasculitis. An elevated creatine kinase may indicate that a more severe muscle disease is present. The possible adverse effects of penicillamine and antimalarial drugs on muscle should also be kept in mind.

BONE DISEASE

The joint manifestations and articular destruction caused by rheumatoid arthritis are covered in detail throughout this book. However, primary articular bone involvement deserves a short mention.

Generalized loss of bone, osteoporosis, in contradistinction to focal erosive loss, is seen regularly in patients with advanced rheumatoid arthritis (Hollingsworth, 1968) (Fig. 14.113). Corticosteroid use, diffuse inflammation with protein catabolism, inactivity,

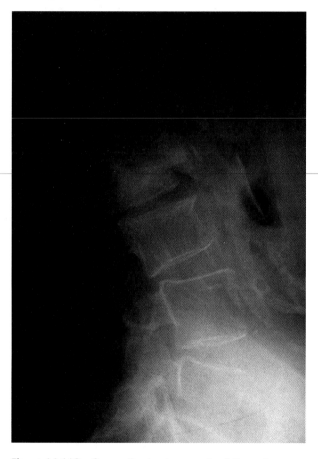 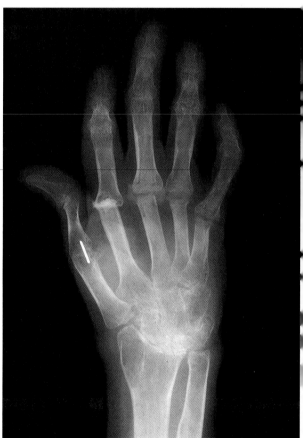

Figure 14.113 Generalized osteoporosis of the spine (*left*). Vertebrae appear to be very dark with very little in the way of cortical bone. These vertebrae are subject to fracture. Diffuse osteoporosis of the hand (*right*) in patient with rheumatoid arthritis. Generalized osteoporosis is not only periarticular but occurs throughout the bones of the hands. Note the absence of cortical bone with the exception of a narrow sharp outline to the metaphyses. The second metacarpal is a perfectly round bone in cross section and can be used as a guidepost to determine the extent of generalized osteopenia because any direction that it might be turned would still show the amount of corticalbone present.

poor nutrition, and loss of anabolic hormones are probably also pathogenic. Pain secondary to microfracture or more gross bone fracture occurs and may dominate the patient's treatment needs. Hip, knee, or any bone may fracture (Fig. 14.114) and crush fracture of the

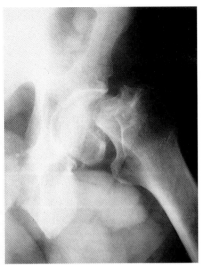

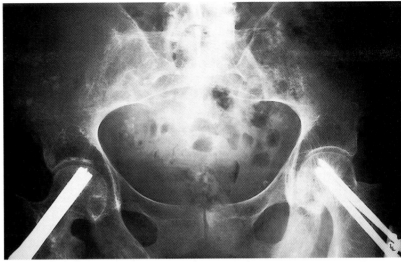

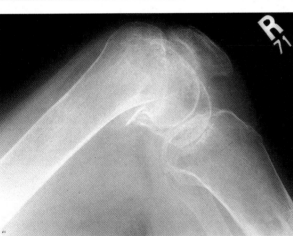

Figure 14.114 Patient with rheumatoid arthritis and osteopenia with spontaneous pathologic fracture of the hip (*top left*). Surgical nailing of hip fractures in a patient with rheumatoid arthritis on corticosteroids (*top right*). Stabilization of such hip fractures is extremely difficult since the weakened osteopenic bone cannot be held in place with metal. Pathologic fracture of the knee in a patient with severe osteopenia and inflammatory arthritis (*bottom left*).

vertebrae (Fig. 14.115) are not uncommon.

Treatment includes the use of analgesics, and, occasionally, narcotics. Short-term bed rest, followed by physical therapy and re-mobilization, or the application of a back brace or cast, may be needed. Occasionally, operative intervention is required. Calcium and vitamin D supplementation and hormone (estrogen plus progesterone) replacement is widely used. The prophylactic use of calcium and vitamin D in steroid-treated patients to prevent drug-induced osteopenia has also been recommended (Hahn and Hahn, 1976).

Rib erosion, consisting of a localized notching or diffuse bone loss, has been re-ported (Anderson et al, 1972) (Fig. 14.116). This may be seen on chest radiographs and may be painful. It has been seen more often in systemic sclerosis.

The geode is a large cavity rarely seen in subchondral areas of patients with rheuma-toid arthritis (Cruickshank et al, 1954) (Fig. 14.117). Jayson et al (1972) suggested that these cystic masses are caused by increased intra-articular pressure around a damaged joint that causes herniation of the joint con-tents into the bone. Collapse of these cysts can lead to severe joint damage and pain. Also, patients being treated with corticoste-

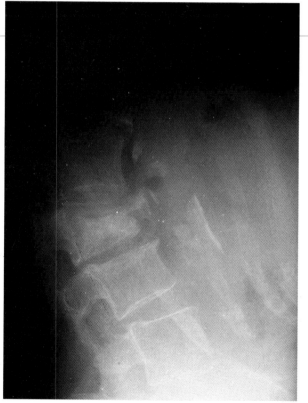

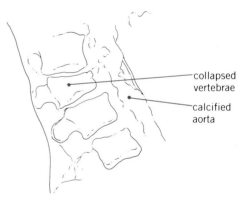

Figure 14.115 Crush fracture secondary to osteoporosis and trauma with anterior wedging and increased density of the involved vertebrae is seen. Some wedging of the inferior vertebra is also present and is probably also frac-tured. The age of the fracture is often difficult to assess without serial radiographs.

collapsed vertebrae

calcified aorta

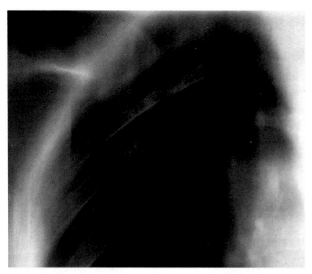

Figure 14.116 Ribs with large erosions on either the second or third rib superiorly. Such rib erosions are infrequently seen in rheumatoid arthritis and may be due to scapular pressure, although their etiology is not known. (Courtesy of Michael Pitt, MD)

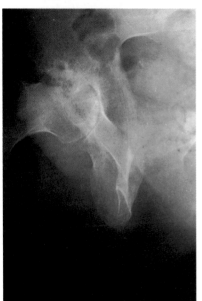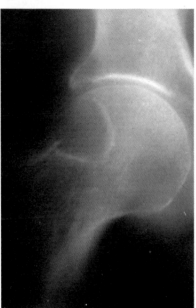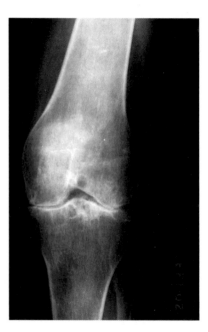

Figure 14.117 Geode formation in the hip. Large subchondral cyst-like formation is seen in the hip and acetabulum. Geodes are subject to pathologic fracture and collapse of bone (*left*). Large geode of the hip in a patient with rheumatoid arthritis (*middle*). Knee with small geodes in the femur and tibia (*right*). These small cyst-like formations can lead to fracture.

roids can develop avascular necrosis of the bone, with collapse (Fig. 14.118).

Severe resorption of bone can occur in patients with rheumatoid joint involvement, which is above and beyond the normal erosive process usually seen (Fig. 14.119).

Why some patients have more severe resorptive bone changes than others is not known. Such resorptive arthropathy is more characteristic of severe psoriatic arthritis than of rheumatoid disease, but a subclass of rheumatoid patients have this syndrome.

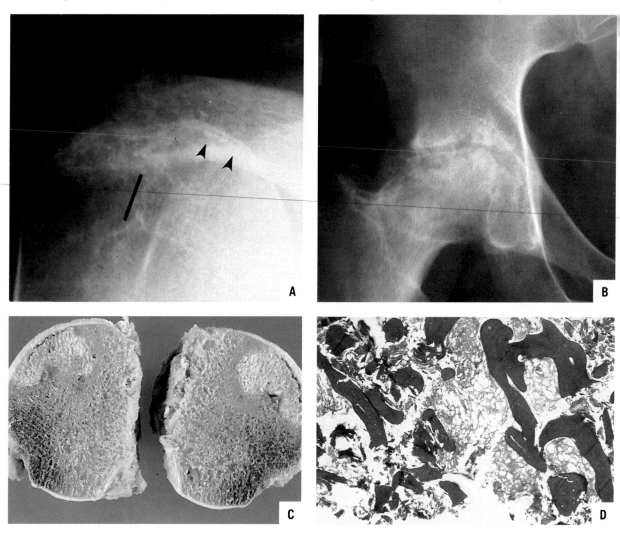

Figure 14.118 Avascular necrosis of the shoulder in inflammatory arthritis **(A)**. Arrows point to subcortical clear space caused by dead bone (the crescent sign). Patients on steroids are particularly susceptible to this complication. Late-stage avascular necrosis of the hip **(B)** shows collapse and flattening of the femoral head. Bilateral avascular necrosis of the hip **(C)** is seen in this cross section of the femoral heads, revealing dead bone and separation from the overlying cortex and cartilage. This dead bone shows as a white, wedge-like abnormality on radiograph. The separation of the cortex from the underlying dead bone shows as a clear space on radiograph (crescent sign). Marked necrosis and fragmentation of the femoral head are seen **(D)**.

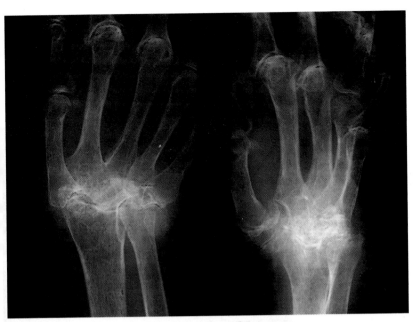

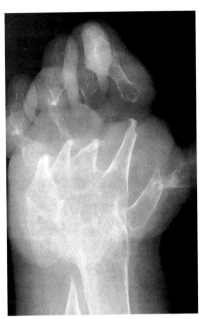

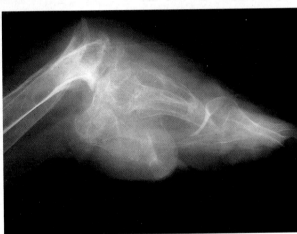

Figure 14.119 Severe resorption of multiple bones of the hand. This is a so-called opera glass hand with floppy fingers that are nonfunctional. This patient has virtually no carpal bones due to the severe resorption with rheumatoid arthritis (*top left*). Tapering of the distal portions of the bone is called "penciling" (*top right*). Some of the phalanges are completely resorbed. This type of resorptive arthropathy can occur in severe rheumatoid arthritis. Lateral view radiograph of severe resorptive opera glass hand of same patient (*bottom left*).

LARYNGEAL OR CRICOARYTENOID JOINT INVOLVEMENT

Although the larynx is not an extra-articular structure per se, its involvement in rheumatoid arthritis is frequently grouped with non-articular diseases. The cricoarytenoid joint is a diarthrodial joint lined with synovium, which allows the vocal cords to open and close (Figs. 14.120 and 14.121). When acute arthritis occurs, the joint may become fixed in a position that closes the vocal cords, and thus obstructs air flow. The joint is tender, swollen, and red, as in peripheral limb joint involvement. Fusion may occur when the joint is in a partially open position. Hoarseness ensues, but breathing is possible. Problems occur, in this instance, after intubation for anesthesia. At the time of extubation, the joint is fractured and the vocal cords are flail; thus air flow is obstructed, and suffocation can occur if immediate treatment by tracheostomy or reintubation is not instituted.

Lofgren and Montgomery (1962) noted an incidence of 26% of cricoarytenoid involvement in 100 patients with rheumatoid arthritis. The symptoms of this disorder, noted in Figure 14.122, are related to phonation, airway obstruction, painful swelling of the joint, and pain on swallowing. Food may not be ingested because of this pain, which also may radiate to the ear. A sensation of a foreign body in the throat is not unusual.

Hoarseness in a rheumatoid patient should always lead the clinician to evaluate the cricoarytenoid joint, at least by indirect laryngoscopy. As obstruction becomes more severe, stridor, particularly at night, may occur. Without intervention, suffocation will eventually occur, and sudden death has been reported in such patients.

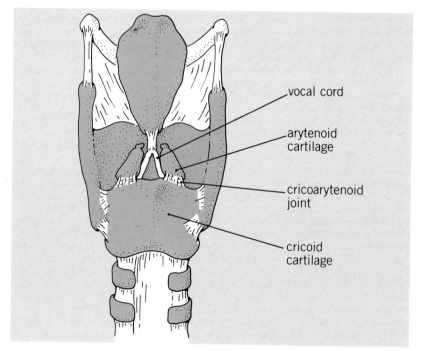

Figure 14.120 The larynx. Note the cricoid cartilage and the arytenoid cartilage. The articulation between these cartilage segments is a true synovial joint.

vocal cord

arytenoid cartilage

cricoarytenoid joint

cricoid cartilage

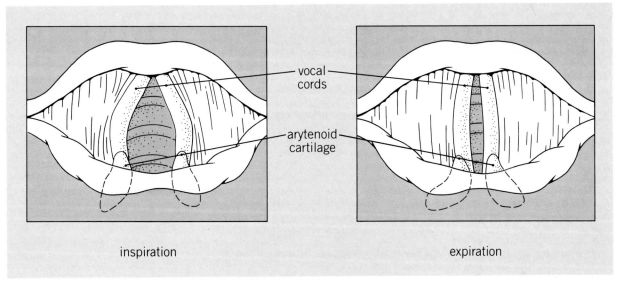

Figure 14.121 The opening and closing of the laryngeal (vocal) cords during breathing and phonation. Indirect laryngoscopy allows the clinician to look at the cords for normal motion. With acute arthritis the cords are fixed and do not move well. In addition redness and swelling can be seen over the cricoarytenoid joint.

SYMPTOMS OF CRICOARYTENOID ARTHRITIS

Symptom	No. of patients	Symptom	No. of patients
Sensation of foreign body	17	Stridor at night	8
Hoarseness	15	Dysphagia	7
Sensation of fullness and tension	14	Odynophagia	4
Dyspnea	10	Pain with speech	4
Radiation of pain to ear	10	Signs but no symptoms	3
		Total	100

100 patients at Massachusetts General Hospital with rheumatoid arthritis

Lofgren and Montgomery, 1962

Figure 14.122 Symptoms of cricoarytenoid arthritis.

Diagnostic testing begins with direct laryngoscopy (Fig. 14.123). Redness and swelling of the joint can be seen by the experienced clinician. Cords may not move easily and may bow on inspiration. Manipulation of the cord with a spatula is painful. In a study of 45 rheumatoid patients with laryngeal involvement, 42% exhibited hoarseness (Lawry et al, 1984). Nodules or polyps were seen in six patients and eight showed bowing of the cords, asymmetry of closure, or decreased mobility. In another study, erythema on the inferior arytenoid, sometimes with edema, was seen (Lawry et al, 1985). This study showed reduced cord mobility in 66% of rheumatoid patients. Structural lesions are seen on high-resolution CAT scans (Lawry et al, 1984; Charlin et al, 1985). Erosion and subluxation of the cricoarytenoid joint, as well as soft tissue swelling, can be easily seen in such studies (Brazeau-Lamontagne et al, 1986).

Treatment is outlined in Figure 14.124. Early hospitalization is encouraged, since the situation can rapidly deteriorate. Local measures, combined with local and/or systemic steroids, are usually successful. Surgical intervention is occasionally needed and may be lifesaving. Heated moist air, local steroid injections, rest of the voice, and comfortable positioning in bed are important.

DIAGNOSIS OF CRICOARYTENOID ARTHRITIS

CAT scan

Laryngoscopy:
Redness or swelling
Bowing of vocal cords on inspiration
Pain on manipulation

Passive mobility test

Pain on palpation of anterior portion, or on compression of superior cornua of thyroid cartilage

Stridor

Figure 14.123   Diagnosis of cricoarytenoid arthritis.

TREATMENT OF CRICOARYTENOID ARTHRITIS

Anti-inflammatory drugs

Voice rest

Humidification

Local heat

Air

Systemic steroids

Steroid injection at cricoarytenoid joint

Emergency tracheostomy

Unilateral arytenoidectomy

Intubation

Figure 14.124   Treatment of cricoarytenoid arthritis.

REFERENCES

Abdou NI, Naombejara C, Balentine L, Abdou NL: Suppressor cell-mediated neutropenia in Felty's syndrome. *J Clin Invest* 1978;61:738–743.

Abel T, Andrews BS, Cunningham PH, et al: Rheumatoid vasculitis; Effect of cyclophosphamide on the clinical course and levels of circulating immune complexes. *Ann Intern Med* 1980;93:407–413.

Adachi JD, Buchanan WW, Kean WF: Sjögren's syndrome. Its clinical and laboratory manifestations and associations, in Utsinger PD, Zvaifler NJ, Ehrlich GE (eds): *Rheumatoid Arthritis*. Philadelphia, JB Lippincott, 1985, pp 465–486.

Adler RH, Norcooss BM, Lockie LM: Arteritis and infarctions of the intestine in rheumatoid arthritis. *JAMA* 1962;180:992–926.

Anderson IF, Corrigan AB, Champion GD: Rib erosions in rheumatoid arthritis. *Ann Rheum Dis* 1972;31:16–21.

Asherman RA, Morgan SH, Hackett D, Montoneo P, Oakley C, Hughes GRV: Rheumatoid arthritis and preliminary hypertension, a report of 3 cases. *J Rheumatol* 1985;12:154–159.

Bacon PA, Gibson DG: Cardiac involvement in rheumatoid arthritis. *Ann Rheum Dis* 1974;33:20–24.

Ball GV, Schrohenloher R, Hester R: Gammaglobulin complexes in rheumatoid pericardial fluid. *Am J Med* 1975;58:123–128.

Balogh K: The histologic appearance of corticosteroid injection sites. *Arch Pathol Lab Med* 1986;110:1168–1172.

Bankhurst AD, Rowe T: Letter: Rheumatoid pleural effusion, the case for a primary glucose transport defect. *J Rheumatol* 1980;7:110–111.

Barnes CG, Turnbull AL, Vernon-Roberts B: Felty's syndrome. A clinical and pathological survey of 21 patients and their response to treatment. *Ann Rheum Dis* 1971;30:359–374.

Barnett EV, Winkelstein A, Weinberger HJ: A gammaglobulinemia with polyarthritis and subcutaneous nodules. *Am J Med* 1970;48:40–47.

Bathon JM, Young MA, Mayes MD, DiBartolomeo AG: Rheumatoid nodules: A reappraisal of incidence and prognostic significance. *Clin Res* 1985;33:786A (Abst).

Benedek TG, Zawadzki ZA, Medsger TA: Serum immunoglobulins, rheumatoid factor and pneumoconiosis in coal miners with rheumatoid arthritis. *Arthritis Rheum* 1976;19:731–736.

Blendis LM, Jones KL, Hamilton EBD, Williams R: Familial Felty's syndrome. *Ann Rheum Dis* 1976;35:279–281.

Blendis LM, Parkinson MC, Shilkin KB, Williams R: Nodular regeneractive hyperplasia of the liver in Felty's syndrome. *Quart J Med* 1974;43:25–32.

Bloch KJ, Buchanan WW, Wohl MJ, Bunim JJ: Sjögren's syndrome. A clinical pathological and serological study of 62 cases. *Medicine* 1965;44:187–231.

Boh LE, Schuna AA, Pitterle ME, Adams EM, Sundstrom WR: Low dose weekly oral methotrexate therapy for inflammatory arthritis. *Clin Pharmacol* 1986;5:503–508.

Bonfiglio T, Atwater EC: Heart disease in patients with seropositive rheumatoid arthritis: A controlled autopsy study and review. *Arch Intern Med* 1969;124:714–719.

Brazeau-Lamontagne L, Charlin B, Levesque RY, Lussier A: Cricoarytenoiditis: CT assessment in rheumatoid arthritis. *Radiology* 1986;158:463–466.

Brun C, Olsen TS, Raaschou F, Sorensen AWS: Renal biopsy in rheumatoid arthritis. *Nephron* 1965;2:65–81.

Bulger RJ, Healy LA, Polinsky P: Renal abnormalities in rheumatoid arthritis. *Ann Rheum Dis* 1968;27:339–344.

Burke MJ: Ocular manifestations, in Utsinger PD, Zvaifler NJ, Ehrlich GE (eds): *Rheumatoid Arthritis*. Philadelphia, JB Lippincott, 1985, pp 357–364.

Burney DP, Martin CE, Thomas CS, Fisher HW: Rheumatoid pericarditis. *J Thorac Cardiovasc Surg* 1979;77:511–515.

Burry H: Renal disorders in rheumatoid arthritis. *Rheum Phys Med* 1971;11:2–9.

Bywaters EGL: The relationship between heart and joint disease including "rheumatoid heart disease" and chronic post rheumatic arthritis (Type Joccond). *Br Heart J* 1950;12:101–131.

Bywaters EGL: Editorial: On two papers dealing with nodules. *J Rheum* 1979;6:243–246.

Caplan A: Certain radiological appearances in the chest of coal miners suffering from rheumatoid arthritis. *Thorax* 1953;8:29–37.

Cerventes-Perez P, Toro-Perez AN, Rodriquez-Jurado P: Pulmonary involvement in rheumatoid arthritis. *JAMA* 1980;243:1715–1719.

Chang LW, James JDC, Granger CV, Millender LH: Entrapment neuropathy of the posterior interosseous nerve. A complication of rheumatoid arthritis. *Arthritis Rheum* 1972;15:350–352.

Charlin B, Brazeau-Lamontagne L, Levesque RY, Lussier A: Cricoarytenoiditis in rheumatoid arthritis: Comparison of fibro-laryngoscopic and high resolution computerized tomographic findings. *J Otolaryngol* 1985;14:381–386.

Chen S-T, Chou C-T, Schumacher HR, Lee J-F, Ho H-H, Murphy B, Liu B-Y: Rheumatoid arthritis (RA): A study comparing Chinese and American patients. *Arthritis Rheum* 1986;30:S40 (Abst).

Clive DM, Staff JS: Renal syndromes associated with non-steroidal antiinflammatory drugs. *N Engl J Med* 1984;310:563–572.

Cohen AS, Canoso JJ: Pericarditis in rheumatological diseases. *Cardiovasc Clin* 1976;7:237–255.

Cohen MD, Ginsburg WW, Allen GL: Nodular regenerative hyperplasia of the liver and bleeding esophageal varices in Felty's syndrome. *J Rheum* 1982;9:716–718.

Comess KA, Fenster PE, Gall EP: Cardiac involvement in rheumatoid arthritis. *Cardiovas Res* 1982;3:533–542.

Conn DL, McDuffie FC, Dyck PJ: Immunopathology of sural nerves in rheumatoid arthritis. *Arthritis Rheum* 1972;15:135–143.

Cruickshank B, Macleod JG, Shearer WG: Subarticular pseudocysts in rheumatoid arthritis. *J Fac Radiol* 1954;5:218–226.

Davies SF, Iber C: Obstructive sleep apnea associated with adult-acquired micrognathia from rheumatoid arthritis. *Am Rev Respir Dis* 1983;127:245–247.

Davis P, Johnston C, Bertouch J, Starkebaum G: Depressed superoxide radical generation by neutrophils from patients with rheumatoid arthritis and neutropenia. *Ann Rheum Dis* 1987;46:51–54.

Davis RF, Engleman EG: Incidence of myocardial infarctions in patients with rheumatoid arthritis. *Arthritis Rheum* 1974;17:527–533.

deWilde PCM, Bakk JPA, Shootseg PJ, Hene RJ, Kater L: Morphometry in the diagnosis of Sjögren's syndrome. *Anal Quant Cytol Histol* 1986;8:49–55.

Dieppe PA: Empyema in rheumatoid arthritis. *Ann Rheum Dis* 1975;34:181–185.

Dietrichson O, From A, Christofferson P, et al: Morphological changes in liver biopsies from patients with rheumatoid arthritis. *Scand J Rheum* 1976;5:65–69.

Dyer NH, Kendall MJ, Hawkins CF: Malabsorption in rheumatoid disease. *Ann Rheum Dis* 1971;30:626–630.

Editorial: Infection in rheumatic disease. *Br Med J* 1972;2:549–550.

Edmonds ME, Jones TC, Saunders WA, et al: Autonomic neuropathy in rheumatoid arthritis. *Br Med J* 1979;2:173–175.

Edstrom L, Nordemar R: Differential changes in type I and type II muscle fibers in rheumatoid arthritis. *Scand J Rheum* 1974;3:155–160.

Edwards JCW: Relationship between pressure and digital vasculitis in rheumatoid arthritis. *Ann Rheum Dis* 1980; 39:138–140.

Empire Rheumatism Council: Report on an inquiry into the aetiology factors associated with rheumatoid arthritis. *Ann Rheum Dis* (Suppl 9) 1950;176.

Eraut D, Evans J, Caplin M: Pulmonary necrobiotic nodules without rheumatoid arthritis. *Br J Dis Chest* 1978;72:301–306.

Erhardt CC, Mumford P, Mani RN: The association of cryoglobulinemia with nodules, vasculitis and fibrosing alveolitis in RA and their relationship to serum Clq binding activity and rheumatoid factor. *Clin Exp Immunol* 1979;38:405–413.

Estes ML, Ewing-Wilson D, Chou SM, et al: Chloroquine neuromyotoxicity. *Am J Med* 1987;82:447–455.

Faurschou P, Francis D, Faarup P: Thoracoscopic histological and clinical findings in nine cases of rheumatoid pleural effusion. *Thorax* 1985;40:371–375.

Flores M, Agosti I, Damlorenca C, Aguirre C: Rheumatoid arthritis with severe aortic insufficiency and prolapse of the mitral valve. *Scand J Rheum* 1984;13:28–32.

Foster CS, Forstot SC, Wilson LA: Mortality rate in rheumatoid arthritis patients developing necrotizing scleritis or peripheral keratitis: Effects of systemic immunosuppression. *Ophthalmology* 1984;91:1253–1262.

Fox RI, Michelson PE, Howell FU: Ocular and oral problems in arthritis. *Postgrad Med* 1985;78:87–97.

Franco AE, Levine HD, Hall AP: Rheumatoid pericarditis. *Ann Intern Med* 1972;77:837–844.

Fye KH, Terrasaki PI, Michalski JP, Daniels TE, Opelz G, Talal N: Relationship of HLA, Dw3 and HLA B8 to Sjögren's syndrome. *Arthritis Rheum* 1978;21:337–342.

Gall EP: Aspirin, a safe drug in treating rheumatoid arthritis. *JAMA* 1982;247:63–64.

Geddes DM, Webley M, Emerson PA: Airways obstruction in rheumatoid arthritis. *Ann Rheum Dis* 1979;38:222–225.

Gibberd FB: Dyspepsia in patients with rheumatoid arthritis. *Acta Rheum Scand* 1966;12:112–121.

Goldberg J, Pinals RS: Felty's syndrome. *Semin Arthritis Rheum* 1980;10:52–65.

Goldman S, Gall EP, Hager D: Rheumatoid pericarditis presenting as a mass lesion. *Chest* 1978;73:550–552.

Good AE, Christopher RP, Koepke GH, Bender LF, Tarter ME: Peripheral neuropathy associated with rheumatoid arthritis. *Ann Intern Med* 1965;63:87–99.

Gordon DA, Hyland RH, Broder I: Clinical presentation and differential diagnosis of pulmonary abnormalities, in Utsinger PD, Zvaifler NJ, Ehrlich GE (eds): *Rheumatoid Arthritis.* Philadelphia, JB Lippincott, 1985, p 934.

Gottlieb NL, Gray RG: Hepatotoxicity from antirheumatic drugs. *Arthritis* 1983;2:2–7.

Granirer LW, Milstein JJ, Schmidt H: The spontaneous rupture of the spleen in Felty's syndrome. *NY State Med J* 1958;58:413–414.

Gray RG, Poppo MJ: Necrotizing vasculitis as the initial manifestation of rheumatoid arthritis. *J Rheum* 1983;10:326–328.

Greening AP: Editorial: Bronchioalveolar lavage. *Br Med J* 1982;284:1896–1897.

Gupta R, Robinson WA, Albrecht D: Granulopoietic activity in Felty's syndrome. *Ann Rheum Dis* 1975;34:156–161.

Haden WB: On dry mouth or suppression of the salivary and buccal secretions. *Trans Clin Soc Lond* 1888;21:176–179.

Hahn BH, Yardley JH, Stevens MB: Rheumatoid nodules in systemic lupus erythematosus. *Ann Int Med* 1970;72:49–58.

Hahn TJ, Hahn BH: Osteopenia in patients with rheumatoid diseases, principles of diagnosis and therapy. *Semin Arthritis* 1976;6:165–188.

Halla JT, Koopman WJ, Fallahis OHSF, Gay RE, Schrohenloher RE, et al: Rheumatoid myositis. *Arthritis Rheum* 1984;27:737–743.

Hart FD, Golding JR: Rheumatoid neuropathy. *Br Med J* 1960;5186:1594–1600.

Helin H, Korpela M, Mustonen J, Pasternack A: Mild mesangial glomerulopathy: a fragment finding in rheumatoid arthritis patients with hematuria or proteinuria. *Nephron* 1986;42:224–230.

Hench PS: The advantages of hepatic injury and jaundice in certain conditions, notably in rheumatic diseases. *Med Clin North Am* 1940;24:1209–1237.

Hollingsworth JW: Amyloidosis, in Hollingsworth JW (ed): *Local and Systemic Complications of Rheumatoid Arthritis.* Philadelphia, WB Saunders, 1968; pp 67–73.

Hollingsworth JW: Local and systemic complications of rheumatoid arthritis, in *Osteoporosis.* Philadelphia, WB Saunders, 1968, pp 74–76.

Hsieh L-F, Didenko B, Schumacher HR, Torg JS: Isokinetic and isometric testing of knee musculature in patients with rheumatoid arthritis with mild knee involvement. *Arch Phys Med Rehabil* 1987;68:294–297.

Hughes JT, Esiri M, Osbury JM, Whilty CWM: Chloroquine myopathy. *Quart J Med* 1971;157:85–93.

Hull S, Mathews J: Pulmonary necrobiotic nodules as a presenting feature of rheumatoid arthritis. *Ann Rheum Dis* 1982;41:21–24.

Hurd ER: Extraarticular manifestations of rheumatoid arthritis *Semin Arthritis Rheum* 1979;8:151–176.

Hyland RH, Gordon DA, Broder I, Davies GM, Russell ML, Hutcheon MA, Reid GD, Cox DW: A systematic controlled study of pulmonary abnormalities in rheumatoid arthritis. 1983;10:395–405.

Jackson CG, Chess RL, Ward JR: A case of rheumatoid nodule formation within the central nervous system and review of the literature. *J Rheum* 1984;11:237–240.

Jaffe IA: The treatment of rtheumatoid arthritis and necrotizing vasculitis with penicillamine. *Arthritis Rheum* 1970;13:436–443.

Jayson MIV, Dixon AS, Dixon J, Yooman P: Unusual geodes (bone cysts) in rheumatoid arthritis. *Ann Rheum Dis* 1972;31:174–178.

Jayson MIV, Jones DIP: Scleritis and rheumatoid arthritis. *Ann Rheum Dis* 1971;30:343–347.

Johnson RL, Fink CW, Ziff M: Lymphotoxic formation by lymphocytes and muscle in polymyositis. *J Clin Invest* 1972; 52:2435–2449.

Jurik AG, Davidsen D, Graudal H: Prevalence of pulmonary involvement in rheumatoid arthritis and its relationship to some characteristics of the patients. *Scand J Rheumatol* 1982;11:217–224.

Jurik AG, Davidsen D, Graudal H: Prevalence of cardiac and aortic enlargement in rheumatoid arthritis and its relationship to some characteristic of patients. *Rheum Int* 1984;5:15–19.

Kassen SS, Thomas TL, Moutsopoulos HM, et al: Increased risk of lymphoma in Sicca syndrome. *Ann Intern Med* 1978;89:888–892.

Kaye BR, Kaye RL, Bobrove A: Rheumatoid nodules:

Review of the spectrum of associated conditions and proposal of a new classification with a report of four seronegative cases. *Am J Med* 1984;76:279–292.

Kim RC, Collins GH: The neuropathology of rheumatoid disease. *Human Pathol* 1981;12:5–15.

Kimura SJ, Hogan MJ, O'Connor GR, Epstein WV: Ureitis and joint diseases. Clinic findings in 191 cases. *Arch Ophthalmol* 1967;77:309–316.

Klofkorn RW, Steigerwald JC, Mills DM, Smyth CJ: Esophageal varices in Felty's syndrome. *Arthritis Rheum* 1976;19:150–154.

Lawry GV, Finerman ML, Hanafee WN, Mancuso AA, Fan PT, Bluestine R: Laryngeal involvement in rheumatoid arthritis. *Arthritis Rheum* 1984;27:873–882.

Lawson AAH, McLean N: Renal disease and drug therapy in rheumatoid arthritis. *Ann Rheum Dis* 1966;25:441–449.

Leading article: Renal disease and rheumatoid arthritis. *Lancet* 1966;2:1451–1452.

Leber: Uber die Entstenhung der Netzhautablosung. *Klin Monatsbl Augenheilkd* 1882;20:115.

Levine MA, Toback AC: Enhancement of granulopoiesis by lithium carbonate in a patient with hairy cell leukemia. *Am J Med* 1987; 82:146–148.

Lewis RB, Sanders LL, Lipsmeyer E: Characteristics of rheumatoid arthritis in a male population. *J Rheum* 1980;7:539–562.

Lofgen RH, Montgomery WW: Incidence of laryngeal involvement in rheumatoid arthritis. *N Engl J Med* 1962;267:193–195.

Logue GL, Huang AT, Shimm DS: Failure of splenectomy in Felty's syndrome: The role of antibodies supporting granulocyte lysis by lymphocytes. *N Engl J Med* 1981;304:580–583.

MacSween RN, Goudie RB, Anderson JR, et al: Occurrence of antibody to salivary duct epithelium in Sjögren's syndrome, rheumatoid arthritis and other arthritides. *Ann Rheum Dis* 1967;26:402–411.

Mandybur TI: Cerebral amyloid angiopathy; Possible relationship to rheumatoid vasculitis. *Neurology* 1979;39:1336–1340.

Marcolongo R, Bayeli PF, Montagnani M: Gastrointestinal involvement in rheumatoid arthritis, a biopsy study. *J Rheum* 1979;6:163–173.

Markenson JA, McDougal JS, Tsairis P, Lockshin MD, Christian CL: Rheumatoid meningitis; A localized immune process. *Ann Intern Med* 1979;90:786–789.

McGavin D, Williamson J, Forrester J, Foulds WS, Buchanan WW, Dick WC, Lee P, McSween RNM, Whaley K: Episcleritis and scleritis. A study of their clinical manifestations and association with rheumatoid arthritis. *Br J Rheum* 1976;60:192–226.

Mickulicz JP, Daniels TE, Talal N, Grey HM: Beta microglobulin and lymphocytic infiltrate in Sjögren's syndrome. *N Engl J Med* 1975;293:1228–1231.

Mickulicz J: In Discussion at Verein für Wissenschaftlicheff. Heilkunde zu Konigsberg. *Berl Klin Wochenschr* 1888;25:759.

Moore RA, Brunner CM, Sandusky WR, et al: Felty's syndrome: Long-term followup after splenectomy. *Ann Intern Med* 1971;75:381–385.

Morales-Piga A, Elena-Ibanez A, Zea-Mendoxa AC, Rocamora-Ripoll A, Beltran-Gutierrez J: Rheumatoid nodulosis: Report of a case with evidence of intraosseous rheumatoid granuloma. *Arthritis Rheum* 1986;29:1278–1283.

Moran H, Chen S-L, Muirden KD, Jiang S-J, Gu Y-Y, Hopper J, Jiang P-L, Lawler G, Chen R-B: A comparison of rheumatoid arthritis in Australia and China. *Ann Rheum Dis* 1986;45:572–578.

Moritz U: Electromyographic studies in adult rheumatoid arthritis. *Acta Rheum Scand* (Suppl 6) 1963;1–123.

Motulsky AG, Weibers S, Saphir O, Rosenberg E: Lymph nodes in rheumatoid arthritis. *Arch Int Med* 1952;90:660–676.

Moutsopoulos HM, Mann DL, Johnson AH, Chused TM: Genetic differences between primary and secondary Sicca syndrome. *N Engl J Med* 1979;301:761–763.

Mueller EE, Mead S: The electromyogram in rheumatoid arthritis. *Am J Phys Med* 1952;31:67–73.

Nasanchuk JS, Schnitzer B: Follicular hyperplasia in lymph nodes from patients with rheumatoid arthritis. *Cancer* 1969; 24:343–354.

Nomier A, Turner R, Watts E, Smith D, West G, Edmonds J: Cardiac involvement in rheumatoid arthritis. *Ann Intern Med* 1973;79:800–806.

Nüsslein HG, Rödl W, Giedel J, et al: Multiple peripheral pulmonary nodules preceding rheumatoid arthritis. *Rheumatol Int* 1987;7:89–91.

Ojeda VJ, Bronwyn GA, Owen OT, Walters MNI: Cardiac rheumatoid nodulosis. *Med J Aust* 1986;144:92–100.

Oribe M, Singu M, Nobunaga M: Serum alkaline ribonuclease derived from vascular endothelial cells is raised in patients with rheumatoid vasculitis. *Ann Rheum Dis* 1986;45:937–940.

Percy JS: Gold in the treatment of Felty's syndrome. *J Rheum* 1981;8:878–879.

Petersen J, Halberg P, Hojgaard K: Penicillamine induced polymyositis-dermatomyositis. *Scand J Rheum* 1978;7:113–117.

Petry H: Silikose und Polyarthritis. *Arch Gewerbepathol* 1954;13:221–236.

Pettersson T, Klockars M, Hellstrom PE: Chemical and immunological features of pleural effusions, comparison between rheumatoid arthritis and other diseases. *Thorax* 1982;37:354–361.

Petterson T, Wegelius O, Skrifuars B: Gastrointestinal disturbances in patients with severe rheumatoid arthritis. *Acta Med Scand* 1970;188:139–144.

Peyronnard J-M, Charron L, Beaudet F, Couture F: Vasculitic neuropathy in rheumatoid disease and Sjögren syndrome. *Neurology* 1982;32:839–845.

Pieterse AS, Aaronis I, Jose JS; Focal prostatic granulomas: Rheumatoid-like, probably iatrogenic in origin. *Pathology* 1984;16:174–177.

Pizarello RA, Goldberg J: The heart in rheumatoid arthritis, in Utsinger PD, Zvaifler NJ, Ehrlich GE (eds): *Rheumatoid Arthritis*. Philadelphia, JB Lippincott, 1985, pp 431–440.

Prakash R, Atassi A, Pokske R, Rosen KM: Prevalence of pericardiac effusion and mitral valve involvement in patients with rheumatoid arthritis without cardiac symptoms. *N Engl J Med* 1973;289:597–600.

Rasker JJ, Kuipers FC: Are rheumatoid nodules caused by vasculitis? A study of 13 early cases. *Ann Rheum Dis* 1983;42:384–388.

Roberts WN, Coblyn JS: Rheumatoid arthritis and granulomatous hepatitis, a new association. *J Rheumatol* 1983;10:969–972.

Robertson MDJ, Hart FD, White WF, Nuki G, Boardman PL: Rheumatoid lymphadenopathy. *Ann Rheum Dis* 1968;27:253–260.

Rosenbaum J, Katz WA, Schumacher HR: Hepatotoxicity associated with the use of D-penicillamine in rheumatoid arthritis. *Ann Rheum Dis* 1980;39:152–154.

Rubin P, Holt JF: Secretory dialography in diseases of the major salivary glands. *Am J Roentgentol* 1957;77:575–598.

Russell AS, Lindstrom JM: Penicillamine induced myasthenia gravis associated with antibodies to acetylcholine receptor. *Neurology* 1978;28:847–849.

Salomon MI, Gallo G, Poon TP, Goldblat MV, Tchertkoff V: The kidney in rheumatoid arthritis. *Nephron* 1974;12:297–310.

Saltzman DA, Gall EP, Robinson SF: Aspirin-induced

hepatic dysfunction in a patient with adult rheumatoid arthritis. *Am J Dig Dis* 1976;9:815–820.

Scharf J, Levy J, Venderly A, Nahir M: Pericardial tamponade in juvenile rheumatoid arthritis. *Arthritis Rheum* 1976;19:760–762.

Schlumpf U, Meyer M, Ulrich J, Friede RL: Neurologic complications induced by gold treatment. *Arthritis Rheum* 1983;26:825–831.

Schorn P, Hough IP, Anderson IF: The heart in rheumatoid arthritis. *S Afr Med J* 1976;3:8–10.

Schrader PL, Peters PA, Dahl DS: Polymyositis and penicillamine. *Arch Neurol* 1972;27:456–457.

Schumacher HR, Carrol E, Taylor F, Shelley WB, Wood WB: Erythema elevatum diutinum; Vasculitis, impaired clot lysis and response to phenformin. *J Rheum* 1977;4:103–112.

Scott DG, Bacon PA, Bothamley JE, et al: Plasma exchange in rheumatoid vasculitis. *J Rheum* 1981a;8:433–439.

Scott DG, Bacon PA, Tribe R: Systemic rheumatoid vasculitis; A clinical and laboratory study of 50 cases. *Medicine (Baltimore)* 1981b;60:288–297.

Shapiro R, Weisner K, McLaughlin GE, Utsinger PO: Evaluation as a prelude to management; Management of patients, in Utsinger PD, Zvaifler NJ, Ehrlich GE (eds): *Rheumatoid Arthritis: Etiology, Diagnosis, Management*, Philadelphia, JB Lippincott, 1985, pp 505–544.

Short Cl, Bauer W, Reynolds WE: *Rheumatoid Arthritis*. Cambridge, MA, Harvard University Press, 1957, p 311.

Shupak R, Bernier V, Rabinovich S. Wright T, Gordon DA: Avascular necrosis of bone with rheumatoid vasculitis. *J Rheum* 1983;10:261–266.

Sienknecht CW, Urowitz MB, Pruzanski W, Stein HB: Felty's syndrome. Clinical and serological analysis of 34 cases. *Ann Rheum Dis* 1977;36:500–507.

Silberman S: A case of rheumatoid hyperviscosity syndrome with characterization of serum immune complexes. *Ann Clin Lab Sci* 1986;16:26–33.

Sjögren H: Zurkenntnis der Keratoconjunctivitis Sicca (Keratits Filiformis bei Hypofuncktion der Tranendrugen). *Acta Ophthalmol (Copenh)* (Suppl 2) 1933;11:1–151.

Sokoloff L: The heart in rheumatoid arthritis. *Am Heart J* 1953;45:635–643.

Sokoloff L, Wilens SL, Bunim JJ, McEwen C: Diagnostic value of histologic lesions of striated muscle in rheumatoid arthritis. *Am J Med Sci* 1950;219:174–182.

Spivak JL: Felty's syndrome: An analytic review.

Johns Hopkins Med J 1977;141:156–162.

Steiner G, Freund HA, Leichtentritt B, Maun ME: Lesions of skeletal muscles in rheumatoid arthritis nodular polymyositis. *Am J Pathol*, 1946;22:103–127.

Still GH: On a form of chronic joint disease in children. *Trans Roy Soc Med Chir* 1897;80:47–59.

Strand V, Talal N: Advances in the diagnosis and concepts of Sjögren's syndrome (autoimmune exocrinopathy). *Bull Rheum Dis* 1980;30:1046–1051.

Sun DCH, Roth SH, Mitchell CS, Englund DW: Upper gastrointestinal disease in rheumatoid arthritis. *Dig Dis* 1974;19:405–410.

Sutton PP, Nadir N, Pavia D, Sheahan NF, Clarke SW: Lung mucociliary clearance in rheumatoid disease. *Ann Rheum Dis* 1982;41:47–51.

Taccari E, Teodori S: Rheumatoid chyliform bursitis: Pathogenetic role of rheumatoid nodules. *Arthritis Rheum* 1984;27:221–226.

Talal N: Sjögren's syndrome and connective tissue disease with other immunologic disorders, in McCarty DJ (ed): *Arthritis and Allied Conditions*, ed 10. Philadelphia, Lea & Febiger, 1985; p 1773.

Talal N, Sylvester RA, Daniels TE, Greenspan JS, Williams RC, Rand B: Lymphocytes in peripheral blood and tissue losses in Sjögren's syndrome. *J Clin Invest* 1974;53:180–189.

Termini TE, Biundo JJ, Ziff M: The rarity of Felty's syndrome in blacks. *Arthritis Rheum* 1979;22:999–1005.

Tessler HH: The eye in rheumatic disease. *Bull Rheum Dis* 1985;35:1–8.

Thadani U, Iveson JMI, Wright V: Cardiac tamponade, constrictive pericarditis and pericardial resection in rheumatoid arthritis. *Medicine (Baltimore)* 1975;54:261–270.

Tomasi TB, Fudenberg HH, Fingy M: Possible relationship of rheumatoid factors and pulmonary disease. *Am J Med* 1962;33:243–248.

Trevor-Ropor PD (ed): Watson PG, Hazelman BL: The sclera and systemic disorders, in *Major Problems in Ophthalmology*, Vol 2. Philadelphia, WB Saunders, 1976, p 458.

Tribe CR, Scott DG, Bacon PA: Rectal biopsy in the diagnosis of systemic vasculitis. *J Clin Pathol* 1981;34:843–850.

Tucker RA: Drugs and liver disease. A tubular compilation of drugs and the histopathologeal changes that can occur in the liver. *Drug Intell Clin Pharmacol* 1982;16:569–580.

Villecco AS, DeLiborali E, Bianchi B, Pisi E: Antibodies to cardiac conducting tissue and abnormalities of cardiac induction in rheumatoid arthritis. *Clin Exp Immunol* 1983;53:536–540.

Voyles WF, Searles RP, Bankhurst AD; Myocardial infarction caused by rheumatoid vasculitis. *Arthritis Rheum* 1980;23:860–862.

Voyles WF, Searles RP, Bankhurst AD: Myocardial infarction caused by rheumatoid vasculitis. *Arthritis Rheum* 1980;23:860–862.

Walker WC, Wright V: Pulmonary lesions and rheumatoid arthritis. *Medicine* 1968;47:501–520.

Wallis WJ, Loughran TP, Kadin ME, Clark EA, Starkebaum GA: Polyarthritis and neutropenia associated with circulating large granular lymphocytes. *Ann Intern Med* 1985;103:357–362.

Walters, MNI, Ojeda, VJ: Pleuropulmonary necrobiotic nodules. *Med J Aust* 1986;144:648–651.

Watson P, Fekete J, Deck J: Central nervous system vasculitis in rheumatoid arthritis. *Canad J Neurol Sci* 1977;4:269–272.

Watson PG, Hayreh SS: Scleritis and episcleritis. *Br J Ophthalmol* 1976;60:163–191.

Watson PG, Hazelman BL: The sclera and systemic disorders, in Trevor-Ropor PD (ed): *Major Problems in Ophthalmology*, Vol 2. Philadelphia, WB Saunders, 1976, p 458.

Webb J, Whaley K, MacSween RNM, Nuki G, Dick WC, Buchanan WW: Liver disease in rheumatoid arthritis and Sjögren's syndrome. *Ann Rheum Dis* 1975;34:70–81.

Weinblatt ME, Tesser JRP, Gilliam JR: The liver in rheumatic diseases. *Semin Arthritis Rheum* 1982;11:399–405.

Whisnant JP, Espinosa RE, Kierland RR, Lambert EG: Chloroquine neuromyopathy. *Mayo Clin Proc* 1963;38:501–513.

White R, Wegnan A, Bolpitt P, Wood G, Fleming A: Facial rash with scarring due to granulomatous vasculitis in rheumatoid disease. *Ann Rheum Dis* 1986;45:75–77.

Winkelstein A, Starz TW, Agarwal A: Efficacy of combined therapy with plasmapheresis and immunosuppressants in rheumatoid vasculitis. *J Rheum* 1984;11:162–166.

Wisnieski JJ, Askari AD: Rheumatoid nodulosis. *Arch Intern Med* 1981;141:515–619.

Yarbrough JW, Sealy WC, Miller JA: Thoracic surgical problems associated with rheumatoid arthritis. *J Thorac Cardiovasc Surg* 1975;69:347–354.

CHAPTER 15

COMPLICATIONS OF RHEUMATOID ARTHRITIS

DANIEL G. BAKER, MD

In addition to the involvement of multiple organ systems by rheumatoid inflammation, complications may occur that are less directly related to rheumatoid arthritis. In fact, the effects of chronic inflammation and drug therapy can lead to both disabling and lethal complications. Awareness of these processes is important since their therapy is significantly different from that of the underlying disease. Indeed, important complications may be secondary to therapy for rheumatoid arthritis.

SEPTIC ARTHRITIS

That the joints of patients with rheumatoid arthritis are more susceptible to infection is well documented (Kellgren et al, 1958). This susceptibility appears to be multifactorial. There is evidence that systemic host defenses may be impaired so that rheumatoid patients may be more prone to generalized infections (Mitchell et al, 1976). Factors involved probably include the presence of chronic immune-mediated disease, drug therapy such as immunosuppressives or corticosteroid preparations, or occasionally the neutropenia of Felty's syndrome. The joints are specifically vulnerable because of several factors. Infectious agents may be more likely to arrive at inflamed joints because of their increased blood flow and be more difficult to eradicate in the diseased tissue (Fig. 15.1). There appears to be decreased polymorphonuclear leukocyte chemotaxis (Mowat and Baum,

Figure 15.1 An inflamed rheumatoid knee joint with possible sites for local infection illustrated.

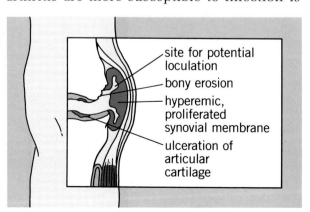

site for potential
loculation

bony erosion

hyperemic,
proliferated
synovial membrane

ulceration of
articular
cartilage

1971) and phagocytosis (Turner et al, 1973), decreased bacteriolytic activity (Pruzanski et al, 1974), and decreased available synovial fluid complement (Pekin and Zvaifler, 1964). The exact contributions of any or all of the findings is unclear. In addition, local steroid injections seem to be related occasionally to the development of joint sepsis in patients with rheumatoid arthritis.

In addition to the susceptibility of rheumatoid joints to infection, prosthetic joint re-placements are common in patients with rheumatoid arthritis. Prosthetic joints are also more susceptible to infection and when infection occurs it can be disastrous (Fig. 15.2).

Diagnosis

Septic joints in patients with rheumatoid arthritis frequently go unrecognized because clinical signs and symptoms are shared by the two diseases. All patients with rheuma-

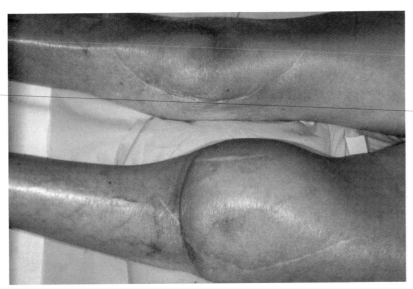

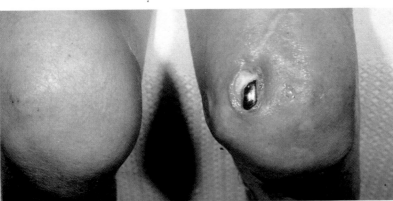

Figure 15.2 An infected prosthetic knee in a patient with rheumatoid arthritis can result in joint swelling (*top*) or fistula formation (*bottom*). In both cases the prosthesis was infected by different organisms. (Courtesy of PA Dieppe, MD).

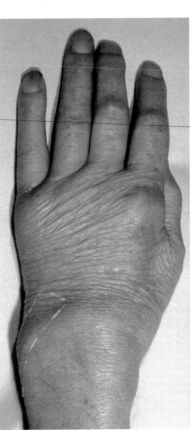

Figure 15.3 Septic arthritis of the index finger MCP joint in a patient with preexisting rheumatoid arthritis. The wrist deformity is due to the rheumatoid disease; the swollen MCP joint developed acutely. Fever and malaise accompanied the joint infection. (Courtesy of PA Dieppe, MD).

toid arthritis appear to be predisposed to infection but there may be an increased incidence in older, more severely affected individuals. Most commonly a single joint is involved but not infrequently there is polyarticular involvement. Involved joints may appear to be flaring with an acute increase in swelling and pain that is similar to and may be mistaken for a flare of rheumatoid arthritis (Fig. 15.3). However there may be more dramatic inflammation that is especially suggestive of infection. Synovial fluid white blood cell counts may be elevated above the usual 20,000 to 40,000/mm³ seen in rheumatoid joints. Fever and peripheral leukocytosis are occasionally helpful indications of infections. However, it should be stressed that none of the above findings are necessary. The absence of systemic findings or even acute articular findings should not preclude the diagnosis since they may be absent in up to 50% of cases of septic joints (Mitchell et al, 1976). Frequently neither peripheral nor synovial fluid white blood cells counts are especially elevated. Fortunately, gram stains are positive in about 70% of cases (Myers et al, 1969) (Fig. 15.4), and cultures are generally positive depending on the organisms involved.

Synovial fluid glucose levels are often not helpful since glucose levels in synovial fluid in rheumatoid arthritis are also often markedly reduced (Cohen et al, 1975). Very low levels such as 5 mg/dL would help favor infection. There has been recent interest in synovial fluid lactate levels as an aid to distinguish sepsis from other causes of inflammation. However, there appears to be too much overlap with rheumatoid synovial fluids levels for there to be any usefulness for differential diagnosis (Arthur et al, 1983).

It should be noted that calcium pyrophosphate deposition disease and apatite crystal deposition can complicate rheumatoid arthritis and can account for some septic-like exacerbations (Fig. 15.5).

Radiologically in septic arthritis there may be a rapidly worsening cortical destruction and erosion (Resnick, 1975). It should be em-

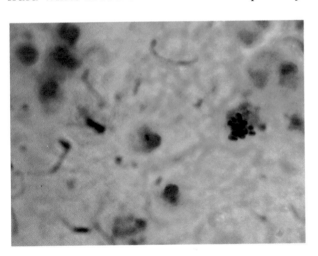

Figure 15.4 A positive gram stain, as seen here, with gram positive cocci indicates presence of joint infection. However, 30% of infected joints in rheumatoid arthritis have negative gram stains.

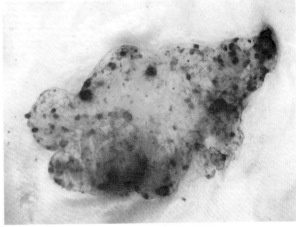

Figure 15.5 Hydroxyapatite crystal deposition increases as secondary osteoarthritis develops in late rheumatoid arthritis. The alizarin red stained crystals seen here accounted for an acute septic-like monoarthritis.

phasized that such changes occur only after 7 to 10 days (Fig. 15.6) and too late to be of real diagnostic benefit at the time when treatment would be most helpful. Radionuclide scanning with technetium pyrophosphate has been shown to be of little value as both rheumatoid arthritis and septic joints show increased uptake (Coleman et al, 1982).

The source of the infection frequently goes unrecognized. Bacteremia from any source, such as pneumonia or meningitis may lead to localized joint involvement. Arthrocentesis has been reported as a cause of infection, but this appears to be an uncommon occurrence (Gowans and Granieri, 1959). Skin ulcers (Fig. 15.7) due to vasculitis or Felty's syndrome, and infected rheumatoid nodules (Fig.

15.8) deserve special mention since such lesions were thought to be the origin of the infection in the majority of identified sources in several series (Mitchell et al, 1976). It is important that such lesions be treated aggressively in any patient with rheumatoid arthritis.

As with the general population, *Staphylococcus aureus* is the most common nongonococcal organism isolated. However, most other organisms, including gonococci, have been reported as well as several uncommon infections including kingella kingae, brucella, saccharomyces, and plesiomonas shigelloides. Mycobacterial and fungal infections have also been documented and should always be considered.

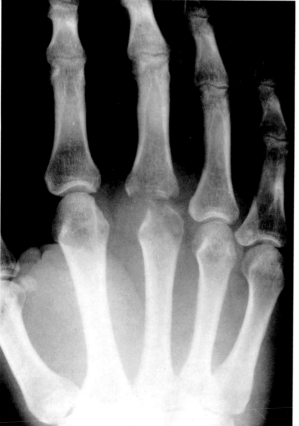

Figure 15.6 Rapidly progressing destructive changes seen on radiographs can suggest superimposed infection in patients with rheumatoid arthritis. Acute septic arthritis of the third MCP joint is seen with soft tissue swelling, osteoporosis, bone destruction, and narrowing of the joint space. (Courtesy of PA Dieppe, MD)

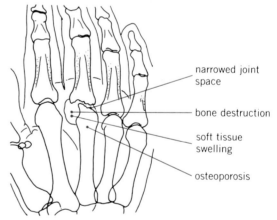

narrowed joint space

bone destruction

soft tissue swelling

osteoporosis

Therapy

Early diagnosis and rapid institution of therapy are the keys to successful treatment. Several series convincingly document that delay in therapy leads to a marked increase in mortality which may be as high as 35% (Karten, 1969). Because rheumatoid joints already have altered anatomy and subchrondral bone damage, they are more susceptible to sequestration of organisms and osteomyelitis. This leads to frequent recurrences especially when the organism is *S aureus*. Prolonged therapy may be needed.

If a septic joint is suspected, therapy should be instituted with broad antimicrobial coverage until an organism is identified or cultures are negative. Parenteral therapy should be continued for at least 4 to 6 weeks. As with non-rheumatoid joints, frequent aspirations, as many as it takes to keep the joint adequately drained, are essential. Removal of purulent fluid (Fig. 15.9) reduces enzymatic damage to articular tissues. If response is not adequate in 48 to 72 hours, surgical intervention may be necessary. Whether surgical drainage should be considered earlier in patients with rheumatoid arthritis is not known. If there has been a long delay in diagnosis, surgical drainage may be indicated promptly as loculation may make needle aspiration difficult. Infected joints should always be immobilized during the acute phase but passive range of motion should be started as soon as pain allows in order to minimize stiffness.

Patients with rheumatoid arthritis are susceptible to septic joints and the mortality of such an event is quite high. The likelihood of such a disastrous outcome can be lessened by a high index of suspicion, aggressive therapy of any infection in a patient with rheumatoid arthritis, low threshold for culture and gram stain of synovial fluid, and early and aggressive antibiotic therapy.

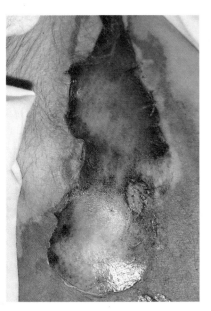

Figure 15.7 Necrotic skin lesions such as this can become infected and lead to joint sepsis.

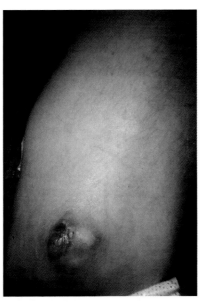

Figure 15.8 This perforating rheumatoid nodule was not infected but required meticulous local care to prevent infection.

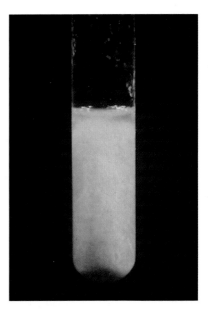

Figure 15.9 Cloudy, purulent synovial fluid removed from a septic rheumatoid knee.

AMYLOIDOSIS

Secondary amyloidosis has long been considered a complication of chronic rheumatoid arthritis (Eingerman and Andrus, 1943). Autopsy studies discovered amyloidosis in 14% of 181 patients with rheumatoid arthritis (Missen and Taylor, 1956). Other authors have reported rates of 26% (Cohen, 1968) and even 61% (Wright and Calkins, 1981). Despite these high percentages there have also been controlled studies showing much lower rates and even reports of no increased incidence of amyloid deposits in rheumatoid arthritis patients (Ozlmir et al, 1971). Studies performed in liv-

ing rheumatoid arthritis patients reveal lower rates compared to autopsy studies (Bland, 1965). The conflicting rates reported by these studies may be explained by different genetic and environmental influences. For instance, the incidence of amyloidosis in Europe is different than the incidence in the United States. In addition, therapy for rheumatoid arthritis and means of detection of amyloid may vary between studies. Good epidemiologic studies are not available, but most authors believe that secondary amyloidosis is associated with rheumatoid arthritis.

Amyloidosis is a syndrome in which insoluble proteinaceous material is deposited in the

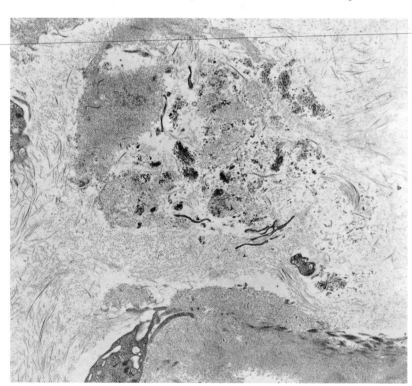

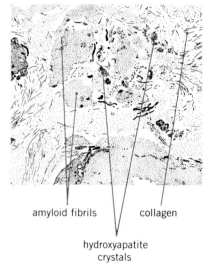

Figure 15.10 Electron micrograph of synovium in a patient with rheumatoid arthritis and secondary amyloidosis.

amyloid fibrils   collagen

hydroxyapatite
crystals

extracellular matrix of several organ systems. Patients with rheumatoid arthritis develop secondary amyloidosis as a result of the chronic inflammation that characterizes the disease. The amyloid protein of secondary amyloidosis (AA protein) is not derived from immunoglobulin light chains (Husby, 1985). It is therefore distinct from the protein of primary disease (AL) which originates from light chains produced by plasma cells. AA proteins vary slightly from patient to patient but the amino acid sequences of the molecules are remarkably similar. AA proteins are probably synthesized in the liver as a precursor protein, termed SAA. SAA is a ubiquitous acute phase reactant found in serum. SAA synthesis can be stimulated by interleukin-1 (McAdams et al, 1982), a peptide known to be elevated in secondary amyloidosis as well as in many chronic inflammatory states. Degradation of SAA has been attributed to neutral proteases from monocytes, polymorphonuclear cells, and serum. The deposition of amyloid protein may therefore depend upon the increased production of SAA coupled with systemic and local alterations in degradation.

The diagnosis of amyloidosis is seldom made during the first two years of disease; mean disease duration before diagnosis is about 16 years. There appears to be an increased incidence in males with rheumatoid arthritis since one study reported a male to female ratio of 1:1, despite the predominance of females with rheumatoid arthritis (Cohen, 1968). The possible predisposing factors therefore may be increased SAA with prolonged inflammation, decreased catabolism of SAA and/or AA, and male sex.

The clinical features of secondary amyloidosis depend upon the location of the protein deposition. Small blood vessels and the parenchyma of organs appear to be preferred sites of deposition of type AA amyloid. The kidneys are involved in the majority of patients who develop secondary amyloidosis. Nephrotic syndrome with eventual renal failure is a major cause of death. Persistent proteinuria should always suggest amyloidosis even if other possibilities exist, such as drug toxicity.

The gastrointestinal tract is also frequently involved. Infiltration of the liver can cause hepatomegaly but rarely functional disturbances. However, infiltration of the intestine can cause malabsorption. Blood vessel involvement can cause serious bleeding. Amyloid deposition in organs such as the spleen or endocrine glands is common but usually not of clinical significance. Cardiac involvement is usually present at autopsy yet only infrequently causes symptoms. Although carpal tunnel syndrome occurs, it is less frequent than with AL-type amyloidosis. Interestingly, clinical evidence of joint involvement is quite rare in secondary amyloidosis, although amyloid fibrils can be seen on synovial biopsies. A synovial biopsy from a rheumatoid patient with renal failure and nephrotic syndrome revealed findings of diffuse amyloidosis. In addition to amyloid fibrils, both calcium hydroxyapatite and calcium oxalate crystals were also found in synovial fluid (Schumacher et al, 1987) (Fig. 15.10).

Diagnosis

The diagnosis of secondary amyloidosis should be suspected in any patient with rheumatoid arthritis who develops proteinuria, hepatosplenomegaly, persistent gastrointestinal bleeding, or malabsorption. The diagnosis can be made by identifying amyloid fibrils by Congo red staining of tissue specimens (Fig. 15.11). One must confirm that Congo red-stained material shows apple-green birefringence with standard polarized light before assuming that red material is amyloid (Fig. 15.12). Rectal biopsies are useful and are positive in 80% of patients, although submucosa must be obtained (Blum and Sohar, 1962). Gingival biopsies and aspiration of subcutaneous fat are easily done and safe but are less frequently positive (Westermark, 1971). Biopsy of liver or kidney can be hazardous since the amyloid-laden tissue may bleed profusely.

Therapy

There is no adequate therapy for secondary amyloidosis except for treatment of the underlying disease. The accumulation of amyloid can be halted if the disease activity is controlled. There is animal data that actually suggests that there may be regression of the amyloid if the primary disease is controlled. Whether this is possible in patients with rheumatoid arthritis is questionable. Al-

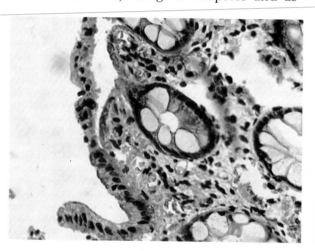

Figure 15.11 Congo red staining of the vessel wall from a rectal biopsy of a rheumatoid patient indicates secondary amyloidosis.

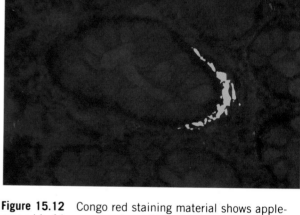

Figure 15.12 Congo red staining material shows apple-green birefringence under polarized light, confirming the presence of amyloid.

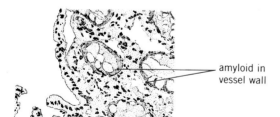

amyloid in vessel wall

though colchicine may be helpful in the amyloidosis associated with familial Mediterranean fever, it has been not shown to be effective in the amyloidosis of rheumatoid arthritis. Dimethylsulfoxide (DMSO) has been used for the secondary amyloidosis of rheumatoid arthritis sucessfully in a single uncontrolled study (Takahashi, 1985).

Dialysis and renal transplantation are indicated in these patients if renal failure ensues. Although not as successful as in some groups of patients with renal failure, results are clearly adequate. Amyloid is deposited in the transplanted kidneys but does not seem to shorten survival.

DRUG COMPLICATIONS IN RHEUMATOID ARTHRITIS

As previously discussed, the chronic inflammation of rheumatoid arthritis can cause complications leading to morbidity and mortality in patients. It is also clear that there are significant risks associated with the drugs used to treat the disease. The variety and amount of different drugs prescribed for one patient for rheumatoid arthritis can easily lead to a myriad of side effects (Fig. 15.13).

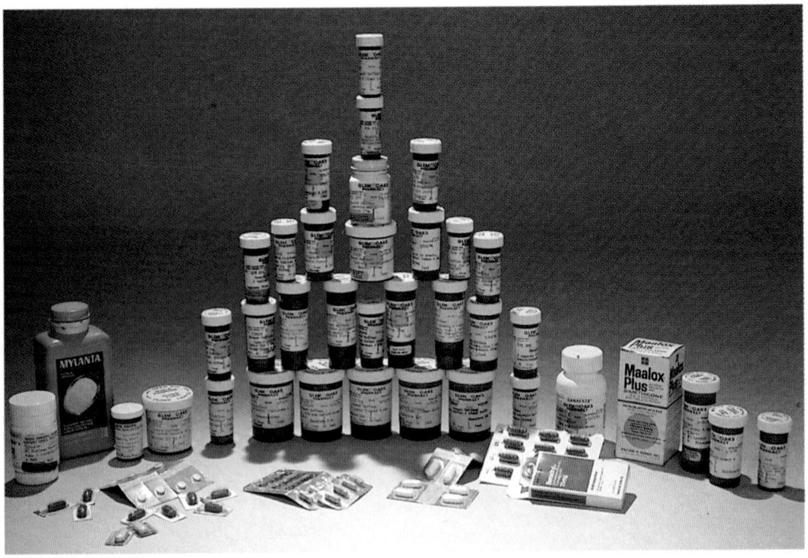

Figure 15.13 Drugs taken over a period of time by a single patient. The possibilities for drug complications and cross reactions are myriad.

Delineation of all the possible occurrences with each drug is beyond the scope of this text, but an overview is possible (Fig. 15.14).

Gastrointestinal toxicity with the possibility of bleeding is universally known. Diffuse gastritis or peptic ulcer with nausea, vomiting, and pain is common with acetylsalicylic acid. Most other nonsteroidal drugs are associated with peptic ulcer disease, probably also on the basis of prostaglandin inhibition. The effects of these drugs are not merely due to local irritation of the gastric lining but can be systemic, occurring frequently with suppository preparations.

MAJOR DRUG TOXICITIES IN RHEUMATOID ARTHRITIS

DRUG GROUP	COMMON AND/OR SERIOUS REACTION	RARE AND/OR MILD REACTION
Acetylsalicylic Acid	Gastrointestinal toxicity Tinnitus/hearing loss Prolonged bleeding time	Lowered glomerular filtration rate Bronchospasm Urticaria Alteration of uric acid Elevated liver enzymes
Other Nonsteroidal drugs	Gastrointestinal toxicity Headache/change in mental status Lowered glomerular filtration rate	Bronchospasm Aseptic meningitis Prolonged bleeding time Elevated liver enzymes
Gold	Proteinuria Leukopenia Thrombocytopenia Pancytopenia Rash	Cholestasis Enterocolitis Nitritoid reactions (gold sodium thiomalate) Diffuse pulmonary infiltrates Corneal or skin chrysiasis
D-Pencillamine	Leukopenia Thrombocytopenia Proteinuria Rash/nail changes	Hypogeusia Autoimmune syndromes: Systemic lupus erythymatosus Goodpasture's syndrome Myasthenia gravis Sjögren's syndrome Pemphigus Polymyositis Obliterative bronchiolitis Alopecia Mammary gigantism Pemphigoid-type reaction Aphthous stomatitis

Figure 15.14 Major drug toxicities in rheumatoid arthritis

However, there are many other side effects from drugs that should not be ignored. Nonsteroidal agents can produce central nervous system effects including headaches, changes in mental status, and depression (Goodwin and Regan, 1982). Nonsteroidal drugs can reduce the glomerular filtration rate and induce renal failure, especially in patients with already impaired function (Kimberly and Plotz, 1979). Bronchospasm may be worsened in patients with asthma. There are minor prolongations of the bleeding time which are usually clinically insignificant but may be important in patients undergoing surgery and

MAJOR DRUG TOXICITIES IN RHEUMATOID ARTHRITIS (cont.)

DRUG GROUP	COMMON AND/OR SERIOUS REACTION	RARE AND/OR MILD REACTION
Antimalarial drugs (chloroquine and hydroxychloroquine)	Retinopathy Corneal deposits	Loss of corneal reflex Weakness of external rectus muscles Weakness of accommodation Lightened hair coloration Neuromyopathy
Methotrexate	Hepatotoxicity Stomatitis Nausea Leukopenia Thrombocytopenia	Pneumonitis (uncommon but dangerous)
Azathioprine	Leukopenia Thrombocytopenia Tumor promotion	Nausea
Cyclophosphamide	Leukopenia Thrombocytopenia Hematuria/bladder tumors Tumor promotion Sterility Immunosuppression	Nausea Alopecia Pulmonary fibrosis

may contribute to cosmetically disturbing ecchymoses (Fig. 15.15). The nonacetylsalicylates seem much less likely to cause many of the above side effects that appear to be related to inhibition of cyclooxygenase.

Gold and penicillamine also have significant toxicities. The most serious complications are renal, including proteinuria, which can progress to nephrotic syndrome, and hematologic, including aplastic anemia (Gottlieb and Gray, 1978; Hill, 1977). The most bothersome side effect of gold is the typically pruritic scaly rash (Fig. 15.16). Gold-induced pneumonitis can be shown by radiograph and electron microscopy can identify the typical electron dense curved deposits of gold in pulmonary macrophages (Fig. 15.17). Gold can also be seen directly in the skin, giving chrysiasis (15.18). Renal lesions seem to be related to immune disturbances, not gold deposits. Penicillamine is unique for its ability to induce other immunologic phenomena such as Goodpasture's syndrome and myasthenia gravis. It has produced rarely an unusual yellow discoloration of the nails (Fig. 15.19). Toxic epidermal necrolysis is a rare complication of penicillamine (Fig. 15.20).

Antimalarials are commonly used to combat rheumatoid arthritis. Although there is a long list of toxicities, they are uncommon and usually mild (Bunch and O'Duffy, 1980). Retinopathy is the most serious complication

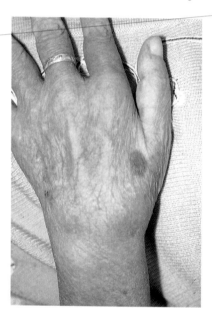

Figure 15.15 Ecchymosis after very minor trauma in a patient with rheumatoid arthritis on aspirin.

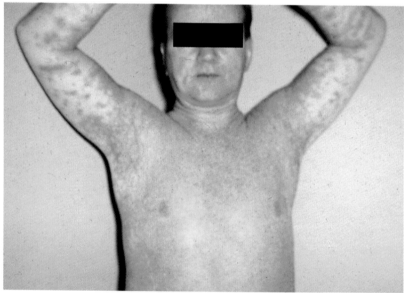

Figure 15.16 A diffuse scaly maculopapular pruritic rash can be seen with gold salt therapy.

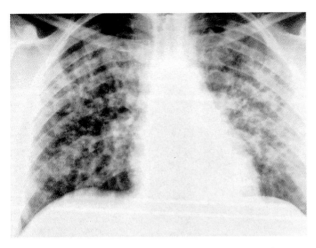

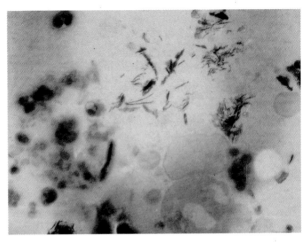

Figure 15.17 Fluffy interstitial pattern shown on chest radiography *(left)* is probably caused by gold deposition.

Electron micrograph *(right)* demonstrates gold particles in the lung of a patient with gold-induced pneumonitis.

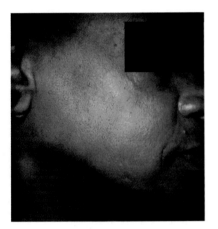

Figure 15.18 Gold deposits in the skin (chrysiasis) can cause a dark discoloration, as shown here.

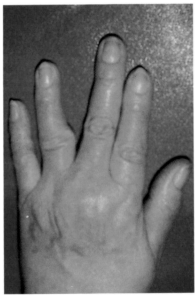

Figure 15.19 Yellow discoloration of the nails is an uncommon complication of D-penicillamine treatment.

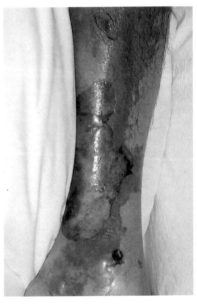

Figure 15.20 Toxic epidermal necrolysis is a rare complication of penicillamine therapy.

but with proper evaluation with frequent opthalmologic exams there is minimal danger (Fig. 15.21). Reversible deposition of hydroxychloroquine in the lens of the eye can also occur (Fig. 15.22). Slit lamp exams and visual fields with a red light should be performed

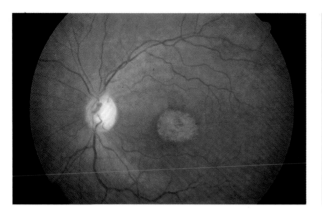

Figure 15.21 Subcapsular deposits of hydroxychloroquine in a patient with rheumatoid arthritis. These deposits will disappear with cessation of therapy.

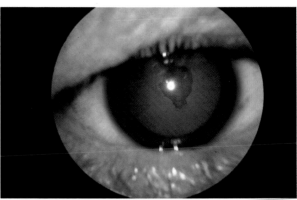

Figure 15.22 Deposits of hydroxycholorquine in the retina of a patient with rheumatoid arthritis.

CORTICOSTEROID SIDE EFFECTS

Body System	Adverse Reactions
Musculoskeletal	Osteoporosis Aseptic necrosis
Gastrointestinal	Peptic ulcer disease Pancreatitis
Ophthalmologic	Posterior subcapsular cataracts
Cardiovascular	Aggravation of hypertension
Metabolic	Hyperglycemia Truncal obesity Secondary adrenal insufficiency
Immunologic	Suppression of delayed hypersensitivity Susceptibility to acute infections

Figure 15.23 Corticosteroid side effects.

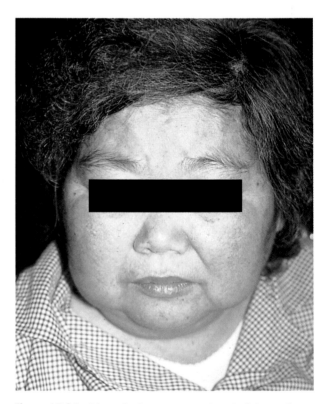

Figure 15.24 Moon facies are secondary to iatrogenic Cushing's syndrome, seen here in an Oriental patient, is a complication of steroid therapy in rheumatoid arthritis.

every six months to minimize any chance of toxicity.

Recent success with the use of methotrexate in rheumatoid arthritis has also renewed the study of its toxicity (Weinblatt et al, 1985). Most worrisome is the hepatotoxicity leading to fibrosis and rarely to cirrhosis. Methotrexate should not be used in anyone with preexisting liver disease, obesity, or in anyone with significant alcohol use. As with all the cytotoxic drugs the long-term potential for development of malignancies must always be taken into account although the amount of risk, if any, for each is unknown.

Corticosteroids have many side effects and proper caution should be used when considering long-term therapy (Fig. 15.23). The use of such agents associated with osteoporosis in patients already susceptible to bone loss is discouraged. The most frequent side effects are Cushing's syndrome with weight gain and cushingoid facies (Fig. 15.24) and thinning of the skin leading to ecchymosis (Fig. 15.25). Avascular necrosis of the hip is a common and devastating complication of high-dose steroid therapy (Fig. 15.26). Local steroids have complications other than predisposing to infection. Extravasation of the steroid

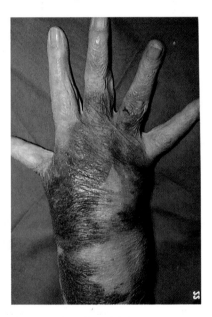

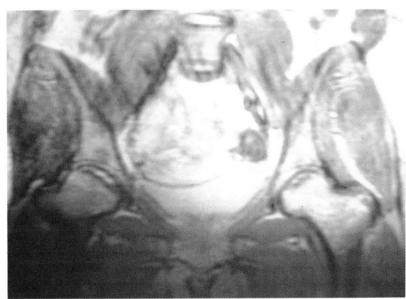

Figure 15.25 Steroid therapy can lead to thinning of the skin and large ecchymoses.

Figure 15.26 Avascular necrosis of the hip, as seen in this MRI, is a frequent and devastating complication of corticosteroid therapy.

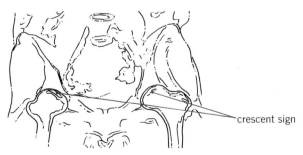

crescent sign

crystals can lead to soft tissue atrophy (Fig. 15.27) and the steroid crystals themselves can be phagocytized and occasionally induce an inflammatory response (Fig. 15.28).

MALIGNANCY IN RHEUMATOID ARTHRITIS

Whether there is an increased incidence of malignancy in patients with rheumatoid arthritis, related to drug therapy or not, remains controversial. Although two reports suggest higher morbidity rates from malignant neoplasms in patients with rheumatoid arthritis than the general population (Moesmann, 1969; Isomaki et al 1978), other studies suggest that the risk is equal or even less (Allebeck, 1982; Vandenbroucke et al, 1984). Studies are confusing because of the drugs used and the increased mortality from other causes in rheumatoid arthritis which shortens the life span and therefore the amount of time for development of neoplasms.

It does appear that there is an increased incidence of neoplasms of the hematopoietic system in rheumatoid patients (Laakso et al, 1986). The overall mortality from all cancer was the same in rheumatoid patients as in the general population in this study, suggesting lower rates of mortality from other neoplasms, specifically gastrointestinal tumors. Sjögren's syndrome, common in rheumatoid arthritis, is associated with a high incidence of lymphoma (Fig. 15.29), although there does not appear to be an increased risk of malignancy developing in the involved parotid glands.

The risk of neoplasms from cyclophosphamide is clear, while, the risk from methotrexate is less established. The risk with azathioprine in renal transplant patients is well documented; however the contribution of simultaneous high-dose steroid in renal transplant patients may be important. Nonetheless, proper caution and patient education should be used before starting cytotoxic drugs, especially in younger individuals.

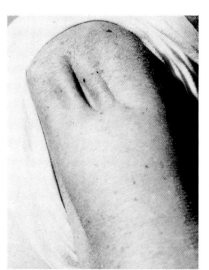

Figure 15.27 Soft tissue atrophy after extravasation of steroid in the tissue after local injection of the shoulder in rheumatoid arthritis.

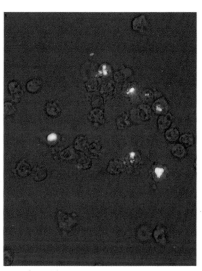

Figure 15.28 Corticosteroid crystals injected into joints can be phagocytized. Such crystals may induce an inflammatory response and temporarily worsen joint symptoms.

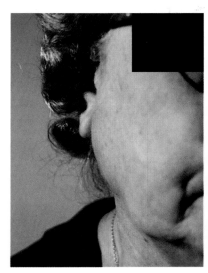

Figure 15.29 Sjögren's syndrome with enlarged parotid glands is associated with an increased risk of lymphoma.

REFERENCES

Allebeck P: Increased mortality in rheumatoid arthritis. *Scand J Rheumatol* 1982;11:81–86.

Arthur RE, Stern M, Galeazzi M, Baldeassre AR, Weiss TD, Rogers JR, Zuckner J: Synovial fluid lactate in septic and nonseptic arthritis. *Arthritis Rheum* 1983;26:1499–1505.

Bland JH: Clinical incidence of renal amyloidosis in rheumatoid arthritis. *J Maine Med Assoc* 1965;56:251–254.

Blum A, Sohar E: Diagnosis of amyloidosis: ancillary procedures. *Lancet* 1962;1:721.

Bunch TW, O'Duffy JD: Disease modifying drugs for progressive rheumatoid arthritis. *Mayo Clin Proc* 1980;55:161–179.

Cohen AS: Amyloidosis associated with rheumatoid arthritis. *Med Clin North Am* 1968;52:643–653.

Cohen AS, Brandt KD, Krey PK: Synovial fluid in laboratory diagnostic procedures in the rheumatic diseases, in Cohen AS (ed): *Laboratory Diagnostic Procedures in the Rheumatic Diseases*, ed 2. Boston, Little Brown & Co, 1975, pp 2–50.

Coleman RE, Samuelson CO, Baim S, Christian PE, Ward JR: Imaging with Tc-99m MDP and Ga-67 citrate in patients with rheumatoid arthritis and suspected septic arthritis: Concise communication. *J Nucl Med* 1982;23:479–482.

Eingerman DL, Andrus FC: Visceral lesions associated with rheumatoid arthritis. *Ann Rheum Dis* 1943;3:168–181.

Goodwin JS, Regan M: Cognitive dysfunction associated with naproxen and ibuprofen in the elderly. *Arthritis Rheum* 1982;25:1013–1015.

Gottlieb NL, Gray RG: Diagnosis and management of adverse reactions from gold. *J Anal Toxicol* 1978;2:173–177.

Gowans JDC, Granieri PA: Septic arthritis: Its relationship to intra-articular injections of hydrocortisone acetate. *NEJM* 1959;261:502–504.

Hill HFH: Treatment of rheumatoid arthritis with penicillamine. *Semin Arthritis Rheum* 1977;6:361–366.

Husby G: Amyloidosis and rheumatoid arthritis. *Clin Exp Rheumatol* 1985;3:173–180.

Isomaki H, Hakulinen T, Joutsenlahti U: Excess risk of lymphomas, leukemia and myeloma in patients with rheumatoid arthritis. *J Chronic Dis* 1978;31:691–696.

Karten I: Septic arthritis complicating rheumatoid arthritis. *Ann Intern Med* 1969;70:1147–1158.

Kellgren JH, Ball J, Fairbrother RW, Barnes KL: Suppurative arthritis complicating rheumatoid arthritis. *Br Med J* 1958;1:1193–1200.

Kimberly RP, Plotz PH: Aspirin induced depression of renal function. *NEJM* 1979;296:1418–1421.

Laakso M, Mutru O, Isomaki H, Koota K: Cancer mortality in patients with rheumatoid arthritis. *J Rheumatol* 1986;13:522–526.

McAdam KPWJ, Li J, Knowles J, Foss NT, Dinarello CA, Rosenwasser LJ, Selinger MI, Kaplan MM, Goodman R: The biology of SAA: Identification of the inducer, in vitro synthesis, and heterogeneity demonstrated with monoclonal antibodies. *Ann NY Acad Sci* 1982;389:126–136.

Missen GAK, Taylor JD: Amyloidosis in rheumatoid arthritis. *J Pathol* 1956;71:179–192.

Mitchell WS, Brooks PM, Stevenson RD, Buchanan WW: Septic arthritis in patients with rheumatoid disease: A still underdiagnosed complication. *J Rheumatol* 1976;3:124–133.

Moesmann G: Malignancy and mortality in subacute rheumatoid arthritis of old age. *Acta Rheum Scand* 1969;15:193–199.

Mowat AG, Baum J: Chemotaxis of polymorphonuclear leukocytes from patients with rheumatoid arthritis. *J Clin Invest* 1971;50:2541–2549.

Myers AR, Miller LM, Pinals RS: Pyoarthrosis complicating rheumatoid arthritis. *Lancet* 1969;2:714–716.

Ozlmir AI, Wright JR, Calins E: Influence of rheumatoid arthritis on amyloidosis of aging. *NEJM* 1971;285:534–538.

Pekin TJ, Zvaifler NJ: Haemolytic complement in synovial fluid. *J Clin Invest* 1964;43:1372–1382.

Pruzanski W, Leers WD, Wardlaw AC: Bacteriolytic and bacteriocidal activity of sera and synovial fluid in rheumatoid arthritis and osteoarthritis. *Arthritis Rheum* 1974;17:207–218.

Resnick D: Pyarthrosis complicating rheumatoid arthritis. *Radiology* 1975;114:581–586.

Schumacher HR, Reginato AJ, Pullman S: Synovial fluid oxalate deposition complicating rheumatoid arthritis with amyloidosis and renal failure. Demonstration of intracellular oxalate crystals. *J Rheumatol* 1987;14:361–366.

Takahashi A, Matsumoto J, Nishimura S, Tanida N, Imura S, Isobe T, Shimoyama T: Improvement of endoscopic and histologic findings of AA-type gastrointestinal amyloidosis by treatment with dimethyl sulfoxide and prednisolone. *Gastroenterol Jpn* 1985;20:143–147.

Turner RA, Schumacher HR, Myers AR: Phagocytic function of polymorphonuclear leukocytes in rheumatic diseases. *J Clin Invest* 1973;52:1632–1635.

Vandenbroucke JP, Hazevoet HM, Cata A: Survival and cause of death in rheumatoid arthritis: A 25 year prospective follow-up. *J Rheumatol* 1984;11:158–161.

Weinblatt ME, Coblyn JS, Fox DA, et al: Efficacy of low dose methotrexate in rheumatoid arthritis. *NEJM* 1985;312:823–827.

Westermark P: Diagnosis of secondary generalized amyloidosis by fine needle biopsy of the skin. *Acta Med Scand* 1971;190:453–454.

Wright JR, Calkins E: Clinicopathologic differentiation of common amyloid syndromes. *Medicine,* 1981;60:429–448.

CHAPTER 16

MANAGEMENT OF RHEUMATOID ARTHRITIS

BRUCE FREUNDLICH, MD

There is as yet no cure for rheumatoid arthritis. Current treatments at best suppress the pathogenetic process and maintain as normal a state as possible for the maximum length of time. Simultaneously, the harmful side effects of therapy are hopefully kept to a minimum. It is important to keep in mind that although drug therapy is critical in the treatment of rheumatoid arthritis patients, a multifaceted approach is necessary for optimal care.

NONDRUG THERAPY

Rheumatoid arthritis is often thought to be a relentless and crippling condition. The wide spectrum of the course of the disease reflecting a more accurate assessment of prognosis should be explained to patients. Only a small percentage of rheumatoid arthritis patients become completely incapacitated and in many cases the disease goes into complete remission (O'Sullivan and Cathcart, 1972).

Patient education should include a discussion of the goals of treatment, ie, maintaining function of the joints and the patient as a whole, and preventing underlying joint destruction. It is important that patients learn to limit or modify their activities to protect their joints, but not by total inactivity. They should be advised not to expect a completely pain-free life, although there is a small chance of this occurring. A mental adjustment is necessary so the patient can minimize the importance of occasional pain while concentrating on living as productively as possible. Narcotics and sedating muscle relaxants should be avoided whenever possible. Peer groups and support groups can be very helpful; mental health professionals are available for consultation and to help patients put their condition in the proper perspective.

Contact with occupational and physical therapists can promote better understanding and awareness of how arthritis effects daily activities and how adjustments can be made to make life easier. Built-up utensils and keys, grip cloths to open jars, and modified door handles to accommodate disabled fingers and wrists, rails for entry and exit from bath tubs, elevated toilet seats, and cookery and cups with adjusted handles are examples of some useful modifications available to the disabled patient. Wrist splints should be used early for wrist disease. Patients may begin wearing these at night to immobilize inflamed joints and take them off during the day when dexterity is necessary. A good general exercise program is also recommended. Whirlpool or hot showers to decrease muscle spasm prior to exercise can improve tolerance.

Localized problems can be managed by orthotics, corrective shoes, joint injections, and surgery. Knee braces may improve a knee with lateral instability in a patient who is not a candidate for surgery. Inserts and molded shoes can greatly improve foot comfort in patients suffering with foot deformities, a frequent problem in rheumatoid arthritis.

When one or several joints are affected, causing significant disability before systemic therapy takes effect, they can be injected with long-acting corticosteroids (Gray et al, 1981). In general it is a good idea to rest joints postinjection for 48 to 72 hrs. A joint can be reinjected every several months if needed and if an objective decrease in inflammation for several weeks is observed. More frequent injections could theoretically weaken ligaments and create joint instability.

Surgery should be considered when the function of a particular joint has deteriorated to such a degree that pain or deformity is incapacitating. For a severely damaged joint the placement of a prosthetic joint can mean the difference between incapacitation and ambulation, or between a functionless and a useful hand. The most commonly replaced joints currently are knees, hips, and metacarpalphalangeal (MCP) joints. Patients can expect that artificial knees and hips are likely to remain functional for 10 to 15 years and possibly longer. Joint replacement may be the preferred management in elderly patients who have a shorter life expectancy and more limited daily activity level. Patients with artificial knees or hips have an 80% chance of being pain-free after surgery and most achieve good to excellent range of motion.

DRUG THERAPY

Medication is the mainstay treatment of rheumatoid arthritis. Regimens can be divided into two categories: the use of aspirin and/or non-steroidal anti-inflammatory drugs (NSAID), and the use of second line agents. Newly diagnosed or suspected rheumatoid arthritis patients are begun on either an aspirin compound or one of the NSAIDs. Agent selection will be discussed below. Several different agents can be tested for a clinical response over time. If the patient has intolerable pain or stiffness that is thought to be due to inflammation (and not merely from a mechanical process), which persists for 4 to 8 weeks after optimal dosages of these medications are tested or if radiographs show erosive changes, a second line agent is begun.

The current second line medications can take weeks to months to begin acting. The selection of a particular agent should be individualized for each patient. Consideration must be given to patient convenience, cost, the need for close follow-up, the urgency for a response, and the side effects. A second line agent is usually given for at least 6 months to evaluate efficacy and allow adjustment of dosage. NSAIDs are frequently continued during treatment with second line agents for a presumed additive effect. Relatively minor flares can be treated by adjusting the dosage of an NSAID or switching to an alternative compound. If only a few joints become affected, local measures such as splints, heat, other physical modalities, and corticosteroid injections should be employed.

When several joints are involved or the above measures have not succeeded in adequately suppressing disease activity, several options are available. First, the dosage or dosage interval of the second line agent can be adjusted to temporarily augment drug levels. For example, gold, if given monthly, can be given biweekly or even weekly. Penicillamine dosage, as another example, can be increased, although this must be done slowly to avoid toxicity. Another approach is to add corticosteroids. This can be accomplished by giving 5 to 10 mg of prednisone daily for recalcitrant disease or by a 1 to 2 week course of prednisone (starting at 20 to 30 mg daily and tapering to 0 to 5 mg) for discrete periods of exacerbation brought on by physical or emotional stress (eg, the patient went on a trip and after considerable walking, stiffness of the lower extremity joints and body developed that has not responded to NSAID increases and local measures).

A third method for confronting disease exacerbation in patients on a second line agent is to discontinue the drug and begin a different second line compound. Over a period of years it is not uncommon for rheumatoid arthritis patients to have been on three or more second line agents. In a given individual it may not be clear whether a medication is actually modifying the disease course or whether a period of spontaneous remission has ensued. Frequently, over time, patients breakthrough periods of disease inactivity attributed to second line drug therapy. Since rheumatoid arthritis does have natural periods of remission and exacerbation, it is imperative to have an organized approach for evaluating the efficacy of medications. Ideally this should consist of both objective and subjective assessments. Periodic reevaluation at intervals of 6 to 12 months may minimize the chance of allowing progressive disease to go unchecked. This need for concern is particularly true in patients with low grade smoldering disease activity without a clear-cut flare subsequent to a period of disease quiescence which would readily be identified as requiring intervention.

It is important to gauge the patient's disease from several viewpoints in order to get a clear picture of its status. It is critical to know how the patient feels in regard to both the arthritis and his or her general systemic and psychological well-being. If there is no feeling of long-term improvement, the patient will lose confidence. Likewise, the physician should attempt to quantify an overall impression of patient progress. Some less subjective measurements include joint counts, a Ritchie index (Ritchie et al, 1968), grip strength (how much the patient can squeeze on a folded cuff inflated to 20 mm Hg attached to a sphygmomanometer, calculated in mm Hg elevation) and 50 foot walking time (with or without cane or walker). These measurements assess both upper and lower extremity joint disease activity. The assessment of activities of daily living (ADL), such as getting dressed, manipulating utensils, and performing personal hygiene, are also useful and can be done by using a questionnaire or by demonstration of activities before a physician, nurse, or therapist using an established grading system. The American Rheumatism Association functional class and ability to work are also important global indicators of patient function. A sample of a useful disease evaluation form is given in Figure 16.1.

Finally, another perspective is necessary to ascertain disease activity at the level of cartilage and bone. The reason for this assessment is that despite functional improvement and the feeling of well being, the cellular reactions in the pannus may undermine the structure of the joints themselves, even dur-

A DISEASE EVALUATION FORM

How do your joints feel?   (worst: 0-10: best) _____

How do you feel in general?   (worst: 0-10: best) _____

How long are you stiff in the morning?   _____

Inflamed swollen joint count   _____

Grip Strength   Right hand   mm/Hg   _____
                   Lefthand   mm/Hg   _____

50 foot walking time   _____

Physician assessment of disease   (worst: 0-10: best) _____

Radiograph findings:

New erosions?   _____

Joints with narrowing?   _____

ARA functional class   _____

Ability to perform job or pursue   (worst: 0-10: best) _____
   premorbid necessary daily activities

PIP circumferences: Right hand digits: Left hand digits:

                        2 _____   2 _____

                        3 _____   3 _____

                        4 _____   4 _____

                        5 _____   5 _____

Figure 16.1 A disease evaluation form is a helpful tool for determining the rheumatoid arthritis patient's physical status.

ing clinical improvement. The best means of assessing this situation is to obtain radiographs of involved joints at defined intervals (every 6 to 12 months in very active disease, every 2 to 5 years if clinically inactive disease is present). Hand films are often sufficient for this purpose since the hands are the most frequently affected joints in rheumatoid arthritis and multiple joints can be assessed with minimal radiation exposure.

Most of the above parameters should be quantified at least every 12 months while a patient is on second line therapy. The use of a new second line agent should be pursued if self and physician assessment scores, physical exam measurements, and life-function scores demonstrate deterioration or if radiographs show significant progression.

Patients who have done well on a particular agent without serious side effects but have sustained a flare of disease activity can be treated by adding a second drug to the preexisting regimen (McCarty and Carrera, 1982; Bitter, 1984). This strategy will be discussed later.

Two issues that need to be addressed concerning which second line drugs to use and in what sequence are efficacy and toxicity. Unfortunately, the evidence for clearcut long-term efficacy of most second line drugs is controversial (Kirwan and Currey, 1983; Wright and Amos, 1980). This controversy is not only about their ability to allay erosive disease, but in some instances also about their effect on functional improvement. Despite the high frequency of rheumatoid arthritis in the general population, the ability to study this disease in an unbiased manner has been hampered by many factors (Fig. 16.2). It is therefore important to be familiar with the original data supporting the use of particular drugs in the treatment of rheumatoid arthritis before deciding what outcome to anticipate. One recent survey of the

Figure 16.2 Several factors which make conclusive drug studies in rheumatoid arthritis patients difficult.

PROBLEMS CONFOUNDING DRUG STUDIES IN RHEUMATOID ARTHRITIS

Rheumatoid arthritis may be a disease involving multiple mechanisms (eg, ± RF, ± HLA-DR4, ± nodules).

The course is highly variable and unpredictable.

There are spontaneous remissions and exacerbations.

There is a potent placebo effect.

The disease often lasts 10 to 20 years, despite therapy.

The effect of NSAID on disease course is undefined.

Corticosteroids are frequently used as adjuvant therapy.

literature examining the ability of second line drugs to prevent the progression of erosive disease in rheumatoid arthritis found that the majority of studies had major methodological flaws. Most of the acceptable studies did not demonstrate an anti-erosive effect (Iannuzzi et al, 1983). Only randomized double-blind placebo studies were evaluated in this survey.

Many studies, on the other hand, show improved functional and subjective assessment of rheumatoid arthritis with second line drugs compared to placebo. There are no unequivocal data in this regard that one agent works better than another. Because of this situation, it is best to use drugs that are least toxic and most acceptable to the patient. Drawbacks for particular regimens may include, for example, the weekly visits, laboratory tests, and injections associated with the use of IM gold; the fear of vision loss in patients using antimalarials; the frequent toxic reactions caused by penicillamine; the potential need for a liver biopsy with long-term methotrexate; and the increased risk of malignancy for some cytotoxic agents. Each physician must decide which medication is most efficacious and least toxic, and work with the patient to decide upon the best treatment strategy. Although gold has tradi-

SIDE EFFECTS OF ASPIRIN AND OTHER NSAIDs

Side effect	Aspirin	NSAID	Comment
Gastric irritation, ulcers	+	+	Less irritation with enteric-coated aspirin, nonacetylated salicylates and some NSAIDs.
Tinnitus	+	+	Associated with toxic salicylate levels.
Allergy	+	+	If history of allergy to aspirin, NSAIDs are not safe (except nonacetylated salicylates).
Fluid retention	+	+	Decreased creatinine clearance, especially in patients with renal disease.
Diarrhea, constipation	−	+	
Allergic interstitial nephritis	−	+	Fenoprofen mostly; also other NSAIDs.
Increases bleeding on Coumadin	+	+	Aspirin should probably be avoided. Use other NSAID cautiously.
Central nervous system (headache, confusion, loss of concentration)	−	+	Particularly indomethacin and tolmetin.

Figure 16.3 Side effects found with the use of aspirin and other nonsteroidal anti-inflammatory drugs (NSAIDs).

tionally been the initial second line agent administered, many rheumatologists begin with other drugs such as hydroxychloroquine or penicillamine. Methotrexate is rapidly entering this category, as experience with its use accumulates. Cyclophosphamide and azathioprine are reserved for more resistant disease because of their more severe side effects. Apheresis, total lymphoid irradiation, and combination therapies are more experimental and their use should probably be confined to studies at academic centers.

SALICYLATES AND NSAIDs

Salicylates have long been the mainstay of treatment for mild rheumatoid arthritis. They have been used for over 100 years for various conditions and there is much information about their side effects and long-term safety. Aspirin is one of the most reliable first line agents in rheumatoid arthritis. Aspirin is an acetylated form of salicylic acid. It works by acetylating proteins, particularly prostaglandin synthetase (Roth and Majerus, 1975), and therefore blocking the production of prostaglandins, important mediators of inflammation. Salicylic acid inhibits cyclooxygenase which is also involved in prostaglandin synthesis. Other mechanisms of action not related to prostaglandins may occur (Smith and Land, 1971). Aspirin is partially absorbed in the stomach but mostly in the intestine. It has a half-life of minutes and is deacetylated to salicylate. Salicylate in contrast to aspirin has a plasma half-life of hours. Salicylate levels are highly variable among individuals for a given dosage (Gupta et al, 1975). It is useful to monitor these levels to gauge effectiveness or toxicity. The anti-inflammatory range is from 20 to 30 mg/dL. Salicylate is metabolized in the liver. Aspirin has both analgesic and anti-inflammatory properties.

Patients can be started on 9 to 12 regular aspirin (3 to 4 g) per day in divided doses (qid). It is helpful to ingest aspirin with meals and snacks to minimize gastrointestinal toxicity. Serum salicylate levels may increase rapidly with small increments of aspirin dose. It is recommended, therefore, to increase the dosage by 1 tablet every 5 to 7 days until optimal clinical improvement is noted, toxicity occurs, or salicylate levels are in the anti-inflammatory range. Tinnitus has been used as a rough indicator of toxicity and, if it appears, warrants a decrease in dosage.

Important side effects of aspirin and other NSAIDs are listed in Figure 16.3. Gastric irritation leading to gastric ulcers is of particular importance. There is a clear increase in the incidence of gastric ulcers and gastritis associated with aspirin intake. Aspirin buffered with antacids does not decrease the incidence of gastritis while enteric-coated aspirin does (Lanza et al, 1980). Patients with a history of aspirin gastrointestinal intolerance, peptic ulcers, or gastrointestinal bleeding are preferably started on an enteric-coated or a nonacetylated preparation. The latter are also less gastrointestinal toxic. Diflunisol, a newer salicylate derivative may also have lower gastrointestinal toxicity and is given twice daily. Asthma is only a relative contraindication to aspirin use unless nasal polyps or prior aspirin-induced bronchospasm or urticaria has been noted, in which case aspirin absolutely should be withheld. Elderly patients in whom loss of high frequency hearing often occurs, may not experience tinnitus at potentially toxic salicylate doses. These patients may also be slower to report serious gastrointestinal toxicity. Therefore, other NSAIDs may be more appropriate in this age group.

There are many nonsalicylate NSAIDs on the market. Some of the most frequently prescribed ones are listed in Figure 16.4. These drugs are derived from several different unrelated chemical groups, all of which inhibit prostaglandin synthesis to some degree and might do so differentially in different tissues. Other inhibitory mechanisms of action have also been proposed including scavenging free hydroxyl radicals, the inhibition of neutro-

phil chemotaxis, cAMP enhancement, and lipoxygenase inhibition. These drugs are well absorbed and should be taken with meals. There is now available a preparation of indomethacin in suppository form for patients who cannot take oral medications.

Clinically, there is no proof that one NSAID is superior to another in treating rheumatoid arthritis. Factors to take into account in choosing a preparation are physician familiarity, cost (the price range of NSAID is wide), and dosing schedule. Patients who have difficulty remembering to take medication might benefit from piroxicam given once daily. Another option is naproxen or sulindac given twice daily. Some patients appear to get a psychological boost by taking drugs frequently during the day, so ibuprofen

CURRENTLY AVAILABLE NSAIDs

DRUG	CHEMICAL TYPE	TRADE NAME (EXAMPLES)	RECOMMENDED DAILY DOSAGE	GIVEN
Indomethacin	Indole	Indocin	75 to 150 mg	bid/tid
Tolmetin	Indole	Tolectin	800 to 2000 mg	qid
Sulindac	Indole	Clinoril	200 to 400 mg	bid
Ibuprofen	Phenylpropionic Acid	Motrin, Rufen, Advil, Nuprin	1.6 to 3.2 g	qid
Naproxen	Phenylpropionic Acid	Naprosyn	500 to 1000 mg	bid
Fenoprofen	Phenylpropionic Acid	Nalfon	2.4 to 3.0 g	bid
Ketoprofen	Phenylpropionic Acid	Orudis	75 to 150 mg	bid
Meclofenamate	Fenamate	Meclomen	200 to 400 mg	bid
Piroxicam	Oxicam	Feldene	10 to 20 mg	qd

Figure 16.4 Nonsteroidal anti-inflammatory drugs (NSAIDs) are listed by name, chemical type, trade name, and frequency given.

given four times daily could be a good choice for such patients. The benefit or risk of giving different NSAIDs simultaneously is controversial. Displacement from protein binding sites will occur, though the clinical implications of this phenomenon are not apparent. One study showed a beneficial effect of combining naproxen with aspirin in rheumatoid arthritis patients (Wilkens and Segre, 1976). However, a second study using aspirin and piroxicam together noted a high incidence of peptic ulcers (Semble et al, 1982). A long-acting preparation such as naproxen or sulindac can occasionally be added at bedtime with a snack to a patient on a short-acting agent such as ibuprofen. This can improve sleep by decreasing waking due to pain and may diminish morning stiffness. None of the nonsalicylate NSAID preparations seem superior to aspirin in preventing gastric ulceration, although symptomatic gastrointestinal tolerance is probably superior to aspirin. NSAID should not be used in aspirin-allergic patients. Although the NSAIDs do not prolong prothrombin times in patients on warfarin, they do displace the anticoagulant from protein binding sites and interfere with platelet function, and so should be used cautiously with patients on this drug. Hepatotoxicity has occasionally been reported with several NSAIDs (Lewis, 1984). Acetaminophen has no significant anti-inflammatory effect in humans but produces good analgesic effect, especially in individual doses of about 1 g 3 to 4 times daily.

SECOND LINE AGENTS

Numerous agents have been tested on rheumatoid arthritis patients after NSAIDs have failed to adequately suppress disease. There is considerable controversy as to which drugs are effective, whether they prevent erosions and in what order to use them. A summary of some of the more important double blind-ed placebo controlled studies appears in Figure 16.5. These drugs represent the most commonly used second line agents in practice today. Most of these studies either do not address the effect of treatment on radiograph changes or come to negative conclusions. The study that comes closest to showing a positive effect using gold (Sigler et al, 1974), has been noted to have serious methodological flaws (Kirwan and Currey, 1983). All the drugs shown in Figure 16.5 have been found to have a beneficial effect on joint inflammation and function. From a clinical standpoint, this is important, since painful, inflamed, functionless joints can limit a patient's quality of life. Since none of these drugs have been proved to be clearly superior, the order in which they are used is based on the experience of the physician and the acceptance by the patient.

Gold is still probably the most widely used initial second line agent in the United States. There are now both intramuscular and oral forms (auranofin). Gold may work by affecting macrophages since it accumulates in tissues enriched with these cells, such as the spleen, liver, and synovium (Gottlieb et al, 1972). It takes weeks to months of therapy for gold to begin working and gold therapy requires frequent monitoring of blood counts and urine. Response is not expected until 2 to 4 months. Injections are given weekly (50 mg per week) until there is dramatic improvement or a total dosage of 1 g is achieved. Injections are then adjusted to a bimonthly schedule and then a monthly schedule, depending on response. It is common practice to continue therapy for years in patients who appear to be responding, although there is some indication that gold should be given for a 5 to 6 month course (Empire Rheumatism Council, 1960).

Side effects of gold are frequent. Rashes are common, often pruritic and pleomorphic. Such side effects require withholding the drug until their disappearance, after which time the gold can be restarted at a low dose

DOUBLE-BLINDED, PLACEBO, CONTROLLED STUDIES

Agent	No. of patients	Duration of study	Disease duration	Comparability of treatment groups	Dose	Significant differences Inflammation*	Function**
Gold	200	18 mo	1 to 5 yr	+ + + +	50 mg/wk × 5 mo.	+ + +	+ + +
Gold	68	27 to 72 wk	1 to 7.5 yr	+ + + +	50 mg/wk	+	+ +
Gold	32	2 yr	2.5 yr mean	+ +	50 mg/wk taper	+ +	+
Gold IM Oral	193	5 mo	5 mo to 36 yr	+ + + +	IM 50 mg/wk PO 6 mg/wk	+ + +	+ +
Chloroquine	107	1 yr	1 to 10 yr	+ +	400 mg/day	+ +	+ +
Chloroquine	134	1 yr	not stated	+ +	250 mg/day	+ +	+ +
Hydroxy-chloroquine	113	6 mo	6 yr mean (1.5 to 21 yr)	+ + +	800 mg/day	+ +	+ + +
Hydroxy-chloroquine	41	6 mo	5.5 yr mean (0.25 to 25 yr)	NA	200 mg/day	+ +	+ +
Penicillamine	105	1 yr	11 yr mean	+ + +	1.5 g/day	+ + +	+ + +
Penicillamine	179	6 mo	most >2 yr	+ +	up to 900 mg/day	+ + +	+ + +
Penicillamine	171	7.5 mo	10 yr mean (1 to 40 yr)	+ + + +	125 mg/day or 500 mg/day	+	+
Methotrexate	14 crossover***	26 wk	14 yr mean (4 to 30 yr)	NA	10 to 25 mg/wk IM	+ + +	+ +
Methotrexate	35 crossover***	24 wk	9 yr mean (1.8 to 30 yr)	NA	7.5 to 15 mg/wk	+ + +	+ + +
Methotrexate	189	18 wk	13.3 yr mean	+ + +	7.5 to 15 mg/day	+ + +	+ + +

Figure 16.5 Important double-blinded placebo controlled studies of second line agents for rheumatoid arthritis.

% Side effects	Radiologic differences from placebo	Comments	Reference
35%	none	Gold given only for 5 mo; Multicenter study.	Empire Rheumatism Council, 1960
33%	none	Few patients remained for full trial.	Coop. Clinics, 1973
9% withdrew	Decreased narrowing & erosions	Placebo group may have had worse disease (by radiograph) at start.	Sigler, 1974
68% 33%	not done	Many parameters (ie, grip strength, patient assessment) showed no difference from placebo.	Ward, 1983
9% withdrew	possible improvement	Erosion healing noted in 2 pts on high dose.	Freedman, 1960
20%	none	No previous eye problems.	Popert, 1961
10% to 20% more than placebo	none	About twice the usual dose used currently.	Mainland, 1962
2% withdrew	none	Low dose, short duration of drug ingestion.	Hamilton, 1962
60% 31% withdrew	none	Side effects were frequent.	Multicenter, 1973
49% 20% withdrew	equivocal	Orthopedist found no radiographic difference. Internists found less erosions.	Shiokawa, 1977
11% withdrew 22% withdrew	not done not done	Treated group did somewhat better than controls on low dose.	Williams, 1983
21% 7% withdrew	not done	Did well 13 wks on drug, compared with placebo.	Anderson, 1985
52% 3% withdrew	not done	HLA-DR2 patients had the best response.	Weinblatt, 1985
32% withdrew	not done	Large number of withdrawals for SLE mostly elevated LFTs.	Williams, 1985

* Drug induced improvement in parameters of inflammation such as Ritchie index, joint count, ring size.
** Improved functional status of patients ie, ability to work, daily activity, grip strength.
*** Each patient received either drug or placebo initially and was switched to the opposite therapy midway through the study.

and slowly increased to maintenance levels. Proteinuria is also frequent and can be the harbinger of a membranous glomerulonephritis. Mild bone marrow suppression occurs commonly and can be addressed by holding the drug until counts return to baseline. Severe suppression is occasionally encountered, and may require high dose steroids or chelators. Less common side effects include myalgias and arthralgias 24 hours postinjection, a vasomotor depression ("nitritoid reaction") within a half hour of injection, cholestatic jaundice, enterocolitis, and stomatitis. Auranofin seems to have less associated renal and bone marrow effects but can cause significant gastrointestinal toxicity (Ward et al, 1983). Auranofin may require less intensive monitoring. While serious toxicity from gold can usually be avoided by close frequent monitoring, the cost and inconvenience of this monitoring must be discussed with the patient before initiating therapy.

Another second line agent, penicillamine, was developed to bind and eliminate rheumatoid factor. Although it does not appear to work via this mechanism and may actually regulate oxide metabolism (Lipsky and Ziff, 1980) and immune antigen expression (Freundlich and Jimenez, 1987), there are several studies which indicate it reduces disease activity in rheumatoid arthritis. It appears that doses above 500 mg/day are more efficacious but it is critical to start with a low dose (eg, 125 to 250 mg daily) and build up slowly over a period of months (eg, 250 mg every 3 to 4 months) to reduce the frequent and sometimes serious side effects (Jaffe, 1978). Although penicillamine is administered orally, it is similar to gold in that both renal and bone marrow toxicity may occur, so frequent monitoring is necessary. Mild rashes or pruritis may occur early during therapy and often respond to antihistamines, while later rashes (after 6 months) require discontinuation of the drug. Less commonly, a glomerulonephritis may occur. As with

gold, HLA-DR3 individuals are at higher risk of developing this problem (Wooley et al, 1980). A potentially fatal bronchiolitis obliterans is a rare but important complication to recognize. Interestingly, penicillamine can provoke several autoimmune syndromes including myasthenia gravis and systemic lupus erythematosus. The mechanism for this is unknown.

The antimalarial compounds hydroxychloroquine and chloroquine are also used as second line drugs and offer the advantage of limited toxicity and convenience. They are given by mouth daily and do not require frequent laboratory monitoring. Their mechanism of action is not clear but they appear to have both immunologic and anti-inflammatory activities (Salmeron and Lipsky, 1983). As with the other second line agents, no clear positive effect can be found on radiograph. The main concern with these medications is potential degenerative retinopathy that can lead to loss of vision if unchecked. This side effect appears to be less frequent with hydroxychloroquine than with chloroquine (Bernstein, 1983) and can essentially be eliminated if the daily dose does not exceed 6.5/mg/Kg per day. Visual field testing should be performed every 6 months by an ophthalmologist to detect early maculopathy which generally resolves upon drug discontinuation.

Finally, the antimetabolite methotrexate has gained recent popularity as a second line drug. This folate antagonist, may work like other cytotoxic agents to kill rapidly dividing cells. In rheumatoid arthritis, such rapidly dividing cells include subsets of activated lymphocytes engaged in the autoimmune response. Methotrexate has a more rapid onset of action than the above-mentioned treatments with statistically significant differences from placebo, noticeable as little as 6 weeks into therapy (Williams et al, 1985). Methotrexate is easy to take once a week orally. A test dose of 2.5 mg/wk is given initially as a control for patients who may have a sudden drop in blood counts due to sensitivity to the drug. The dose may then be raised to 7.5 mg/wk and then increased as needed every few weeks. No blind study to date has examined the question of radiograph progression, although a report of erosion improvement in 7 of 11 patients over 2 years was recently published (Kremer and Lee, 1986). Perhaps the major limiting factor in methotrexate usage is its toxicity, particularly hepatic damage and bone marrow suppression. The large doses of methotrexate that have been used in psoriasis can lead to hepatic fibrosis (Weinstein, 1977). However, the risk of this complication on the lower doses used to treat rheumatoid arthritis, although apparently less, has not been completely defined. Little long-term toxicity so far has been noted (Kremer and Lee, 1986). While liver enzymes do not correlate with fibrotic changes they still must be followed. Liver biopsies should probably be obtained after a cumulative dose of 1 to 2 gms is reached to rule out moderate to marked fibrosis, an indication for discontinuing the drug. Cytopenias may also occur and, though usually reversible, can be severe if undetected. Other complications include acute pneumonitis, pulmonary fibrosis, infections, transient oligospermia, mouth ulcers, nausea, and rashes. Since the drug is excreted via the kidneys it is important to withhold methotrexate from patients with renal failure. Also it is better not to give this therapy to patients who are prone to fatty livers such as alcohol abusers, obese people, and diabetics.

Other agents used on a more experimental basis to treat rheumatoid arthritis include cyclophosphamide, azathioprine, levamisole, sulfasalazine, and cyclosporine. One of the most important causes for concern using these drugs is toxicity. For example, cyclophosphamide, which appears to be active in reducing symptoms of rheumatoid arthritis, may produce a small increase in malignancy, serious cytopenias, and hemorrhagic cystitis. Its use is warranted in cases where severe disease is resistant to conventional therapy and is disrupting a patient's life. Sulfasalazine, which has shown promise in a recent double-blind study (Pinals et al, 1986), has a small incidence of agranulocytosis.

FUTURE DIRECTIONS

Future developments in drug therapy will undoubtedly produce more effective treatment for rheumatoid arthritis. NSAIDs that effectively block not only the cyclooxygenase but also the lipoxygenase pathway are likely to have more potent anti-inflammatory effects. A similar result could be obtained by giving patients oils such as the omega-3 fatty acid precursors. This approach takes advantage of the fact that different precursors eventuate the production of different cyclooxygenase and lipoxygenase products. For example, certain fish and plant oils will stimulate the production of LTB5, a much less potent inflammatory mediator than LTB4 (from arachidonic acid) which is produced by mononuclear cells from people on the usual Western culture meat diet. Fish oil diets have been used successfully to treat mice with a lupus-like syndrome (Robinson et al, 1986).

Therapy targeted at more specific points of the immune response could potentially alter the intense intrasynovial immune response. Drugs that could block interleukin-1 (IL-1) production or function might be quite effective. Interleukin-1 is not only a key initiator of the immune response, but also stimulates PGE and collagenase secretion, two mediators which appear to effect both inflammation and joint destruction via collagen catabolism. Several human cytokines produced by genetic engineering, such as gamma interferon, tumor necrosis factor, and colony stimulating factor, are now available and are being given to cancer patients for various reasons. Some of these effect the immune response, and suppressive effects that could be beneficial in autoimmune states are currently being studied.

An even more precisely directed approach could be applied if cross reactive idiotypic lymphocytes can be isolated from the synovium of different patients. It may be presumed that at least a percentage of rheumatoid arthritis patients are responding to a specific organism (such as a virus) or antigen (such as a peptidoglycan from a bacterial cell wall). These patients are likely to have T cells in common with receptors that specifically bind to the same antigenic determinant. These antigen specific T cells would form an important component of the cell population of affected joints and could initiate the immune response occurring in rheumatoid synovium. Synthesis of an antibody (called an anti-idiotype) directed against this T cell receptor (called an idiotype) could be engineered by immunizing mice with rheumatoid synovial T cells. Resultant anti-idiotypes would be tested on synovial lymphocytes of multiple rheumatoid arthritis patients. Those antibodies that reacted with T cells from multiple patients or "cross-reactive" anti-idiotypes, could be tagged with a poison such as ricin to kill these specific T cells. Alter-natively, these antibodies could be given without a poison in the hope of dampening the specific immune response, something anti-idiotype antibodies probably do naturally. Once an anti-idiotype is obtained, methods could be developed for phoresis of the critical T cell on anti-idiotype lined surfaces.

The success of combined chemotherapy regimens in multiple neoplastic conditions has spurred interest in a similar treatment approach in rheumatoid arthritis. Theoretically, combinations of second line drugs in low doses could curtail the toxicities of each medication and increase their effectiveness by attacking multiple pathways simultaneously. Initial trials of such regimens have met with great success in one report (McCarty et al, 1982) and less enthusiasm in another (Bitter, 1984).

Whatever innovative therapy is tested in the treatment of rheumatoid arthritis, it is clear that randomized double-blind groups need to be studied in order to assess the efficacy of a particular regimen. Since rheumatoid arthritis is a chronic process, it is necessary to observe long-term effects, including toxicity of each treatment.

REFERENCES

Anderson PA, West SG, O'Dell JR, et al: Weekly pulse methotrexate in rheumatoid arthritis: Clinical and immunologic effects in a randomized double-blind study. *Ann Intern Med* 1985;103:489–496.

Bernstein HM: Ophthalmologic consideration and testing in patients receiving long-term antimalarial therapy. *Am J Med* 1983;75S:25–34.

Bitter T: Combined disease modifying chemotherapy for intractable rheumatoid arthritis. *Clin Rheum Dis* 1984;10:417–429.

The Cooperative Clinics Committee of the ARA: A controlled trial of gold salt therapy in rheumatoid arthritis. *Arthritis Rheum* 1973;16:353–358.

Empire Rheumatism Council: Gold therapy in rheumatoid arthritis. *Ann Rheum Dis* 1960;19:95–119.

Freedman A, Steinberg VL: Chloroquine in rheumatoid arthritis: A double blindfold trial of treatment for one year. *Ann Rheum Dis* 1960;19:243–250.

Freundlich B, Jimenez SA: Phenotype of peripheral blood lymphocytes of patients with progressive systemic sclerosis. *Clin Exp Imm* 1987, 69:375-384.

Gottlieb NL, Smith PM, Smith EM: Tissue gold concentration in a rheumatoid arthritic receiving chrysotherapy. *Arthritis Rheum* 1972;15:16–22.

Gray RG, Tenenbaum J, Gottlieb NL: Local corticosteroid injection treatment in rheumatic disorders. *Semin Arthritis Rheum* 1981;10:231–254.

Gupta N, Sarkissian E, Paulus HE: Correlation of plateau serum salicylate level with rate of salicylate metabolism. *Clin Pharmocol Ther* 1975; 18:350.

Hamilton EBD, Scott JT: Hydroxychloroquine sulfate (Plaquenil) in treatment of rheumatoid arthritis. *Arthritis Rheum* 1962;5:502–512.

Iannuzzi L, Dawson N, Zein N, et al: Does drug therapy slow radiographic deterioration in rheumatoid arthritis? *N Engl J Med* 1983;17:1023–1028.

Jaffe IA: D-penicillamine. *Bull Rheum Dis* 1978; 28:948–952.

Kremer JM and Lee JR: The safety and efficacy of the use of methotrexate in long-term therapy for rheumatoid arthritis. *Arthritis Rheum* 1986;29:822–831.

Kirwan JR, Currey HL: Rheumatoid arthritis: Disease modifying antirheumatic drugs. *Clin Rheum Dis* 1983;9:581–599.

Lanza FL, Royer GL, Nelson RS: Endoscopic evaluation of the effects of aspirin, buffered aspirin and enteric coated aspirin on gastric and duodenal mucosa. *N Engl J Med* 1980;303:136–138.

Lewis JH: Hepatic toxicity of nonsteroidal antiinflammatory drugs. *Clin Pharmacy* 1984;3:128–138.

Lipsky PE, Ziff M: Inhibition of human helper T cell function *in vitro* by D-penicillamine and $CuSO_4$. *J Clin Invest* 1980;65:1069.

Mainland D, Sutcliffe MI: Hydroxychloroquine sulfate in rheumatoid arthritis: A six month, double-blinded trial. *Bull Rheum Dis* 1962;13:287–290.

McCarty DJ, Carrera GF: Intractable rheumatoid arthritis: Treatment with combined cyclophosphamide azathioprine and hydroxychloroquine. *JAMA* 1982;248:1718–1723.

Multicenter Trial Group: Controlled trial of D-penicillamine in severe rheumatoid arthritis. *Lancet* 1973;1:275–280.

O'Sullivan JB, Cathcart ES: The prevalance of rheumatoid arthritis: Follow-up evaluation of the effect of criteria on rates in Sudbury, Mass. *Ann Int Med* 1972;76:573–580.

Pinals RS, Kaplan SB, Lawson JG, et al: Sulfasalazine in rheumatoid arthritis: A double blind, placebo-controlled trial. *Arthritis Rheum* 1986;29:1427–1434.

Popert AJ, Meijers KAE, Sharp J, et al: Chloroquine diphosphate in rheumatoid arthritis. A controlled study. *Ann Rheum Dis* 1961;20:18–35.

Ritchie DM, Boyle JA, McInnes JM, et al: Clinical studies with an articular index for the assessment of joint tenderness in patients with rheumatoid arthritis. *Quart J Med* 1968;37:393–406.

Robinson DR, Prickett JD, Makoul GT, Steinberg AD, Colvin B: Dietary fish oil reduces progression of established renal disease in $(NZBxNZW)F_1$ mice and delays renal disease in BxSB and $MRL/_1$ strains. *Arthritis Rheum* 1986;29:539–546.

Roth GJ, Majerus PW: The mechanism of the effect of aspirin on human platelets. *J Clin Invest* 1975;56:624.

Salmeron G, Lipsky PE: Immunosuppressive potential of antimalarials. *Am J Med* 1983;75:19–24.

Semble E, Metcalf D, Turner R, et al: Genetic predictors of patient response amd side effects in the treatment of rheumatoid arthritis with a high dose of nonsteroidal anti-inflammatory drug regimen. *Arthritis Rheum* 1982;25:370–381.

Shiokawa Y, Horiuchi Y, Hohma M, et al: Clinical evaluation of D-penicillamine by multicenter double blind comparative study in chronic rheumatoid arthritis. *Arthritis Rheum* 1977;20:1464–1472.

Sigler JW, Bluhm GB, Duncan H, et al: Gold salts in

the treatment of rheumatoid arthritis: A double-blind study. *Ann Intern Med* 1974;80:21–26.

Smith WL, Land WE: Stimulation and blockade of prostaglandin biosynthesis. *J Biol Chem* 1971;246:6702.

Steinbroker O, Traeger CH, Batterman RC: Therapeutic criteria in rheumatoid arthritis. *JAMA* 1949;140:659.

Ward JR, Williams HJ, Egger MJ, et al: Comparison of auranofin, gold sodium thiomalate, and placebo in the treatment of rheumatoid arthritis. *Arthritis Rheum* 1983;26:1303–1315.

Weinblatt ME, Coblyn JS, Fox DA, et al: Efficacy of low-dose methotrexate in rheumatoid arthritis. *N Engl J Med* 1985;312:818–822.

Weinstein G: Methotrexate. *Ann Int Med* 1977;86:199–204.

Wilkens RF, Segre EJ: Combination therapy with naproxen and aspirin in rheumatoid arthritis. *Arthritis Rheum* 1976;19:677–682.

Williams HJ, Ward JR, Reading JC, et al: Low dose D-penicillamine therapy in rheumatoid arthritis. *Arthritis Rheum* 1983;26:581–592.

Williams HJ, Wilkens RF, Samuelson CO, et al: Comparison of low dose pulse methotrexate and placebo in the treatment of rheumatoid arthritis. *Arthritis Rheum* 1985;28:721–730.

Wooley PH, Griffin J, Panayi GS, et al: HLA-DR antigens and toxic reaction to sodium thiomalate and D-penicillamine in patients with rheumatoid arthritis. *N Engl J Med* 1980;303:300–305.

Wright V, Amos R: Do drugs change the course of rheumatoid arthritis? *Br Med J* 1980;1:964–966.

INDEX